Clinical Application of Ultra-High Frequency Ultrasound:
Emerging Trends

Clinical Application of Ultra-High Frequency Ultrasound: Emerging Trends

Editors

Rossana Izzetti
Marco Nisi

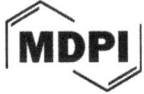

Basel • Beijing • Wuhan • Barcelona • Belgrade • Novi Sad • Cluj • Manchester

Editors

Rossana Izzetti
Department of Surgical,
Medical and Molecular
Pathology and Critical
Care Medicine
University of Pisa
Pisa
Italy

Marco Nisi
Department of Surgical,
Medical and Molecular
Pathology and Critical
Care Medicine
University of Pisa
Pisa
Italy

Editorial Office
MDPI
St. Alban-Anlage 66
4052 Basel, Switzerland

This is a reprint of articles from the Special Issue published online in the open access journal *Diagnostics* (ISSN 2075-4418) (available at: www.mdpi.com/journal/diagnostics/special_issues/7292GQR8Z8).

For citation purposes, cite each article independently as indicated on the article page online and as indicated below:

Lastname, A.A.; Lastname, B.B. Article Title. *Journal Name* **Year**, *Volume Number*, Page Range.

ISBN 978-3-7258-1052-9 (Hbk)
ISBN 978-3-7258-1051-2 (PDF)
doi.org/10.3390/books978-3-7258-1051-2

© 2024 by the authors. Articles in this book are Open Access and distributed under the Creative Commons Attribution (CC BY) license. The book as a whole is distributed by MDPI under the terms and conditions of the Creative Commons Attribution-NonCommercial-NoDerivs (CC BY-NC-ND) license.

Contents

Rossana Izzetti and Marco Nisi
Imaging the Micron: New Directions in Diagnosis with Ultra-High-Frequency Ultrasound
Reprinted from: *Diagnostics* **2024**, *14*, 735, doi:10.3390/diagnostics14070735 1

Arzu Alan, Ayse Isil Orhan and Kaan Orhan
Evaluation of the Breastfeeding Dynamics of Neonates with Ankyloglossia via a Novel Ultrasonographic Technique
Reprinted from: *Diagnostics* **2023**, *13*, 3435, doi:10.3390/diagnostics13223435 9

Marco Nisi, Stefano Gennai, Filippo Graziani and Rossana Izzetti
The Reliability of Ultrasonographic Assessment of Depth of Invasion: A Systematic Review with Meta-Analysis
Reprinted from: *Diagnostics* **2023**, *13*, 2833, doi:10.3390/diagnostics13172833 23

Giammarco Granieri, Alessandra Michelucci, Flavia Manzo Margiotta, Bianca Cei, Saverio Vitali and Marco Romanelli et al.
The Role of Ultra-High-Frequency Ultrasound in Pyoderma Gangrenosum: New Insights in Pathophysiology and Diagnosis
Reprinted from: *Diagnostics* **2023**, *13*, 2802, doi:10.3390/diagnostics13172802 37

Giovanni Fulvio, Rossana Izzetti, Giacomo Aringhieri, Valentina Donati, Francesco Ferro and Giovanna Gabbriellini et al.
UHFUS: A Valuable Tool in Evaluating Exocrine Gland Abnormalities in Sjögren's Disease
Reprinted from: *Diagnostics* **2023**, *13*, 2771, doi:10.3390/diagnostics13172771 50

Tobias Erlöv, Tebin Hawez, Christina Granéli, Maria Evertsson, Tomas Jansson and Pernilla Stenström et al.
A Computer Program for Assessing Histoanatomical Morphometrics in Ultra-High-Frequency Ultrasound Images of the Bowel Wall in Children: Development and Inter-Observer Variability
Reprinted from: *Diagnostics* **2023**, *13*, 2759, doi:10.3390/diagnostics13172759 59

Giorgia Salvia, Nicola Zerbinati, Flavia Manzo Margiotta, Alessandra Michelucci, Giammarco Granieri and Cristian Fidanzi et al.
Ultra-High-Frequency Ultrasound as an Innovative Imaging Evaluation of Hyaluronic Acid Filler in Nasolabial Folds
Reprinted from: *Diagnostics* **2023**, *13*, 2761, doi:10.3390/diagnostics13172761 68

Valentina Dini, Michela Iannone, Alessandra Michelucci, Flavia Manzo Margiotta, Giammarco Granieri and Giorgia Salvia et al.
Ultra-High Frequency UltraSound (UHFUS) Assessment of Barrier Function in Moderate-to-Severe Atopic Dermatitis during Dupilumab Treatment
Reprinted from: *Diagnostics* **2023**, *13*, 2721, doi:10.3390/diagnostics13172721 78

Alessandra Michelucci, Valentina Dini, Giorgia Salvia, Giammarco Granieri, Flavia Manzo Margiotta and Salvatore Panduri et al.
Assessment and Monitoring of Nail Psoriasis with Ultra-High Frequency Ultrasound: Preliminary Results
Reprinted from: *Diagnostics* **2023**, *13*, 2716, doi:10.3390/diagnostics13162716 91

Edoardo Marrani, Giovanni Fulvio, Camilla Virgili, Rossana Izzetti, Valentina Dini and Teresa Oranges et al.
Ultra-High-Frequency Ultrasonography of Labial Glands in Pediatric Sjögren's Disease: A Preliminary Study
Reprinted from: *Diagnostics* **2023**, *13*, 2695, doi:10.3390/diagnostics13162695 . . . . **102**

Maria Evertsson, Christina Graneli, Alvina Vernersson, Olivia Wiaczek, Kristine Hagelsteen and Tobias Erlöv et al.
Design of a Pediatric Rectal Ultrasound Probe Intended for Ultra-High Frequency Ultrasound Diagnostics
Reprinted from: *Diagnostics* **2023**, *13*, 1667, doi:10.3390/diagnostics13101667 . . . . **113**

Xin Liu, Jingxi Wang, Yanglu Liu, Shuang Luo, Gaowu Yan and Huaqi Yang et al.
High Intensity Focused Ultrasound Ablation for Juvenile Cystic Adenomyosis: Two Case Reports and Literature Review
Reprinted from: *Diagnostics* **2023**, *13*, 1608, doi:10.3390/diagnostics13091608 . . . . **128**

Jian Yu, Hong Wang, Meijing Zhou, Min Zhu, Jing Hang and Min Shen et al.
A Hypothesis on the Progression of Insulin-Induced Lipohypertrophy: An Integrated Result of High-Frequency Ultrasound Imaging and Blood Glucose Control of Patients
Reprinted from: *Diagnostics* **2023**, *13*, 1515, doi:10.3390/diagnostics13091515 . . . . **140**

Marco Di Battista, Simone Barsotti, Saverio Vitali, Marco Palma, Giammarco Granieri and Teresa Oranges et al.
Multiparametric Skin Assessment in a Monocentric Cohort of Systemic Sclerosis Patients: Is There a Role for Ultra-High Frequency Ultrasound?
Reprinted from: *Diagnostics* **2023**, *13*, 1495, doi:10.3390/diagnostics13081495 . . . . **151**

Tebin Hawez, Christina Graneli, Tobias Erlöv, Emilia Gottberg, Rodrigo Munoz Mitev and Kristine Hagelsteen et al.
Ultra-High Frequency Ultrasound Imaging of Bowel Wall in Hirschsprung's Disease—Correlation and Agreement Analyses of Histoanatomy
Reprinted from: *Diagnostics* **2023**, *13*, 1388, doi:10.3390/diagnostics13081388 . . . . **159**

Saeed Jerban, Victor Barrère, Michael Andre, Eric Y. Chang and Sameer B. Shah
Quantitative Ultrasound Techniques Used for Peripheral Nerve Assessment
Reprinted from: *Diagnostics* **2023**, *13*, 956, doi:10.3390/diagnostics13050956 . . . . **171**

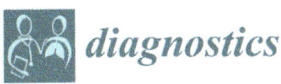

Editorial

Imaging the Micron: New Directions in Diagnosis with Ultra-High-Frequency Ultrasound

Rossana Izzetti *[ ] and Marco Nisi

Department of Surgical, Medical and Molecular Pathology and Critical Care Medicine, University of Pisa, 56126 Pisa, Italy; marco.nisi@unipi.it
* Correspondence: rossana.izzetti@unipi.it

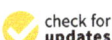

Citation: Izzetti, R.; Nisi, M. Imaging the Micron: New Directions in Diagnosis with Ultra-High-Frequency Ultrasound. *Diagnostics* 2024, 14, 735. https://doi.org/10.3390/diagnostics14070735

Received: 30 January 2024
Accepted: 26 March 2024
Published: 29 March 2024

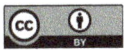

Copyright: © 2024 by the authors. Licensee MDPI, Basel, Switzerland. This article is an open access article distributed under the terms and conditions of the Creative Commons Attribution (CC BY) license (https://creativecommons.org/licenses/by/4.0/).

1. Introduction

In recent decades, advancements in medical imaging technologies have revolutionized diagnostic and therapeutic approaches, enhancing the precision and efficacy of healthcare interventions [1,2]. Among these cutting-edge technologies, ultra-high-frequency ultrasonography (UHFUS) has emerged as a powerful tool, offering unprecedented resolution and depth for imaging biological tissues [3]. This sophisticated ultrasound technique has gained an increasingly important role in several medical fields since its introduction into the clinical setting in the early 2000s [4–7]. Indeed, the technique has undergone significant changes due to the implementation of devices enabling the use of frequencies up to 100 MHz, which has led to a widespread application of UHFUS in all branches of medicine in which imaging of superficial structures at submillimeter resolution is required [8]. According to the current definition, UHFUS employs frequencies above 30 MHz, providing high-resolution imaging of anatomical structures at a microscopic level [9]. The applications of ultra-high-frequency ultrasonography in medicine are diverse and span various medical disciplines, including dermatology, rheumatology, pediatrics, and oral medicine. Recent studies have demonstrated how UHFUS can play a role in the diagnosis, management, surgical treatment, and follow-up of various pathologic conditions.

Hence, we provide a brief review on the applications of UHFUS and on the treatment opportunities related to this technique.

2. Uses of UHFUS Imaging by Medical Specialty

2.1. Dermatology

Dermatology was one of the first fields of application of ultrasonography; the technique was first employed in the late 1970s for the assessment of skin thickness [10–12] and has since then been used for the study of normal skin as well as several diseases and conditions with various etiologies. A recent systematic review by Lintzeri and coll. [13] summarized the evidence from the literature on epidermal thickness evaluated with different techniques, including UHFUS, and provided a stratification depending on the anatomic area investigated, gender, age, and ethnicity of the subjects, method of assessment, and skin phototype. Dini and coll. (Contributor 1) employed UHFUS to assess atopic dermatitis (AD) and its treatment outcomes. Importantly, in diagnosing AD, UHFUS can detect the pathognomonic sign of a subepidermal low-echogenic band (SLEB), which has been found to correlate with disease severity and treatment response. Moreover, SLEB measurement, along with the assessment of vascularity and epidermal thickness, might serve as an objective criterion to track responses to treatment. Additionally, detecting SLEB in non-lesional skin could indicate the presence of subclinical inflammation, potentially predicting the emergence of clinical lesions and emphasizing the need for proactive therapeutic intervention. Similarly, the assessment of pyoderma gangrenosum, a dermatosis of unknown origin, may benefit from UHFUS, as the technique may allow for the early identification of imaging biomarkers of lesion inflammatory status, as reported by Granieri and coll.

(Contributor 2). Such biomarkers can support the detection, differential diagnosis, and treatment monitoring of PG and include epidermal and dermal morphology, vascularity, presence of edema, and aliasing phenomena.

UHFUS is also extremely valuable in the diagnostic algorithm of cutaneous autoimmune diseases [14]. Interestingly, the assessment and treatment monitoring of psoriasis represent a promising novel field of investigation [15]. Michelucci and coll. (Contributor 3) describe the use of UHFUS to evaluate psoriatic onychopathy severity.

When considering skin tumors, UHFUS may support the diagnosis and surgical treatment of several neoplastic conditions. Laverde-Saad and coll. [16] report that UHFUS provided accurate depth measurements of basal-cell carcinomas, especially if the lesions were above 1 mm. More specifically, the technique allowed for the assessment of tumor depth and margins, as well as for discriminating between aggressive and non-aggressive subtypes. Regarding melanoma skin lesions, a Cochrane systematic review by Dinnes and coll. [17] reported derived sensitivities of at least 83% and combined the assessment of three qualitative features, namely hypoechogenicity, homogeneity, and well-defined margins. In fact, UHFUS has been found to correlate the Breslow scale with ultrasonographic thickness [18,19]. The good correspondence between UHFUS and histology may improve the surgical treatment of these lesions, increasing the capability to obtain clear resection margins, which is of utmost importance in prognosis and in recurrence prevention. However, it should not be forgotten that UHFUS, combined with dermoscopy, can also prove beneficial in the diagnostic work-up of non-melanoma skin tumors [20–22].

Finally, additional evidence for using UHFUS to support clinical practice is provided by its role in esthetic medicine, where the technique is employed to monitor and assess treatment effects following anti-cellulite therapies, volumetric treatments, and discoloration correction [23,24]. Salvia and coll. (Contributor 4) utilized UHFUS to monitor hyaluronic acid filler distribution and nasolabial fold amelioration, potentially improving the outcomes of esthetic procedures.

2.2. Rheumatology

Most of the evidence on the applications of UHFUS in rheumatology revolves around the diagnosis and management of Sjögren's syndrome [25]. The role of conventional ultrasonography of major salivary glands has been extensively investigated and was eventually recognized to improve the performance of the 2016 American College of Rheumatology/EUropean League Against Rheumatism (ACR/EULAR) classification criteria [26,27]. The application of UHFUS has permitted the evaluation of minor salivary glands, giving insights into a direct correlation between imaging and histology. Moreover, UHFUS-guided minor salivary gland biopsies have been proven to improve sampling accuracy and to reduce the risk of postoperative complications [28,29].

It is recognized that Sjögren's syndrome incidence has two peaks, namely one after menarche (20–40 years of age) and one after menopause (50–60 years of age) [30]. However, some juvenile forms of Sjögren's syndrome have been identified in patients below 18 years of age. Interestingly, in these cases, the presentation differs from that observed in adults, as xerostomia is significantly more common, while recurrent parotitis is often an early symptom [31–33]. Using diagnostic imaging for the evaluation of salivary glands in pediatric patients with suspected Sjögren's syndrome may support the assessment of parenchymal and ductal damage, parenchymal inhomogeneity, and the presence of hypoechoic areas [34].

Indeed, the study by Marrani and coll. (Contributor 5) supports the usage of UHFUS in the monitoring of disease progression without exposing pediatric patients to surgical procedures. Another interesting aspect is the fact that UHFUS can be used to assess both the salivary and the lachrymal glands, which are both involved in the course of Sjögren's syndrome [35–37]. Interestingly, symptoms of dry eye correlate poorly with clinical signs. While several techniques have been proposed for the assessment of lachrymal gland function, only recently has diagnostic imaging been introduced to evaluate glandular size and inflammation [38].

According to Fulvio and coll. (Contributor 6), assessing the lachrymal glands by means of UHFUS may improve the phenotyping of affected patients, providing a more comprehensive understanding of overall glandular involvement.

A pivotal role of UHFUS has also been proposed in the measurement of epidermal thickness and echogenicity in evaluating patients with systemic sclerosis as a complementary method to standard assessment, as reported by Di Battista and coll. (Contributor 7).

2.3. Pediatrics

UHFUS finds several applications in pediatric dermatological medicine due to the lack of ionizing radiation, which is extremely important when managing young patients [39]. As reported by the pictorial review by Ait Ichou et al. [40], the technique can be utilized for the assessment of cutaneous lesions, musculoskeletal imaging, and vascular malformations. UHFUS has been reported to help in the evaluation of soft tissues and superficial structures, and it can potentially be employed intraoperatively to evaluate tumor margins and small structures.

It appears noteworthy that abdominal imaging may also benefit from UHFUS application. In fact, previous evidence supports the use of UHFUS for the study of the bowel wall in the course of Hirschsprung disease, a congenital disorder which compromises distal bowel innervation [41]. In these patients, nerve fiber hypertrophy as well as absent or impaired ganglia are observed as a result of an anomaly in neural crest cell migration during fetal development [42]. While the gold standard for diagnosis is rectal suction biopsy, it has been hypothesized that ultrasonography may help to rule out the presence of the disease [22]. Erlöv et al. (Contributor 8) employed UHFUS to study the bowel wall in Hirschsprung's disease to assess the thickness of bowel wall layers. In the study by Hawez and coll. (Contributor 9), UHFUS was able to discriminate between bowel wall muscular layers in children with Hirschsprung's disease, with a good correlation with histology. Previous research focused on the ability of UHFUS to discriminate between aganglionic and ganglionic bowel wall [36]. However, the study by Evertsson and coll. (Contributor 10) highlights that as of now, a dedicated UHFUS probe for rectal ultrasound is not available, thus highlighting the unmet need for a specific device for bowel assessment in pediatric patients.

Functional imaging, aimed at detecting the physiology and dynamics of anatomical structures, is gaining increasing importance. Interestingly, Alan and coll. (Contributor 11) applied UHFUS to study the dynamics of breastfeeding in neonates to detect variations in tongue positioning and movement in subjects with ankyloglossia versus healthy ones. In this field, UHFUS can prove beneficial in evaluating the severity of ankyloglossia and thus provide indication for frenotomy by specifically assessing the amplitude of anterior tongue movement and sucking efficacy during breastfeeding.

From this perspective, the ability to study the dynamics of the digestive system represents an advance in terms of diagnostic performance. Moreover, UHFUS may be helpful not only in assessing the presence of disease or impaired function, but also in providing guidance for surgical procedures. As reported by Guo et al. [43], the performance of UHFUS-guided endoscopic retrograde appendicitis therapy may improve treatment outcomes by allowing for real-time monitoring during stent placement.

The evidence in the field of pediatrics thus supports a growing application of UHFUS both for diagnostic and surgical purposes due to it having the major advantage of avoiding radiation exposure to pediatric patients.

2.4. Oral Medicine

Research on intraoral ultrasound has seen an increasing interest since the late 1990s, when the technique started to be employed for the assessment of tongue cancer [44–47]. Importantly, the parameter of depth of invasion was established as a predictor of the presence of lymph node metastases [48–50] and was added as a T-category modifier to the 8th edition of the American Joint Committee on Cancer criteria in 2017 [51–53]. Several studies have investigated the ability of diagnostic imaging to evaluate tumor dimensions [54–56]; a recent systematic review compared the diagnostic accuracy of magnetic resonance, computed tomography, and ultrasonography in assessing tumor dimensions preoperatively [57]. For magnetic resonance, the sensitivity was >80% and the specificity was >75% in all the studies included in the review, while computed tomography was reported in one study to have a sensitivity of 68.75% and a specificity of 77.78%. Ultrasonography showed the highest mean values for both sensitivity (>91%) and specificity (100%). It is noteworthy that ultrasonography proves extremely valuable in the case of small lesions (<4 mm) that may not be detectable with other techniques [58].

Although different ultrasound frequencies and protocols have been employed in the literature, the systematic review by Nisi and coll. (Contributor 12) confirms that ultrasonography to assess the depth of invasion is a sensitive tool with good correlation with histology. Indeed, UHFUS has the unique advantage of providing a higher resolution compared to conventional ultrasonographic techniques, thus improving diagnostic accuracy [59]. Indeed, its reduced invasiveness, repeatability, and the absence of exposure to ionizing radiation make the technique widely applicable to oral lesions. While research on oral cancer appears extremely robust, it should be highlighted that the versatility of UHFUS also allows for the investigation of other oral diseases and conditions, thus supporting the diagnosis, treatment, and follow-up of several oral lesions [60].

2.5. Other Applications

The UHFUS technique has been reported to effectively provide imaging of peripheral nerves [61,62]. Apart from structural analysis, UHFUS can be employed to characterize nerve echogenicity, which can help to discriminate between normal and abnormal nerves by applying the nerve density index, as reported by Jerman and coll. (Contributor 13).

UHFUS can also support the monitoring of lipohypertrophy onset in patients with diabetes treated with insulin injections. According to Yu and coll. (Contributor 14), these lesions can be detected earlier when using UHFUS, allowing practitioners to correct the injection method and to avoid injection at the lesion site.

The application of high-intensity focused ultrasound for surgical purposes is described by Liu and coll. (Contributor 15), with a focus on the ablation of juvenile cystic adenomyosis lesions. Ablation is the technique of choice as surgery may damage the muscular tissues surrounding the cystic adenomyosis lesions, potentially contributing to an increase in the risk of uterine rupture during pregnancy and causing iatrogenic endometriosis. Treatment with high-intensity focused ultrasound allows for the safe treatment of cystic adenomyosis, decreasing lesion dimensions and vascularization while also resolving lesion-associated dysmenorrhea.

3. Conclusions

UHFUS holds promise for several medical fields due to its advantages of providing real-time imaging, avoiding exposure to ionizing radiation, and offering repeatability in the follow-up examination of lesions. As highlighted by the contributions to this Special Issue, the current research supports the increasing use of this technique in the diagnosis, prognosis, treatment, and follow-up of several diseases and conditions.

Conflicts of Interest: The authors declare no conflict of interest.

List of Contributions

1. Dini, V.; Iannone, M.; Michelucci, A.; Manzo Margiotta, F.; Granieri, G.; Salvia, G.; Oranges, T.; Janowska, A.; Morganti, R.; Romanelli, M. Ultra-High Frequency UltraSound (UHFUS) Assessment of Barrier Function in Moderate-to-Severe Atopic Dermatitis during Dupilumab Treatment. *Diagnostics* **2023**, *13*, 2721.

2. Granieri, G.; Michelucci, A.; Manzo Margiotta, F.; Cei, B.; Vitali, S.; Romanelli, M.; Dini, V. The Role of Ultra-High-Frequency Ultrasound in Pyoderma Gangrenosum: New Insights in Pathophysiology and Diagnosis. *Diagnostics* **2023**, *13*, 2802.
3. Michelucci, A.; Dini, V.; Salvia, G.; Granieri, G.; Manzo Margiotta, F.; Panduri, S.; Morganti, R.; Romanelli, M. Assessment and Monitoring of Nail Psoriasis with Ultra-High Frequency Ultrasound: Preliminary Results. *Diagnostics* **2023**, *13*, 2716.
4. Salvia, G.; Zerbinati, N.; Manzo Margiotta, F.; Michelucci, A.; Granieri, G.; Fidanzi, C.; Morganti, R.; Romanelli, M.; Dini, V. Ultra-High-Frequency Ultrasound as an Innovative Imaging Evaluation of Hyaluronic Acid Filler in Nasolabial Folds. *Diagnostics* **2023**, *13*, 2761.
5. Marrani, E.; Fulvio, G.; Virgili, C.; Izzetti, R.; Dini, V.; Oranges, T.; Baldini, C.; Simonini, G. Ultra-High-Frequency Ultrasonography of Labial Glands in Pediatric Sjögren's Disease: A Preliminary Study. *Diagnostics* **2023**, *13*, 2695.
6. Fulvio, G.; Izzetti, R.; Aringhieri, G.; Donati, V.; Ferro, F.; Gabbriellini, G.; Mosca, M.; Baldini, C. UHFUS: A Valuable Tool in Evaluating Exocrine Gland Abnormalities in Sjögren's Disease. *Diagnostics* **2023**, *13*, 2771.
7. Di Battista, M.; Barsotti, S.; Vitali, S.; Palma, M.; Granieri, G.; Oranges, T.; Aringhieri, G.; Dini, V.; Della Rossa, A.; Neri, E.; et al. Multiparametric Skin Assessment in a Monocentric Cohort of Systemic Sclerosis Patients: Is There a Role for Ultra-High Frequency Ultrasound? *Diagnostics* **2023**, *13*, 1495.
8. Erlöv, T.; Hawez, T.; Granéli, C.; Evertsson, M.; Jansson, T.; Stenström, P.; Cinthio, M. A Computer Program for Assessing Histoanatomical Morphometrics in Ultra-High-Frequency Ultrasound Images of the Bowel Wall in Children: Development and Inter-Observer Variability. *Diagnostics* **2023**, *13*, 2759.
9. Hawez, T.; Graneli, C.; Erlöv, T.; Gottberg, E.; Munoz Mitev, R.; Hagelsteen, K.; Evertsson, M.; Jansson, T.; Cinthio, M.; Stenström, P. Ultra-High Frequency Ultrasound Imaging of Bowel Wall in Hirschsprung's Disease—Correlation and Agreement Analyses of Histoanatomy. *Diagnostics* **2023**, *13*, 1388.
10. Evertsson M, Graneli C, Vernersson A, Wiaczek O, Hagelsteen K, Erlöv T, Cinthio M, Stenström P. Design of a Pediatric Rectal Ultrasound Probe Intended for Ultra-High Frequency Ultrasound Diagnostics. *Diagnostics.* **2023**, *13*, 1667. https://doi.org/10.3390/diagnostics13101667.
11. Alan, A.; Orhan, A.I.; Orhan, K. Evaluation of the Breastfeeding Dynamics of Neonates with Ankyloglossia via a Novel Ultrasonographic Technique. *Diagnostics* **2023**, *13*, 3435.
12. Nisi, M.; Gennai, S.; Graziani, F.; Izzetti, R. The Reliability of Ultrasonographic Assessment of Depth of Invasion: A Systematic Review with Meta-Analysis. *Diagnostics* **2023**, *13*, 2833.
13. Jerban, S.; Barrère, V.; Andre, M.; Chang, E.Y.; Shah, S.B. Quantitative Ultrasound Techniques Used for Peripheral Nerve Assessment. *Diagnostics* **2023**, *13*, 956.
14. Yu, J.; Wang, H.; Zhou, M.; Zhu, M.; Hang, J.; Shen, M.; Jin, X.; Shi, Y.; Xu, J.; Yang, T. A Hypothesis on the Progression of Insulin-Induced Lipohypertrophy: An Integrated Result of High-Frequency Ultrasound Imaging and Blood Glucose Control of Patients. *Diagnostics* **2023**, *13*, 1515.
15. Liu, X.; Wang, J.; Liu, Y.; Luo, S.; Yan, G.; Yang, H.; Wan, L.; Huang, G. High Intensity Focused Ultrasound Ablation for Juvenile Cystic Adenomyosis: Two Case Reports and Literature Review. *Diagnostics* **2023**, *13*, 1608.

References

1. Fogante, M.; Carboni, N.; Argalia, G. Clinical application of ultra-high frequency ultrasound: Discovering a new imaging frontier. *J. Clin. Ultrasound* **2022**, *50*, 817–825. [CrossRef] [PubMed]
2. Brollo, P.P.; Bresadola, V. Enhancing visualization and guidance in general surgery: A comprehensive and narrative review of the current cutting-edge technologies and future perspectives. *J. Gastrointest. Surg.* **2024**, *28*, 179–185. [CrossRef] [PubMed]
3. Russo, A.; Reginelli, A.; Lacasella, G.V.; Grassi, E.; Karaboue, M.A.A.; Quarto, T.; Busetto, G.M.; Aliprandi, A.; Grassi, R.; Berritto, D. Clinical Application of Ultra-High-Frequency Ultrasound. *J. Pers. Med.* **2022**, *12*, 1733. [CrossRef] [PubMed]
4. Lavaud, J.; Henry, M.; Coll, J.L.; Josserand, V. Exploration of melanoma metastases in mice brains using endogenous contrast photoacoustic imaging. *Int. J. Pharm.* **2017**, *532*, 704–709. [CrossRef] [PubMed]
5. Carotenuto, A.R.; Cutolo, A.; Petrillo, A.; Fusco, R.; Arra, C.; Sansone, M.; Larobina, D.; Cardoso, L.; Fraldi, M. Growth and in vivo stresses traced through tumor mechanics enriched with predator-prey cells dynamics. *J. Mech. Behav. Biomed. Mater.* **2018**, *86*, 55–70. [CrossRef] [PubMed]
6. Fernandes, D.A.; Kolios, M.C. Intrinsically absorbing photoacoustic and ultrasound contrast agents for cancer therapy and imaging. *Nanotechnology* **2018**, *29*, 505103. [CrossRef] [PubMed]

7. Foster, F.S.; Hossack, J.; Adamson, S.L. Micro-ultrasound for preclinical imaging. *Interface Focus* **2011**, *1*, 576–601. [CrossRef] [PubMed]
8. Izzetti, R.; Oranges, T.; Janowska, A.; Gabriele, M.; Graziani, F.; Romanelli, M. The Application of Ultra-High-Frequency Ultrasound in Dermatology and Wound Management. *Int. J. Low. Extrem. Wounds* **2020**, *19*, 334–340. [CrossRef] [PubMed]
9. Izzetti, R.; Vitali, S.; Aringhieri, G.; Nisi, M.; Oranges, T.; Dini, V.; Ferro, F.; Baldini, C.; Romanelli, M.; Caramella, D.; et al. Ultra-High Frequency Ultrasound, A Promising Diagnostic Technique: Review of the Literature and Single-Center Experience. *Can. Assoc. Radiol. J.* **2021**, *72*, 418–431. [CrossRef]
10. Alexander, H.; Miller, D.L. Determining skin thickness with pulsed ultrasound. *J. Invest. Dermatol.* **1979**, *72*, 17–19. [CrossRef]
11. Schmid-Wendtner, M.H.; Dill-Müller, D. Ultrasound technology in dermatology. *Semin. Cutan. Med. Surg.* **2008**, *27*, 44–51. [CrossRef]
12. Wortsman, X. Top applications of dermatologic ultrasonography that can modify management. *Ultrasonography* **2023**, *42*, 183–202. [CrossRef]
13. Lintzeri, D.A.; Karimian, N.; Blume-Peytavi, U.; Kottner, J. Epidermal thickness in healthy humans: A systematic review and meta-analysis. *J. Eur. Acad. Dermatol. Venereol.* **2022**, *36*, 1191–1200. [CrossRef]
14. Turner, V.L.; Wortsman, X. Ultrasound Features of Nail Lichen Planus. *J. Ultrasound Med.* **2024**, *43*, 781–788. [CrossRef] [PubMed]
15. Dini, V.; Janowska, A.; Faita, F.; Panduri, S.; Benincasa, B.B.; Izzetti, R.; Romanelli, M.; Oranges, T. Ultra-high-frequency ultrasound monitoring of plaque psoriasis during ixekizumab treatment. *Skin Res. Technol.* **2021**, *27*, 277–282. [CrossRef] [PubMed]
16. Laverde-Saad, A.; Simard, A.; Nassim, D.; Jfri, A.; Alajmi, A.; O'Brien, E.; Wortsman, X. Performance of Ultrasound for Identifying Morphological Characteristics and Thickness of Cutaneous Basal Cell Carcinoma: A Systematic Review. *Dermatology* **2022**, *238*, 692–710. [CrossRef]
17. Dinnes, J.; Bamber, J.; Chuchu, N.; Bayliss, S.E.; Takwoingi, Y.; Davenport, C.; Godfrey, K.; O'Sullivan, C.; Matin, R.N.; Deeks, J.J.; et al. High-frequency ultrasound for diagnosing skin cancer in adults. *Cochrane Database Syst. Rev.* **2018**, *12*, CD013188. [CrossRef] [PubMed]
18. Oranges, T.; Janowska, A.; Scatena, C.; Faita, F.; Lascio, N.D.; Izzetti, R.; Fidanzi, C.; Romanelli, M.; Dini, V. Ultra-High Frequency Ultrasound in Melanoma Management: A New Combined Ultrasonographic-Histopathological Approach. *J. Ultrasound Med.* **2023**, *42*, 99–108. [CrossRef]
19. Reginelli, A.; Russo, A.; Berritto, D.; Patane, V.; Cantisani, C.; Grassi, R. Ultra-High-Frequency Ultrasound: A Modern Diagnostic Technique for Studying Melanoma. *Ultraschall Med.* **2023**, *44*, 360–378. [CrossRef]
20. Oranges, T.; Janowska, A.; Vitali, S.; Loggini, B.; Izzetti, R.; Romanelli, M.; Dini, V. Dermatoscopic and ultra-high frequency ultrasound evaluation in cutaneous postradiation angiosarcoma. *J. Eur. Acad. Dermatol. Venereol.* **2020**, *34*, e741. [CrossRef]
21. Janowska, A.; Oranges, T.; Granieri, G.; Romanelli, M.; Fidanzi, C.; Iannone, M.; Dini, V. Non-invasive imaging techniques in presurgical margin assessment of basal cell carcinoma: Current evidence. *Skin Res. Technol.* **2023**, *29*, e13271. [CrossRef]
22. Chauvel-Picard, J.; Tognetti, L.; Cinotti, E.; Habougit, C.; Suppa, M.; Lenoir, C.; Rubegni, P.; Del Marmol, V.; Berot, V.; Gleizal, A.; et al. Role of ultra-high-frequency ultrasound in the diagnosis and management of basal cell carcinoma: Pilot study based on 117 cases. *Clin. Exp. Dermatol.* **2023**, *48*, 468–475. [CrossRef]
23. Dopytalska, K.; Sobolewski, P.; Mikucka-Wituszyńska, A.; Gnatowski, M.; Szymańska, E.; Walecka, I. Noninvasive skin imaging in esthetic medicine-Why do we need useful tools for evaluation of the esthetic procedures. *J. Cosmet. Dermatol.* **2021**, *20*, 746–754. [CrossRef]
24. Manzaneda Cipriani, R.M.; Cárdenas Larenas, J.P.; Viaro, M.S.S.; Flores González, E.A.; Adrianzen, G.; Babaitis, R.; Duran Vega, H.; Stefanelli, M.; Ventura, R. Jawline Aesthetic Definition: Enhancement with Masseteric Augmentation Using Ultrasound-Guided Fat Transfer. *Plast. Reconstr. Surg. Glob. Open* **2024**, *12*, e5695. [CrossRef]
25. Aringhieri, G.; Izzetti, R.; Vitali, S.; Ferro, F.; Gabriele, M.; Baldini, C.; Caramella, D. Ultra-high frequency ultrasound (UHFUS) applications in Sjogren syndrome: Narrative review and current concepts. *Gland. Surg.* **2020**, *9*, 2248–2259. [CrossRef]
26. Jousse-Joulin, S.; Gatineau, F.; Baldini, C.; Baer, A.; Barone, F.; Bootsma, H.; Bowman, S.; Brito-Zerón, P.; Cornec, D.; Dorner, T.; et al. Weight of salivary gland ultrasonography compared to other items of the 2016 ACR/EULAR classification criteria for Primary Sjögren's syndrome. *J. Inter. Med.* **2020**, *287*, 180–188. [CrossRef]
27. Lee, K.A.; Kim, S.H.; Kim, H.R.; Kim, H.S. Impact of age on the diagnostic performance of unstimulated salivary flow rates and salivary gland ultrasound for primary Sjögren's syndrome. *Front. Med.* **2022**, *9*, 968697. [CrossRef]
28. Saruhanoğlu, A.; Atikler, M.; Ergun, S.; Ofluoğlu, D.; Tanyeri, H. Comparison of two different labial salivary gland biopsy incision techniques: A randomized clinical trial. *Med. Oral Patol Oral Cir. Bucal.* **2013**, *18*, e851–e855. [CrossRef]
29. Izzetti, R.; Ferro, F.; Vitali, S.; Nisi, M.; Fonzetti, S.; Oranges, T.; Donati, V.; Caramella, D.; Baldini, C.; Gabriele, M. Ultra-high frequency ultrasonography (UHFUS)-guided minor salivary gland biopsy: A promising procedure to optimize labial salivary gland biopsy in Sjögren's syndrome. *J. Oral Pathol. Med.* **2021**, *50*, 485–491. [CrossRef]
30. Fox, R.I. Sjögren's syndrome. *Lancet* **2005**, *366*, 321–331. [CrossRef]
31. Takagi, Y.; Sasaki, M.; Eida, S.; Katayama, I.; Hashimoto, K.; Nakamura, H.; Shimizu, T.; Morimoto, S.; Kawakami, A.; Sumi, M. Comparison of salivary gland MRI and ultrasonography findings among patients with Sjögren's syndrome over a wide age range. *Rheumatology* **2022**, *61*, 1986–1996. [CrossRef]
32. Gong, Y.; Liu, H.; Li, G.; Zhang, T.; Li, Y.; Guan, W.; Zeng, Q.; Lv, Q.; Zhang, X.; Yao, W.; et al. Childhood-onset primary Sjögren's syndrome in a tertiary center in China: Clinical features and outcome. *Pediatr. Rheumatol. Online J.* **2023**, *21*, 11. [CrossRef]

33. Narazaki, H.; Akioka, S.; Akutsu, Y.; Araki, M.; Fujieda, M.; Fukuhara, D.; Hara, R.; Hashimoto, K.; Hattori, S.; Hayashibe, R.; et al. Epidemiology conduction of paediatric rheumatic diseases based on the registry database of the Pediatric Rheumatology Association of Japan. *Mod. Rheumatol.* **2023**, *33*, 1021–1029. [CrossRef]
34. Krumrey-Langkammerer, M.; Haas, J.P. Salivary gland ultrasound in the diagnostic workup of juvenile Sjögren's syndrome and mixed connective tissue disease. *Pediatr. Rheumatol. Online J.* **2020**, *18*, 44. [CrossRef]
35. Cornec, D.; Jamin, C.; Pers, J.O. Sjögren's syndrome: Where do we stand, and where shall we go? *J. Autoimmun.* **2014**, *51*, 109–114. [CrossRef]
36. Romão, V.C.; Talarico, R.; Scirè, C.A.; Vieira, A.; Alexander, T.; Baldini, C.; Gottenberg, J.E.; Gruner, H.; Hachulla, E.; Mouthon, L.; et al. Sjögren's syndrome: State of the art on clinical practice guidelines. *RMD Open* **2018**, *4*, e000789. [CrossRef]
37. Vehof, J.; Utheim, T.P.; Bootsma, H.; Hammond, C.J. Advances, limitations and future perspectives in the diagnosis and management of dry eye in Sjögren's syndrome. *Clin. Exp. Rheumatol.* **2020**, *38*, 301–309.
38. Vora, Z.; Hemachandran, N.; Sharma, S. Imaging of Lacrimal Gland Pathologies: A Radiological Pattern-Based Approach. *Curr. Probl. Diagn. Radiol.* **2021**, *50*, 738–748. [CrossRef] [PubMed]
39. Li, L.; Xu, J.; Wang, S.; Yang, J. Ultra-High-Frequency Ultrasound in the Evaluation of Paediatric Pilomatricoma Based on the Histopathologic Classification. *Front. Med.* **2021**, *8*, 673861. [CrossRef]
40. Ait Ichou, J.; Gauvin, S.; Faingold, R. Ultra-high-frequency ultrasound of superficial and musculoskeletal structures in the pediatric population. *Pediatr. Radiol.* **2021**, *51*, 1748–1757. [CrossRef]
41. Granéli, C.; Erlöv, T.; Mitev, R.M.; Kasselaki, I.; Hagelsteen, K.; Gisselsson, D.; Jansson, T.; Cinthio, M.; Stenström, P. Ultra-high frequency ultrasonography to distinguish ganglionic from aganglionic bowel wall in Hirschsprung disease: A first report. *J. Pediatr. Surg.* **2021**, *56*, 2281–2285. [CrossRef]
42. Beltman, L.; Windster, J.D.; Roelofs, J.J.T.H.; van der Voorn, J.P.; Derikx, J.P.M.; Bakx, R. Diagnostic accuracy of calretinin and acetylcholinesterase staining of rectal suction biopsies in Hirschsprung disease examined by unexperienced pathologists. *Virchows Arch.* **2022**, *481*, 245–252. [CrossRef]
43. Guo, X.; Yang, H.; Li, J.; Zeng, L.; Wang, C.; Yang, R.; Yang, Y. Application value of high-frequency ultrasonography in endoscopic retrograde appendicitis therapy for pediatric acute appendicitis. *Surg. Endosc.* **2023**, *37*, 3814–3822. [CrossRef]
44. Ong, C.K.; Chong, V.F. Imaging of tongue carcinoma. *Cancer Imaging* **2006**, *6*, 186–193. [CrossRef]
45. DeJohn, C.R.; Seshadri, M. Ultra-high frequency ultrasound as a clinical adjunct for imaging the oral cavity: Added value of quantitative analysis. *Dentomaxillofac. Radiol.* **2020**, *49*, 20200314. [CrossRef]
46. Wong, K.T.; Tsang, R.K.; Tse, G.M.; Yuen, E.H.; Ahuja, A.T. Biopsy of deep-seated head and neck lesions under intraoral ultrasound guidance. *AJNR Am. J. Neuroradiol.* **2006**, *27*, 1654–1657.
47. Izzetti, R.; Fantoni, G.; Gelli, F.; Faggioni, L.; Vitali, S.; Gabriele, M.; Caramella, D. Feasibility of intraoral ultrasonography in the diagnosis of oral soft tissue lesions: A preclinical assessment on an ex vivo specimen. *Radiol. Med.* **2018**, *123*, 135–142. [CrossRef]
48. Fukano, H.; Matsuura, H.; Hasegawa, Y.; Nakamura, S. Depth of invasion as a predictive factor for cervical lymph node metastasis in tongue carcinoma. *Head Neck* **1997**, *19*, 205–210. [CrossRef]
49. Shintani, S.; Nakayama, B.; Matsuura, H.; Hasegawa, Y. Intraoral ultrasonography is useful to evaluate tumor thickness in tongue carcinoma. *Am. J. Surg.* **1997**, *173*, 345–347. [CrossRef]
50. Pires Duarte, L.C.; Teixeira, K.; Dias, B.M.F.; Fonseca, F.P.; Travassos, D.V.; Smit, C.; Castro, M.A.A.; Sampaio, A.A. Ultrasonography use for tongue cancer management: A scoping review. *J. Oral Pathol. Med.* **2024**, *53*, 107–113. [CrossRef]
51. Pollaers, K.; Hinton-Bayre, A.; Friedland, P.L.; Farah, C.S. AJCC 8th Edition oral cavity squamous cell carcinoma staging—Is it an improvement on the AJCC 7th Edition? *Oral Oncol.* **2018**, *82*, 23–28. [CrossRef]
52. Kowalski, L.P.; Köhler, H.F. Relevant changes in the AJCC 8th edition staging manual for oral cavity cancer and future implications. *Chin. Clin. Oncol.* **2019**, *8*, S18. [CrossRef]
53. Kim, Y.; Lee, D.J. The updated AJCC/TNM staging system (8th edition) for oral tongue cancer. *Transl. Cancer Res.* **2019**, *8*, S164–S166. [CrossRef]
54. Konishi, M.; Fujita, M.; Shimabukuro, K.; Wongratwanich, P.; Kakimoto, N. Predictive Factors of Late Cervical Lymph Node Metastasis Using Intraoral Sonography in Patients with Tongue Cancer. *Anticancer Res.* **2022**, *42*, 287–292. [CrossRef]
55. Konishi, M.; Fujita, M.; Shimabukuro, K.; Wongratwanich, P.; Verdonschot, R.G.; Kakimoto, N. Intraoral Ultrasonographic Features of Tongue Cancer and the Incidence of Cervical Lymph Node Metastasis. *J. Oral Maxillofac. Surg.* **2021**, *79*, 932–939. [CrossRef]
56. Mourad, M.A.F.; Higazi, M.M. MRI prognostic factors of tongue cancer: Potential predictors of cervical lymph nodes metastases. *Radiol Oncol.* **2019**, *53*, 49–56. [CrossRef]
57. Marcello Scotti, F.; Stuepp, R.T.; Leonardi Dutra-Horstmann, K.; Modolo, F.; Gusmão Paraiso Cavalcanti, M. Accuracy of, M.R.I.; CT, and Ultrasound imaging on thickness and depth of oral primary carcinomas invasion: A systematic review. *Dentomaxillofac. Radiol.* **2022**, *51*, 20210291. [CrossRef]
58. Caprioli, S.; Giordano, G.G.; Pennacchi, A.; Campagnari, V.; Iandelli, A.; Parrinello, G.; Conforti, C.; Gili, R.; Giannini, E.; Marabotto, E.; et al. Can High-Frequency Intraoral Ultrasound Predict Histological Risk Factors in Oral Squamous Cell Carcinoma? A Preliminary Experience. *Cancers* **2023**, *15*, 4413. [CrossRef]
59. Izzetti, R.; Nisi, M.; Gennai, S.; Oranges, T.; Crocetti, L.; Caramella, D.; Graziani, F. Evaluation of Depth of Invasion in Oral Squamous Cell Carcinoma with Ultra-High. Frequency Ultrasound: A Preliminary Study. *Appl. Sci.* **2021**, *11*, 7647. [CrossRef]

60. Izzetti, R.; Nisi, M.; Aringhieri, G.; Vitali, S.; Oranges, T.; Romanelli, M.; Caramella, D.; Graziani, F.; Gabriele, M. Ultra-high frequency ultrasound in the differential diagnosis of oral pemphigus and pemphigoid: An explorative study. *Skin. Res. Technol.* **2021**, *27*, 682–691. [CrossRef]
61. Puma, A.; Grecu, N.; Badea, R.Ș.; Morisot, A.; Zugravu, R.; Ioncea, M.B.; Cavalli, M.; Lăcătuș, O.; Ezaru, A.; Hacina, C.; et al. Typical CIDP, distal variant CIDP, and anti-MAG antibody neuropathy: An ultra-high frequency ultrasound comparison of nerve structure. *Sci. Rep.* **2024**, *14*, 4643. [CrossRef] [PubMed]
62. Poelaert, J.; Coopman, R.; Ureel, M.; Dhooghe, N.; Genbrugge, E.; Mwewa, T.; Blondeel, P.; Vermeersch, H. Visualization of the Facial Nerve with Ultra-high-Frequency Ultrasound. *Plast. Reconstr. Surg. Glob. Open* **2023**, *11*, e5489. [CrossRef] [PubMed]

Disclaimer/Publisher's Note: The statements, opinions and data contained in all publications are solely those of the individual author(s) and contributor(s) and not of MDPI and/or the editor(s). MDPI and/or the editor(s) disclaim responsibility for any injury to people or property resulting from any ideas, methods, instructions or products referred to in the content.

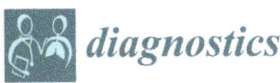

Article

Evaluation of the Breastfeeding Dynamics of Neonates with Ankyloglossia via a Novel Ultrasonographic Technique

Arzu Alan [1], Ayse Isil Orhan [2] and Kaan Orhan [3,*]

1. Ankara 75th Year Oral and Dental Health Hospital, Ministry of Health, Ankara 06230, Türkiye; arzudogruyol@yahoo.com
2. Department of Pediatric Dentistry, Faculty of Dentistry, Ankara Yildirim Beyazit University, Ankara 06220, Türkiye; isilcihan@yahoo.com
3. Department of Dentomaxillofacial Radiology, Faculty of Dentistry, Ankara University, Ankara 06560, Türkiye
* Correspondence: knorhan@dentistry.ankara.edu.tr

Abstract: To effectively address breastfeeding issues for neonates and mothers, one must understand the physiology of breastfeeding and the anatomical components involved in sucking, swallowing, and respiration. This study compared the tongue position and movement of neonates with tongue ties versus healthy controls during sucking. A new objective ultrasonography diagnostic approach was also introduced for the orofacial region. This retrospective study evaluated B-mode and M-mode ultrasonography images from 30 neonates clinically diagnosed with tongue tie, and a control group of 30 neonates. B-mode ultrasound images were used to examine several characteristics to locate the nipple in the oral cavity during breastfeeding. Anatomic M-mode ultrasound images were used to assess tongue movement during sucking. The nipple moved farther from the intersection of the hard and soft palates during the sucking cycle in the ankyloglossia group than in the control group ($p < 0.05$). Compared to the control group, neonates with ankyloglossia have a lower capacity to lift the anterior tongue toward the palate when sucking ($p < 0.05$). There was no significant difference in tongue movement metrics between the two groups ($p > 0.05$). Our findings were consistent with earlier research. The novel measurement method will offer a new perspective on breastfeeding.

Keywords: breastfeeding; ankyloglossia; ultrasonography; diagnostic imaging; tongue movement; sucking function

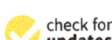

Citation: Alan, A.; Orhan, A.I.; Orhan, K. Evaluation of the Breastfeeding Dynamics of Neonates with Ankyloglossia via a Novel Ultrasonographic Technique. Diagnostics 2023, 13, 3435. https://doi.org/10.3390/diagnostics13223435

Academic Editors: Elina A. Genina, Rossana Izzetti and Marco Nisi

Received: 15 July 2023
Revised: 3 October 2023
Accepted: 11 November 2023
Published: 13 November 2023
Corrected: 13 March 2024

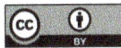

Copyright: © 2023 by the authors. Licensee MDPI, Basel, Switzerland. This article is an open access article distributed under the terms and conditions of the Creative Commons Attribution (CC BY) license (https://creativecommons.org/licenses/by/4.0/).

1. Introduction

The rooting, sucking, and swallowing reflexes of a healthy neonate become active shortly after birth. These reflexes, commonly referred to as sucking physiology, emerge during the prenatal period of development. A newborn infant possesses the innate ability to execute the sucking reflex without any difficulty. However, they must acquire the requisite abilities to effectively utilize these reflexes. The process of milk ejection from the breast is considered a learned ability that necessitates the proper attachment of the infant's mouth to the breast and the comprehensive adaptation of anatomical structures, such as the tongue and lips, for feeding [1]. To achieve successful breastfeeding, the infant must possess the capability to effectively and securely ingest the milk bolus before it enters the digestive system. To execute this particular function, the infant must possess the capability to synchronize the processes of swallowing and respiration, all the while ensuring the maintenance of cardiovascular stability [2]. Symptoms indicating dysfunctions in these processes include breast and nipple pain, challenges with latching and sucking, crying during breastfeeding, refusal of the breast, extended and frequent feeding, inadequate weight gain, crying due to insufficient satiety, and difficulties with milk transfer [3]. Numerous challenges prompt a significant number of women to prematurely cease the practice of breastfeeding [4].

A comprehensive comprehension of the physiology of breastfeeding and an in-depth examination of the anatomical structures of the jaw, palate, hyoid bone, pharynx, and tongue involved in sucking, swallowing, and respiratory actions can enhance the efficacy of therapeutic interventions aimed at addressing breastfeeding difficulties experienced by newborns and mothers [5,6]. The execution of these functions is heavily reliant on the movements of the tongue [7,8]. The examination of literary works reveals the presence of two discernible perspectives regarding the movement of the tongue during the process of sucking. Based on the stripping action theory, the act of extracting milk from the breast is facilitated by peristaltic tongue movements and the application of sucking pressure through the infant's mandible, compressing the breast [8–12]. According to the theory of intra-oral vacuum, the primary mechanism involved in the extraction of milk from the breast is the generation of negative pressure or a vacuum through the downward movement of the tongue [7,13]. Based on the findings of the study assessing milk outflow and sucking dynamics during breastfeeding, it was observed that the posterior tongue exhibits peristaltic movements, effectively guiding the milk bolus toward the esophagus. Furthermore, it should be noted that the anterior tongue tip, located beneath the nipple, applies pressure to the entire breast through periodic mandibular movements without exhibiting peristaltic motion [14]. There is a lack of consensus within the scientific literature regarding the specific role and function of the tongue during the lactation process.

The presence of anatomical variations in the structures involved in the act of sucking may potentially exert detrimental impacts on the process of breastfeeding. Ankyloglossia, also known as tongue tie, is a congenital anomaly that restricts the range of motion of the tongue. This particular condition exerts a significant impact on the suction capacity and may also modify the structure of the dental arches, consequently influencing occlusion [1,15,16]. The occurrence rate of ankyloglossia in newborns varies between 4% and 16%, with a greater frequency observed in males compared to females at a ratio of 2.5 to 1.2 [17]. Despite divergent opinions among healthcare professionals, the condition known as tongue tie has been widely acknowledged as a prevalent issue affecting breastfeeding, as evidenced by numerous studies. According to the findings of Messner et al. (2000), approximately 90% of pediatricians and 70% of otolaryngologists believe that ankyloglossia rarely causes feeding difficulties, while approximately 70% of lactation consultants reported that ankyloglossia often causes feeding difficulties [18]. Research findings indicate that ankyloglossia is linked to a substantial percentage of breastfeeding-related challenges in neonates, with prevalence estimates ranging from 25% to 60%. The aforementioned concerns encompass inadequate milk production, hindered growth and development, nipple injury, breast discomfort, engorgement, and maternal rejection [18–20]. The main contributing factor to these issues, as identified by Marmet et al. (2000) and Segal et al. (2007), is the neonate's inability to maintain a secure latch on the breast, which can be attributed to ankyloglossia [20,21]. According to reports, the rate of breastfeeding cessation as a result of the enduring pain encountered by mothers during the initial three weeks of breastfeeding ranges from 10% to 26% [22,23]. The crucial factor for successful breastfeeding in healthy neonates, as determined through the use of ultrasonography, is appropriate tongue mobility, as indicated by the findings of Smith et al. (1985) [24]. In the case of neonates diagnosed with ankyloglossia, it has been observed that traditional positioning and suckling techniques do not yield satisfactory results in terms of restoring tongue mobility. Consequently, surgical intervention may become necessary [19]. In recent years, there has been an increasing prevalence of frenotomy procedures aimed at facilitating the continuity of breastfeeding in neonates. The existing literature does not provide a consensus on the effectiveness of frenotomy in lactation. There is still a lack of consensus regarding the appropriate course of action for addressing this abnormality, including the timing of treatment and the optimal surgical approach to be employed [25,26].

Therefore, implementing a comprehensive, accurate, and unbiased approach to assess the intraoral modifications occurring during the sucking reflex in newborns would effectively mitigate the need for unnecessary surgical interventions in early infancy. In their study, Geddes and Sakalidis (2016) presented a thorough elucidation of the ultrasound imaging technique employed for observing the tongue's movements during the act of breastfeeding [27]. In their study, McClellan et al. (2010) utilized morphological metrics to illustrate the precise positioning of the nipple within the oral cavity and the tongue's role during breastfeeding, as observed through B-mode ultrasonography images taken in the midsagittal plane [28].

The objective of this study was to conduct a comparative analysis between neonates diagnosed with clinically confirmed tongue ties and a control group of healthy individuals. The comparison was conducted in terms of tongue position and movement during sucking. Additionally, the study aimed to assess the effectiveness and applicability of ultrasound imaging techniques in this context. The main objectives of this study are to present a new and unbiased ultrasound diagnostic approach that has not yet been proven effective in the orofacial region and to establish innovative and unbiased diagnostic criteria to assist in the identification of neonates with tongue tie.

2. Materials and Methods

The research was carried out in compliance with the principles outlined in the Declaration of Helsinki and received approval from the Ethics Committee of Health Sciences at Ankara Yildirim Beyazit University in Ankara, Turkey (04/13 April 2023).

The sample size was calculated for the effect size (d, effect size = 0.85), type I error (α = 0.05), and 85% power values; the sample size was determined to be 30 for the two independent groups.

The current study entailed a retrospective examination of ultrasonography images acquired using B-mode (brightness mode) and M-mode (motion mode) techniques. These images were obtained from a cohort of sixty neonates between May 2022 and December 2022. The researchers conducted a review of the file records of the neonates included in this study, focusing on two key pieces of information: the severity of tongue tie, as assessed using the Bristol Tongue Assessment Tool, and whether a frenotomy procedure had been carried out. Based on the scoring system of the Bristol Tongue Assessment Tool, the participants were categorized into two distinct groups: a group of 30 individuals with ankyloglossia, characterized by a tongue tie score of 5 or less, and a group of 30 healthy individuals, characterized by a tongue tie score exceeding 5. During the course of breastfeeding, ultrasonography images were obtained from full-term neonates aged 5–15 days. All USG evaluations were conducted by a single dentomaxillofacial radiologist observer with 14 years of experience (A.A). The radiologist employed a GE Medical System Verasana Active (Wuxi, Jiangsu, China) mobile ultrasonography device equipped with a 6–10 MHz 8C-RS microconvex probe. This instrument was used to capture 2D real-time, B-mode, and M-mode images of the oral cavity of the neonates. The imaging was performed using a submental approach in the midsagittal plane. The examinations were conducted using Parker Ultrasonic Gel (Fairfield, NJ, USA). The data collection commenced when the infant began to latch onto the breast and concluded when the feeding came to an end. The recording captured by the scan was specifically intended for subsequent academic investigation. The study excluded recordings that exhibited artifacts resulting from movements of the mother–newborn pair or the operator, as well as recordings in which the presence of nutritive sucking could not be observed. All measurements were conducted in recorded ultrasonography images. Before starting the measurement in the study, the observer was calibrated to recognize as well as to identify the neonate maxillofacial and oral anatomy; for such purpose, 10 different neonate ultrasonography images other than the study were used. The observer was blinded to any patient data.

During the act of breastfeeding, the nipple is positioned in such a way that it rests on the anterior region of the tongue, while the tip of the anterior tongue is elevated above the inferior alveolar ridge. The visibility of the tip of the tongue on ultrasonography is hindered by mandibular superposition. The process of sucking begins with the tongue-up posture (Figure 1a–c), wherein the middle portion of the tongue is near the roof of the mouth. This occurs when a newborn is properly attached to the breast and the tongue occupies the entire oral cavity. The sucking cycle is characterized by a downward motion of the tongue towards its lowest point, known as the tongue-down position (Figure 2a–c). In this position, the middle portion of the tongue descends to the floor of the mouth. The cycle concludes when the tongue reverts to its original position adjacent to the palate. The downward movement of the tongue results in the flow of breast milk into the interstitial space created between the surface of the tongue and the palate. In the ultrasonography image, milk boluses are observed as areas of increased echogenicity within the hypoechoic region [28]. Upon the tongue's elevation towards the palate, the milk bolus is introduced into the pharynx. The ultrasound image depicts the process of sucking, where milk is transferred into the oral cavity, referred to as nutritive sucking (Figure 2a–c). Conversely, the act of sucking without milk outflow is termed non-nutritive sucking [29].

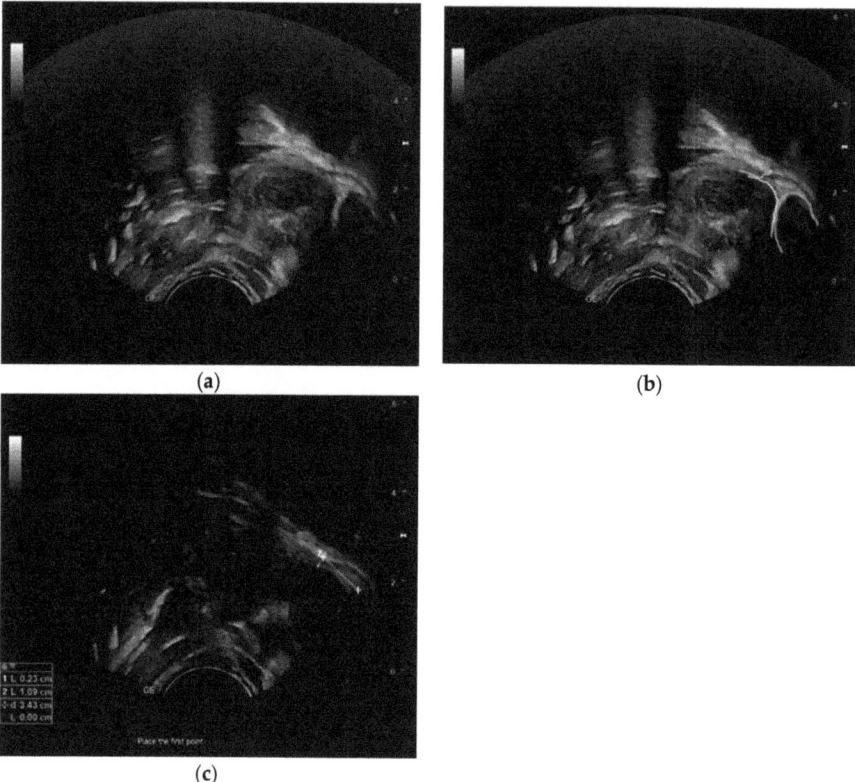

Figure 1. Ultrasonographic image of breastfeeding: (**a**) nipple view, tongue up; (**b**) nipple: dark blue line, hard–soft palate junction (HSPJ): light blue line, tongue: yellow line; (**c**) depth of intraoral space, cm: yellow line 1; nipple–HSPJ distance, cm: green line 2.

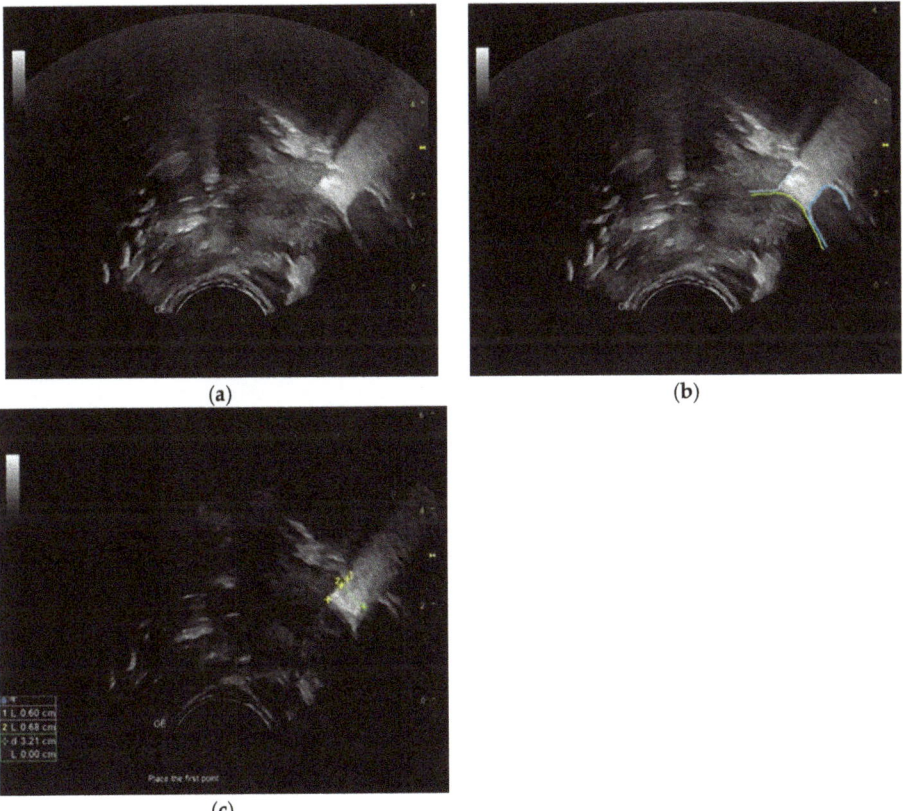

Figure 2. Ultrasonographic image of breastfeeding: (**a**) nipple view, tongue down; (**b**) nipple: dark blue line, HSPJ: light blue line, tongue: yellow line; (**c**) depth of intraoral space, cm: yellow line 1; nipple–HSPJ distance, cm: green line 2.

Frame-by-frame analysis of B-mode ultrasonography recordings was conducted to examine three consecutive sucking cycles during nutritive sucking in both groups. The determination of the nipple's position in the mouth during each cycle involved measuring the distance between the HSPJ and the nipple as well as the depth of the intra-oral space created during the sucking function, as outlined by McClellan et al. (2010) (Figures 1c and 2c) [28]. In ultrasonography images, the hard palate is visualized as a line with high echogenicity, while the soft palate is observed as a structure of intermediate gray shades with a distinct echogenic upper boundary (see Figures 1b and 2b). The observation of the soft palate's motion during the sucking process facilitated the identification and validation of the HSPJ through the analysis of real-time ultrasonography video footage. To determine the alteration in size of the tongue during the act of sucking, measurements of the anterior and middle sections of the tongue were taken in both the tongue-up and tongue-down orientations. The researchers obtained measurements from the dorsal surface of the tongue to the inferior border of the genioglossus muscle, as depicted in Figure 3a,b.

In this study, we employed the measurement technique previously employed by Schleifer et al. (2021) and Boussuges et al. (2020) to evaluate tongue movements and the duration of a sucking cycle during breastfeeding [30,31]. The M-mode cursor was placed at a perpendicular angle to the mid-tongue in ultrasonography images acquired from both groups of neonates utilizing anatomical M-mode. The utilization of anatomical M-mode imaging resulted in improved visualization of the echogenic representation of tongue motility (Figure 4a,b). In M-mode tongue movement images obtained during nutritive feeding, the tongue is hypoechoic. The milk bolus is viewed as hyperechoic on the hypoechoic image of the tongue. In this diagram, the initial caliper was designated at the apex corresponding to the placement of the tongue, while the subsequent caliper was designated at the nadir of the incline formed by the tongue's downward motion. Ultrasonographic measurements were conducted to assess tongue excursion from the palate to the floor of the mouth (in centimeters), excursion time (in seconds), and tongue velocity during movement (in centimeters per second). Furthermore, the initial caliper was positioned at the apex of the hypoechoic diagram representing tongue movement, specifically when the tongue was situated above. Similarly, the second caliper was placed at the subsequent peak of the hypoechoic diagram, also indicating tongue positioning above. Subsequently, the duration (in seconds) of a single sucking cycle was determined. The mean values of the data obtained in M-mode were determined by conducting repetitive measurements over four sucking cycles (Figure 5). Using this novel ultrasonographic measurement technique, the researchers determined the mean duration of the nutritive sucking cycle and the average velocity of tongue movement. The analysis of frenotomy status among neonates diagnosed with tongue tie in our study group was conducted concerning the remaining parameters.

All measurements were taken twice by the same observer, and the mean values of all measurements were included in the statistical analysis. The observer also performed the study twice with an interval of 2 weeks to detect intra-observer variability. Intra-observer reliability was conducted. To assess intra-observer reliability, the Wilcoxon matched pairs signed rank test was used for repeat measurements.

The data for this study were analyzed utilizing IBM SPSS Statistics V22.0 (New York, NY, USA). The Shapiro–Wilk test was utilized to assess normality. The variables nipple-HSPJ distance intraoral space depth, anterior and mid-tongue height, tongue excursion from the palate to the floor of the mouth (cm), excursion time (sec), tongue velocity (cm/sec), and one sucking cycle duration (sec) obtained in the tongue tie and control groups exhibited a non-normal distribution. Therefore, the Mann–Whitney U test was employed to assess the association between the two groups. The frenotomy status data were subjected to a t-test to compare them with other variables as they exhibited a normal distribution. The values are presented in terms of the mean and standard deviation (SD). The chosen level of significance for this study was 0.05. A p-value less than 0.05 is indicative of a statistically significant difference or correlation, while a p-value greater than 0.05 suggests the absence of a statistically significant difference or correlation.

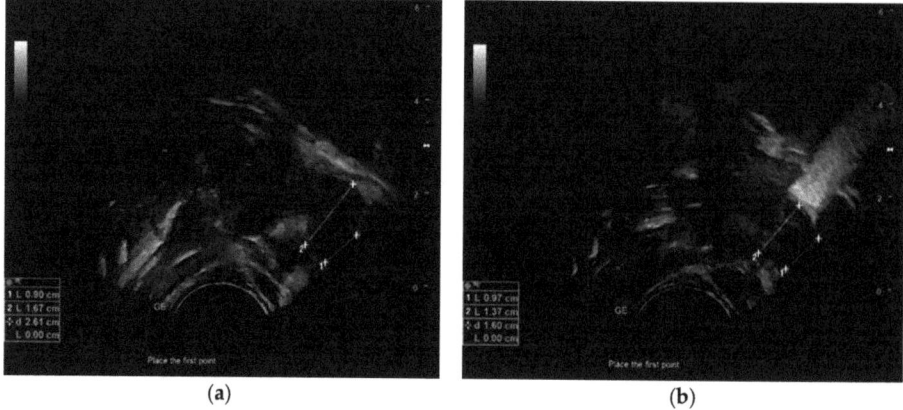

Figure 3. Ultrasonographic image of the tongue during breastfeeding: (**a**) tongue up; anterior tongue height, mm: yellow line 1; posterior tongue height, mm: yellow line 2; (**b**) tongue down; anterior tongue height, cm: yellow line 1; posterior tongue height, cm: yellow line 2.

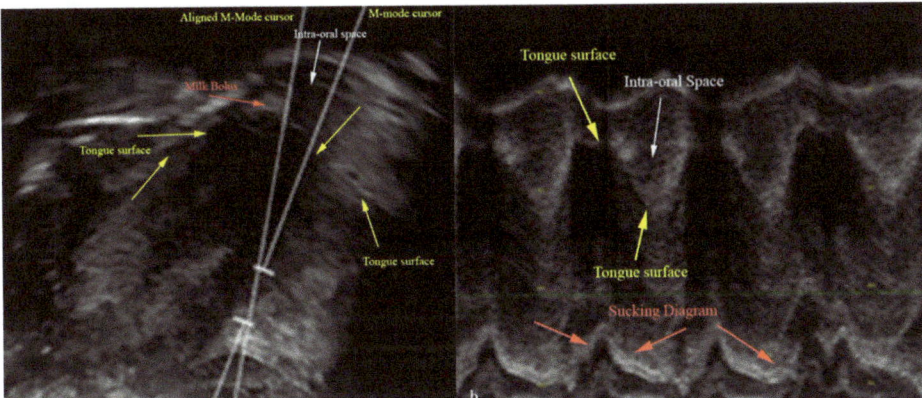

Figure 4. Ultrasound sonographic image of the tongue movement during sucking cycle in B-mode and M-mode. (**a**) The yellow arrow shows the tongue surface, the red arrow milk bolus, the white arrow intra-oral space, and white lines show M-mode cursor lines; (**b**) the yellow arrow shows the tongue surface, the red arrow shows the sucking cycle diagram, and white arrow intra-oral space.

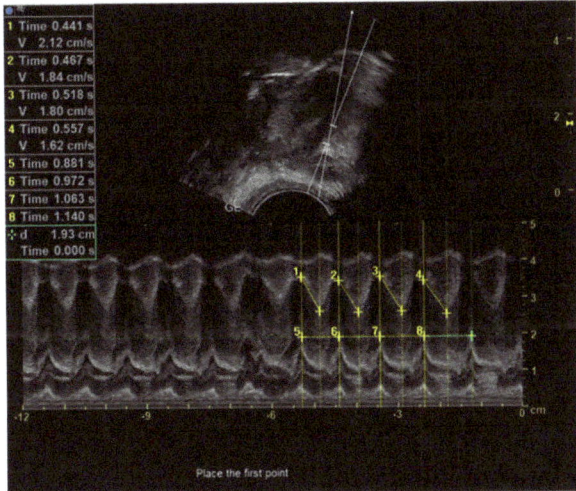

Figure 5. M-mode ultrasonography of tongue movement during breastfeeding. Slope measurement: yellow line 1, 2, 3 and 4; sucking cycle duration: yellow line 5, 6, 7 and 8.

3. Results

Repeated measurements indicated no significant intra-observer difference for the observer ($p > 0.05$). Overall intra-observer consistency was rated among the measurements between 92 and 95%. All measurements were found to be highly reproducible for the observer and no significant difference was obtained from two measurements of the observer ($p > 0.05$). Thus, the mean values of these measurements from the three points were considered to be the final data.

The present study analyzed ultrasonography images obtained from a sample of 30 neonates who were diagnosed with ankyloglossia. This sample consisted of 13 female neonates and 17 male neonates. The mean age of the neonates in this study was determined to be 12 days. By contrast, the mean age of a sample of 30 neonates who were in good health was found to be 11 days.

The findings from our examination of ultrasonography images indicate that, during the process of newborns attaching to the breast, the tongue assumes a resting position on the palate in conjunction with the nipple. The nutrient extraction process began in a state of quiescence. The observation of anechoic milk ducts in the nipple and the subsequent movement of the nipple towards the HSPJ can be attributed to the downward displacement of the middle tongue. At the point of closest proximity between the nipple and the HSPJ, the tongue reached its lowest position while the intraoral space was filled with milk. The movement of the milk bolus towards the pharynx was noted when the middle tongue returned to the palate, causing the cessation of milk flow due to the pressure exerted by the tongue on the nipple. Upon adjusting the position of the tongue against the palate, it was noted that the nipple exhibited a displacement away from the HSPJ in both experimental groups. The data collected in this study were employed to ascertain the location of the nipple within the oral cavity as well as the dimensional fluctuations in the vertical movements of the tongue during the sucking process for both experimental groups.

In the tongue-up position during the sucking cycle, it was observed that, in the ankyloglossia group, the nipple exhibited a greater distance from the HSPJ compared to the control group ($p < 0.05$) (Table 1). There was a statistically significant difference in the anterior tongue height in the tongue-up position between the control group and the ankyloglossia group ($p < 0.05$) (Table 1). In contrast to neonates diagnosed with ankyloglossia, neonates in the control group demonstrated greater ability to elevate the anterior tongue in proximity to the palate during the act of sucking. While there was no statistically significant disparity observed between the two groups regarding anterior tongue height in the tongue-down position, it was observed that healthy neonates exhibited greater anterior tongue height compared to those diagnosed with ankyloglossia ($p > 0.05$). The neonates in the control group exhibited greater proficiency in the act of latching onto and maintaining the breast within their oral cavity compared to the neonates in the ankyloglossia group, as indicated by the data presented in Table 1. Both groups exhibited similar measurements for intraoral space depth and mid-tongue height, as shown in Table 1.

Table 1. Nipple and tongue measurements. Ankyloglossia and control group comparisons.

			Nipple–HSPJ Distance, cm	Depth of Intraoral Space, cm	Anterior Tongue Height, cm	Mid-Tongue Height, cm
Tongue up	Ankyloglossia	n	30 *	30	30 *	30
		mean	0.81 *	0.33	1.08 *	1.66
		SD	0.32 *	0.13	0.29 *	0.26
	Control	n	30 *	30	30 *	30
		mean	0.64 *	0.28	1.26 *	1.76
		SD	0.18 *	0.08	0.23 *	0.18
Tongue down	Ankyloglossia	n	30	30	30	30
		mean	0.51	0.74	1.06	1.33
		SD	0.25	0.29	0.18	0.21
	Control	n	30	30	30	30
		mean	0.43	0.43	1.17	1.36
		SD	0.23	0.26	0.2	0.22

* Statistical analysis performed using Mann–Whitney U test ($p < 0.05$). n: number of participants; SD: standard deviation.

This study aimed to assess the tongue movements observed during the sucking cycle. There was no statistically significant difference observed between neonates diagnosed with ankyloglossia and those in the control group in terms of the duration of tongue movement from the palate to the floor of the mouth, the pace of the tongue during this movement, or the duration of a sucking cycle ($p > 0.05$; Table 2).

Table 2. Tongue movement variables. Ankyloglossia and control group comparisons.

		The Velocity of Transition from the Palate to the Mouth's Floor, cm/s	The Duration of the Transition from the Palate to the Mouth's Floor, s	Sucking Cycle Duration, s
Ankyloglossia	n	30	30	30
	mean	2.07	0.44	0.77
	SD	0.65	0.15	0.19
Control	n	30	30	30
	mean	2.03	0.44	0.81
	SD	0.44	0.13	0.19

Statistical analysis performed using Mann–Whitney U test ($p < 0.05$). n: number of participants; SD: standard deviation.

A decision was made to conduct frenotomies on 16 out of 30 neonates diagnosed with ankyloglossia based on the presence of ultrasonography records and the persistence of breastfeeding difficulties. The average score for the lingual frenulum in neonates who received frenotomy was 3.75 ($\pm$1.06), while the average score for neonates who did not receive frenotomy was 4.29 ($\pm$1.14) ($p > 0.05$) (Table 3). There was no statistically significant difference observed in the scores between the two groups. Furthermore, there was no statistically significant distinction observed between neonates who received intervention and those who did not regarding the extent of nipple approach to the HSPJ, depth of intraoral space, or heights of the tongue ($p > 0.05$) (Table 4). When assessing the variables related to the duration of tongue displacement from the palate to the floor of the mouth, the velocity of the tongue during this motion, and the duration of a complete sucking cycle, no statistically significant distinction was observed between two groups of neonates ($p > 0.05$) (Table 5).

Table 3. Lingual frenulum score and frenotomy decision.

		Lingual Frenulum Score
Frenotomy (−)	n	14
	mean	4.29
	SD	1.14
Frenotomy (+)	n	16
	mean	3.75
	SD	1.06

Statistical analysis performed using Mann–Whitney U test ($p < 0.05$). n: number of participants; SD: standard deviation.

Table 4. Nipple–tongue measurements and frenotomy decision groups comparisons.

			Nipple–HSPJ Junction Distance, cm	Depth of Intraoral Space, cm	Anterior Tongue Height, cm	Mid-Tongue Height, cm
Tongue up	Frenotomy (−)	n	14	14	14	14
		mean	0.81	0.36	1.18	1.64
		SD	0.31	0.15	0.23	0.21
	Frenotomy (+)	n	16	16	16	16
		mean	0.82	0.31	1	1.71
		SD	0.34	0.10	0.32	0.31
Tongue down	Frenotomy (−)	n	14	14	14	14
		mean	0.43	0.82	1.08	1.28
		SD	0.16	0.31	0.17	0.20
	Frenotomy (+)	n	16	16	16	16
		mean	0.57	0.68	1.05	1.37
		SD	0.3	0.28	0.19	0.21

Statistical analysis performed using Mann–Whitney U test ($p < 0.05$). n: number of participants; SD: standard deviation.

Table 5. Tongue movement variables and frenotomy decision groups comparisons.

		The Velocity of Transition from the Palate to the Mouth's Floor, cm/s	The Duration of the Transition from the Palate to the Mouth's Floor, s	Sucking Cycle Duration, s
Frenotomy (−)	n	14	14	14
	mean	2.16	0.47	0.82
	SD	0.68	0.18	0.18
Frenotomy (+)	n	16	16	16
	mean	2	0.41	0.73
	SD	0.63	0.12	0.19

Statistical analysis performed using Mann–Whitney U test ($p < 0.05$). n: number of participants; SD: standard deviation.

4. Discussion

This study introduces a novel and objective measurement technique for assessing tongue movements in neonates during breastfeeding.

Furthermore, we evaluated the differences between neonates with ankyloglossia and healthy neonates regarding the positioning of the nipple within the oral cavity and the positioning and movements of the tongue during the sucking process. Additionally, we compared these parameters between individuals in the ankyloglossia group who underwent frenotomy and those who did not.

According to a study conducted by Li et al. (2008), the primary factor leading to the cessation of early breastfeeding is the challenge faced by neonates in terms of sucking and latching onto the breast [4]. However, at present, there is a lack of a clinically feasible and objective measurement method that elucidates the intricacies of sucking action, specifically the movements of the tongue.

The measurement techniques in the literature that utilize ultrasonography to diagnose based on the extent of muscle movement have garnered considerable interest [30,31]. The applicability of these techniques to the orofacial region has not yet been demonstrated. The studies conducted by Schleifer et al. (2021) and Boussuges et al. (2020) employed the M-mode imaging technique to evaluate the functionality of the diaphragm during both expiration and inspiration. To assess the rate of displacement of the diaphragm during expiration or inspiration, the researchers placed the initial caliper at the lower end of the diaphragmatic echoic slope generated by diaphragmatic motion and the second caliper at the highest point of the slope. As a result, the researchers computed the diaphragmatic excursion in centimeters (cm) during both inspiration and expiration. They also determined the duration of the excursion in seconds (s) and the mean velocity of the excursion in centimeters per second (cm/s). Furthermore, the authors showcased the temporal extent of a single respiratory cycle, encompassing both the inhalation and exhalation phases [30,31].

In our study, adjustments were made to the measurements on M-mode ultrasonography recordings to account for the movements of the tongue during the sucking cycle. The introduction of this novel measurement technique is expected to offer an objective and replicable means of assessing the physiological aspects of sucking. This technique enables the interpretation of both the duration and velocity of tongue displacement during the sucking function. This study utilized a novel measurement technique to compare the parameters of tongue movement between neonates diagnosed with ankyloglossia and neonates who were deemed healthy. Based on the findings, there was no discernible disparity observed in the rate and duration of lingual movements among neonates diagnosed with ankyloglossia in comparison to those belonging to the control group. The results of this study indicate that ankyloglossia does not have a detrimental impact on the vertical movement of the tongue or the flow of milk in neonates. In their research on the effectiveness of ultrasonography studies in examining breastfeeding and sucking dynamics, Douglas et al. (2018) observed that the tongue and mandible exhibit synchronized movement without any independent motion. Furthermore, they found that the lingual frenulum does not exert any influence on the tongue's movement during sucking [3]. The outcome obtained confirms the conclusions drawn from our research. In a study conducted by Geddes et al. (2008), an examination was carried out on tongue movements during breastfeeding. The researchers discovered that the downward motion of the tongue creates a suction effect on the nipple, resulting in the release of milk from the breast [32]. Elad et al. (2014) conducted a biomechanical investigation to examine the mechanics of sucking. Their study revealed the coordinated movement of the anterior tongue with the mandibular motion, specifically positioning itself beneath the nipple. Additionally, the middle and posterior portions of the tongue were found to generate a vacuum effect, facilitating the outflow of milk [14]. The results suggest that the anterior tongue's role in the sucking process may be more pronounced and effective in achieving the necessary oral isolation needed to create a vacuum, thereby aiding in the attachment to the breast and the ejection of milk. In their study, Geddes et al. (2021) conducted a comprehensive examination of breastfeeding and observed that the application of frenotomy to the anterior tongue tie resulted in an increase in milk output and a decrease in nipple pain. Conversely, the application of frenotomy to the posterior tongue tie did not have any impact on milk production but did lead to a reduction in nipple pain [33]. When assessing the severity of ankyloglossia and the necessity of frenotomy, it is hypothesized that conducting further investigations to examine the impact of tongue extension towards the anterior crest of the mandible on breastfeeding latch and sucking functionality would offer a novel insight into tongue function.

Tongue movement was assessed using M-mode in the context of these innovative ultrasonography measurements. Previous studies have reported that there may be a discrepancy between the M-mode cursor and the true axis of the structure being imaged. This discrepancy has raised concerns regarding the potential for inaccurate measurements [30]. Ensuring axis alignment during real-time ultrasonography on breastfeeding neonates poses a significant challenge, primarily attributable to the inherent difficulty in controlling the movements of both the mother and the infant. The angle-independent M-mode, also known as anatomical or post-processing M-mode, allows for unrestricted rotation and movement of the M-mode cursor to capture M-mode images from any desired angle [30]. In the present study, the determination of the examination line was conducted utilizing anatomic M-mode, whereby the cursor was positioned along the vertical axis of the tongue in its elevated position. This enhancement resulted in improved visual clarity of M-mode measurement images.

In their study, Jacobs et al. [34] conducted an investigation using diverse ultrasound transducers to observe the intraoral anatomy of infants during breastfeeding. Their findings led them to determine that a frequency range of 8–10 MHz would be adequate for infants under 12 weeks of age in the context of evaluating contemporary technological devices. In the aforementioned study, the researchers also underscored the appropriateness of convex long-handled transducers (specifically endocavity transducers) for assessing intraoral tissues while the subject is engaged in sucking activities. In our investigation, we opted for a 6–10 MHz 8C-RS microconvex probe that possesses imaging capabilities comparable to endocavitary probes. The image recordings were conducted at a frequency of 8 MHz. The study revealed that the microconvex probe, characterized by its expansive visual scope and elevated frequency spectrum, effectively captures images of intraoral tissues during breastfeeding. Moreover, its compact, convex surface and slender grip area make it particularly suitable for imaging in confined spaces.

According to the findings of Douglas et al. (2018) and Elad et al. (2014), it has been observed that, in healthy neonates, during the sucking process, the anterior tongue tip is situated below the nipple and on the inferior alveolar ridge [3,14]. The analysis of B-mode ultrasonography images revealed that healthy neonates, when in the tongue-up position, exhibited a closer proximity of the nipple to the HSPJ and demonstrated a more pronounced anterior expansion of the tongue compared to neonates with ankyloglossia. There was no statistically significant difference observed in the measured parameters between neonates with ankyloglossia and those without this condition. Based on the findings of our study, it was observed that neonates with ankyloglossia possess the ability to bring the nipple closer to the HSPJ at a comparable rate to that of healthy neonates. This phenomenon occurs due to the creation of a vacuum within the oral cavity when breastfeeding in the tongue-down position. When the tongue is elevated, the loss of the nipple's position in the mouth occurs as a result of a decrease in oral vacuum. However, in neonates with ankyloglossia, the nipple moves further away from the HSPJ compared to healthy neonates. It is hypothesized that the presence of ankyloglossia in neonates hinders their ability to extend their tongue toward the inferior alveolar ridge. Thus, it is postulated that they encounter challenges in successfully latching onto the breast and maintaining proper nipple placement within the oral cavity, consequently leading to frequent disruption of the initial sucking required for proper attachment. Based on the ultrasonography measurements and the observations conducted on a substantial sample size within our study, it has been determined that the anterior tongue exhibits an active role in the retention of the nipple within the oral cavity. There is a belief that conducting additional research on the role of the anterior tongue can provide insights into the challenges faced by neonates with ankyloglossia in latching onto the breast as well as the early breast pain experienced by mothers.

Previous studies have presented divergent viewpoints regarding the requisite nature of frenotomy and its impact on sucking and latching difficulties in neonates diagnosed with ankyloglossia [25,26]. A subset of the neonates whose images were utilized in our study were found to necessitate frenectomies as a result of enduring difficulties with breastfeeding. The pre-procedural ultrasonography measurements of neonates who underwent frenotomy and those who did not undergo frenotomy were found to be statistically similar. This suggests that there were no significant disparities in tongue movements that would influence the decision to pursue surgical intervention. While the diagnosis of ankyloglossia typically indicates the need for a frenotomy procedure, it is important to consider the impact of neonatal development and the family's decision making process on the effectiveness of this intervention. The level of objectivity regarding the decision remains uncertain.

The present study is subject to several limitations. The inability to conduct follow-up assessments on neonates with ankyloglossia, both with and without frenotomy, was a result of the study's retrospective design. Hence, the impact of surgical intervention on breastfeeding outcomes, as assessed through the use of ultrasound imaging, could not be ascertained. The absence of both short- and long-term follow-up studies creates uncertainty regarding the persistence of breastfeeding difficulties associated with ankyloglossia. The examination of subsequent records within this study will enable us to effectively illustrate the effectiveness of the novel ultrasonography measurement technique employed in the oral region.

The implementation of further research endeavors aimed at assessing the effectiveness of frenotomy will furnish healthcare professionals with essential benchmarks for making informed decisions regarding diagnosis and treatment. Additionally, these studies will yield practical diagnostic instruments that can be readily employed to evaluate nipple pain in mothers and breastfeeding difficulties, such as impaired latching and sucking, in neonates diagnosed with ankyloglossia. Consequently, neonates will be safeguarded from undergoing unnecessary surgical procedures at an early stage.

5. Conclusions

This study presents a novel approach in the field of ultrasonography measurement techniques, which offers a valuable and applicable means of objectively evaluating tongue function in the context of breastfeeding. The measurement methodology utilized produced findings that aligned with the outcomes of prior research. There is no significant difference in tongue movements in the middle tongue region between neonates diagnosed with ankyloglossia and neonates who are considered healthy. This methodology enables the assessment of different areas of the tongue and other movable organs implicated in the sucking process during breastfeeding.

Author Contributions: Conceptualization, A.A. and K.O.; methodology, A.A., K.O. and A.I.O.; formal analysis, A.A., A.I.O. and K.O.; investigation, A.A., A.I.O. and K.O.; resources, A.A. and A.I.O.; writing—original draft preparation, A.A. and A.I.O.; writing—review and editing, A.A., A.I.O. and K.O.; visualization, A.A.; supervision, A.I.O. and K.O.; project administration, K.O. All authors have read and agreed to the published version of the manuscript.

Funding: This research received no external funding.

Institutional Review Board Statement: The study was conducted in accordance with the Declaration of Helsinki and approved by the Ethics Committee of Health Sciences Ankara Yildirim Beyazit University Ankara, Türkiye (04/13 April 2023).

Informed Consent Statement: Not applicable.

Data Availability Statement: The datasets generated and analyzed during the study are available from the corresponding author upon reasonable request.

Acknowledgments: We would like to thank GE Health Care Türkiye for providing and demonstrating their ultrasound equipment. We would also like to thank Gozde Alpay for her help and support.

Conflicts of Interest: The authors declare no conflict of interest.

References

1. Patel, J.; Anthonappa, R.P.; King, N.M. All Tied Up! Influences of Oral Frenulae on Breastfeeding and their Recommended Management Strategies. *J. Clin. Pediatr. Dent.* **2018**, *42*, 407–413. [CrossRef] [PubMed]
2. McClellan, H.L.; Hartmann, P.E. Evolution of lactation: Nutrition v. protection with special reference to five mammalian species. *Nutr. Res. Rev.* **2008**, *21*, 97–116. [CrossRef] [PubMed]
3. Douglas, P.; Geddes, D. Practice-based interpretation of ultrasound studies leads the way to more effective clinical support and less pharmaceutical and surgical intervention for breastfeeding infants. *Midwifery* **2018**, *58*, 145–155. [CrossRef] [PubMed]
4. Li, R.; Fein, S.B.; Chen, J.; Grummer-Strawn, L.M. Why mothers stop breastfeeding: Mothers' self-reported reasons for stopping during the first year. *Pediatrics* **2008**, *122* (Suppl. S2), S69–S76. [CrossRef]
5. Arvedson, J. Swallowing and feeding in infants and young children. *GI Motil. Online* **2006**. [CrossRef]
6. Tamura, Y.; Matsushita, S.; Shinoda, K.; Yoshida, S. Development of perioral muscle activity during suckling in infants: A cross-sectional and follow-up study. *Dev. Med. Child. Neurol.* **1998**, *40*, 344–348.
7. Geddes, D.T.; Kent, J.C.; Mitoulas, L.R.; Hartmann, P.E. Tongue movement and intra-oral vacuum in breast-feeding infants. *Early Hum. Dev.* **2008**, *84*, 471–477. [CrossRef]
8. Ardran, G.; Kemp, F.; Lind, J. A cineradiographic study of breastfeeding. *Br. J. Radiol.* **1958**, *31*, 156–162. [CrossRef]
9. Colley, J.R.T.; Creamer, B. Sucking and swallowing in infants. *Br. Med. J.* **1958**, *2*, 422–423. [CrossRef]
10. Woolridge, M. The anatomy of infant sucking. *Midwifery* **1986**, *2*, 164–171. [CrossRef]
11. Weber, J.; Woolridge, M.; Baum, J. An ultrasonographic study of the organization of sucking and swallowing by newborn infants. *Dev. Med. Child. Neurol.* **1986**, *28*, 19–24. [CrossRef] [PubMed]
12. Burton, P.; Deng, J.; McDonald, D.; Fewtrell, M.S. Real-time 3D ultrasound imaging of infant tongue movements during breast-feeding. *Early Hum. Dev.* **2013**, *89*, 635–641. [CrossRef] [PubMed]
13. Smith, W.L.; Erenberg, A.; Nowak, A. Imaging evaluation of the human nipple during breast-feeding. *Am. J. Dis. Child.* **1988**, *142*, 76–78. [CrossRef] [PubMed]
14. Elad, D.; Kozlovsky, P.; Blum, O.; Laine, A.F.; Po, M.J.; Botzer, E.; Dollberg, S.; Zelicovich, M.; Sira, L.B. Biomechanics of milk extraction during breast-feeding. *Proc. Natl. Acad. Sci. USA* **2014**, *111*, 5230–5235. [CrossRef] [PubMed]
15. Siegel, S. Aerophagia Induced Reflux in Breastfeeding Infants with Ankyloglossia and Shortened Maxillary Labial Frenula (Tongue and Lip Tie). *Int. J. Clin. Pediatr.* **2016**, *5*, 6–8. [CrossRef]
16. Ghaheri, B.A.; Cole, M.; Fausel, S.C.; Chuop, M.; Mace, J.C. Breastfeeding improvement following tongue-tie and lip-tie release: A prospective cohort study. *Laryngoscope* **2017**, *127*, 1217–1223. [CrossRef]
17. Pompéia, L.E.; Ilinsky, R.S.; Ortolani, C.L.F.; Faltin, K., Jr. Ankyloglossia and Its Influence on Growth and Development of the Stomatognathic System. *Rev. Paul. Pediatr.* **2017**, *35*, 216–221. [CrossRef]
18. Messner, A.H.; Lalakea, M.L.; Aby, J.; Macmahon, J.; Bair, E. Ankyloglossia: Incidence and associated feeding difficulties. *Arch. Otolaryngol. Head Neck Surg.* **2000**, *126*, 36–39. [CrossRef]
19. Marmet, C.; Shell, E.; Marmet, R. Neonatal frenotomy may be necessary to correct breastfeeding problems. *J. Hum. Lact.* **1990**, *6*, 117–121. [CrossRef]
20. Segal, L.M.; Stephenson, R.; Dawes, M.; Feldman, P. Prevalence, diagnosis, and treatment of ankyloglossia: Methodologic review. *Can. Fam. Physician.* **2007**, *53*, 1027–1033.
21. Marmet, C.; Shell, E.; Aldana, S. Assessing infant suck dysfunction: Case management. *J. Hum. Lact.* **2000**, *16*, 332–336. [CrossRef] [PubMed]

22. Schwartz, K.; D'Arcy, H.J.; Gillespie, B.; Bobo, J.; Longeway, M.; Foxman, B. Factors associated with weaning in the first 3 months postpartum. *J. Fam. Pract.* **2002**, *51*, 439–444. [PubMed]
23. Genna, C.W.; Coryllos, E.V. Breastfeeding and tongue-tie. *J. Hum. Lact.* **2009**, *25*, 111–112. [CrossRef] [PubMed]
24. Smith, W.L.; Erenberg, A.; Nowak, A.; Franken, E.A., Jr. Physiology of sucking in the normal term infant using real-time US. *Radiology* **1985**, *156*, 379–381. [CrossRef]
25. Hooda, A.; Rathee, M.; Yadav, S.P.S.; Gulia, J.S. Ankyloglossia: A review of current status. *Internet J. Otorhinolaryngol.* **2010**, *12*, 1–7.
26. Johnson, P. Tongue tie: Exploding the myths. *Infant* **2006**, *2*, 96–99.
27. Geddes, D.T.; Sakalidis, V.S. Ultrasound imaging of breastfeeding—A window to the inside: Methodology, normal appearances, and application. *J. Hum. Lact.* **2016**, *32*, 340–349. [CrossRef]
28. McClellan, H.L.; Sakalidis, V.S.; Hepworth, A.R.; Hartmann, P.E.; Geddes, D.T. Validation of nipple diameter and tongue movement measurements with B-mode ultrasound during breastfeeding. *Ultrasound Med. Biol.* **2010**, *36*, 1797–1807. [CrossRef]
29. Sakalidis, V.S.; Williams, T.M.; Garbin, C.P.; Hepworth, A.R.; Hartmann, P.E.; Paech, M.J.; Geddes, D.T. Ultrasound imaging of infant sucking dynamics during the establishment of lactation. *J. Hum. Lact.* **2013**, *29*, 205–213. [CrossRef]
30. Schleifer, J.; Shokoohi, H.; Selame, L.A.J.; Liteplo, A.; Kharasch, S. The Use of Angle-Independent M-Mode in the Evaluation of Diaphragmatic Excursion: Towards Improved Accuracy. *Cureus* **2021**, *13*, e17284. [CrossRef]
31. Boussuges, A.; Rives, S.; Finance, J.; Brégeon, F. Assessment of diaphragmatic function by ultrasonography: Current approach and perspectives. *World J. Clin. Cases* **2020**, *8*, 2408–2424. [CrossRef] [PubMed]
32. Geddes, D.T.; Langton, D.B.; Gollow, I.; Jacobs, L.A.; Hartmann, P.E.; Simmer, K. Frenulotomy for breastfeeding infants with ankyloglossia: Effect on milk removal and sucking mechanism as imaged by ultrasound. *Pediatrics* **2008**, *122*, e188–e194. [CrossRef] [PubMed]
33. Geddes, D.T.; Gridneva, Z.; Perrella, S.L.; Mitoulas, L.R.; Kent, J.C.; Stinson, L.F.; Lai, C.T.; Sakalidis, V.; Twigger, A.J.; Hartmann, P.E. 25 Years of Research in Human Lactation: From Discovery to Translation. *Nutrients* **2021**, *13*, 3071. [CrossRef]
34. Jacobs, L.A.; Dickinson, J.E.; Hart, P.D.; Doherty, D.A.; Faulkner, S.J. Normal nipple position in term infants measured on breastfeeding ultrasound. *J. Hum. Lact.* **2007**, *23*, 52–59. [CrossRef] [PubMed]

Disclaimer/Publisher's Note: The statements, opinions and data contained in all publications are solely those of the individual author(s) and contributor(s) and not of MDPI and/or the editor(s). MDPI and/or the editor(s) disclaim responsibility for any injury to people or property resulting from any ideas, methods, instructions or products referred to in the content.

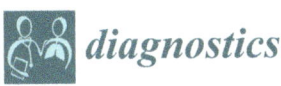

Systematic Review

The Reliability of Ultrasonographic Assessment of Depth of Invasion: A Systematic Review with Meta-Analysis

Marco Nisi, Stefano Gennai, Filippo Graziani and Rossana Izzetti *

Department of Surgical, Medical and Molecular Pathology and Critical Care Medicine, University of Pisa, 56123 Pisa, Italy
* Correspondence: rossana.izzetti@unipi.it

Abstract: Depth of invasion (DOI) has been recognized to be a strong prognosticator for oral squamous cell carcinoma (OSCC). Several diagnostic techniques can be employed for DOI assessment, however intraoral ultrasonography has been increasingly applied for the intraoral evaluation of OSCCs. The aim of the present study is to review the evidence on the application of intraoral ultrasonography to the assessment of DOI in patients affected by OSCC. A systematic electronic and manual literature search was performed, and data from eligible studies were reviewed, selected, and extracted. The studies had to report the correlation between DOI estimated with ultrasonography versus histopathology. A meta-analysis was conducted on the quantitative data available. Sixteen articles were included in the review following the screening of the initial 228 studies retrieved from the literature. The meta-analysis showed a significant correlation between ultrasonographic and histopathologic measurements ($p < 0.01$). The studies were all at low/moderate risk of bias. Ultrasonography appears a valuable tool for DOI assessment.

Keywords: oral neoplasm; ultrasonography; oral squamous cell carcinoma; intraoral ultrasound; systematic review; meta-analysis

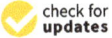

1. Introduction

The parameter of depth of invasion (DOI), defined as the distance between the normal mucosal surface and the deepest margin of a neoplastic lesion in the tissues, has been proven to be a valid prognosticator of oral squamous cell carcinoma, and is recognized as a T-stage modifier by the eighth edition of the American Joint Committee on Cancer (AJCC) criteria [1,2]. The assessment of DOI can be predictive of cervical lymph nodes involvement, as well as facilitating the achievement of clear surgical margins, allowing an improved local disease control and preventing recurrence [3].

DOI can be assessed either on diagnostic imaging datasets prior to tumor excision or on histopathological samples following surgical resection [4]. While pathologic DOI is considered the reference standard for tumor depth assessment, previous evidence has highlighted how magnetic resonance and ultrasonography perform extremely well in preoperative DOI assessment, showing high correspondence with histology [5,6]. Importantly, intraoral ultrasonography has been reported to have the highest correlation with pathological DOI compared to other diagnostic techniques [7].

The aim of the present systematic review is to analyze the evidence behind the application of intraoral ultrasonography to the assessment of DOI in patients affected by oral squamous cell carcinoma.

2. Materials and Methods

2.1. Protocol Development and Eligibility Criteria

The protocol for the present study was prepared according to the Preferred Reporting Items Systematic review and Meta-Analyses (PRISMA) [8–10] and registered in PROSPERO (CRD42023446434). The following focused question was phrased:

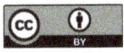

"What is the reliability of ultrasonography in the assessment of depth of invasion of oral squamous cell carcinoma?"

Articles to be included had to follow the following PICO:

(P) Type of participants: patients with a diagnosis of oral squamous cell carcinoma eligible for surgical treatment;

(I) Type of interventions: assessment of depth of invasion with intraoral ultrasonography;

(C) Comparison between interventions: depth of invasion measurement on histology;

(O) Type of outcome measures: correlation between ultrasonographic DOI and pathologic DOI.

Systematic reviews and review articles were not included. No time limitations were applied. Only articles in English were included.

2.2. Literature Search

The electronic search was applied to the Cochrane Oral Health Group specialist trials, MEDLINE via PubMed, and EMBASE (SG) up to June 2023. A combination of MeSH terms and free text words was employed:

((("Mouth Neoplasm"[Mesh] OR "Oral Neoplasm" OR "Oral squamous cell carcinoma" OR "Oral Carcinoma" OR "Oral Cancer") AND ("Ultrasonography"[Mesh] OR "Ultrasound" OR "Intraoral ultrasonography" OR "Intraoral Ultrasound") AND ("Neoplasm Invasiveness"[Mesh] OR "Depth of Invasion"))

Trials databases such as clinicaltrials.gov were searched. The bibliographies of review articles and relevant papers were checked (RI, MN).

2.3. Study Selection and Data Collection

Eligibility assessment was performed through title and abstract analysis of the search results, with an initial screening performed by two reviewers (RI, MN) for possible inclusion in the review. The two reviewers were calibrated for study screening against a third reviewer expert in systematic reviews (SG). Calibration consisted in the independent validity assessment of 20 titles and abstracts retrieved from the search until a κ-score > 0.8 was achieved. The articles selected through title and abstract analysis were then assessed through full text analysis. Unclear abstracts were included in the full text analysis to avoid the exclusion of potentially relevant articles. Title and abstract analysis was performed in June 2023.

Inclusion criteria for the title and abstract analysis were the following:

- Patients with a diagnosis of OSCC and eligible for surgery;
- Patients evaluated with intraoral ultrasound for DOI assessment;
- Studies reporting histological DOI evaluation and correlation with ultrasonographic DOI;
- Manuscripts published in English.

Exclusion criteria for the title and abstract analysis were the following:

- Subjects with conditions other than OSCC;
- Patients not evaluated with ultrasound;
- Assessment of imaging parameters other than DOI;
- Lack of reporting of histopathologic DOI;
- Descriptive studies not reporting the correlation between ultrasonographic and pathologic DOI;
- Studies that could not be classified as case–control studies, cohort studies, cross-sectional studies, case-series trials, controlled trials, or randomized controlled trials.

Full texts of the selected articles were then retrieved and independently assessed by two reviewers against the stated inclusion criteria (RI, MN). The articles had to follow the inclusion criteria to be included in the systematic review. The same exclusion criteria were employed for the full text analysis, together with absence of reporting of any of the studied outcomes. In cases of disagreement, the full text was discussed with a third experienced reviewer (SG). Data of the included articles were extracted and collected through an ad hoc extraction sheet (RI, MN). Full text inclusion was performed in June 2023 and full text data extraction by mid-July 2023. The reviewers conducted all quality assessments independently.

2.4. Risk of Bias in the Included Studies and Quality Assessment

The quality assessment and the risk of bias of the included studies was performed following the criteria of the ROBINS-I tool (Risk Of Bias In Non-randomized Studies—of Interventions) evaluating selection, comparability, and outcome domains for each study [11]. In cases of critical or serious judgment, the study was considered at high risk of bias.

2.5. Summary Measures and Synthesis of the Results

Data synthesis was presented through evidence tables addressing study characteristics and main conclusions. The performance of possible meta-analysis was decided on the basis of the similarity and availability of quantitative data. Results were expressed as weighted mean difference (WMD) and 95% confidence interval (CI) for continuous outcomes using both random and fixed models.

The meta-analysis was performed with the Fisher r-to-z transformed correlation coefficient as the outcome measure. Heterogeneity was assessed via Q-test, I^2, and tau^2, the latter assessed through the restricted maximum likelihood estimator [12]. If $tau^2 > 0$ was detected, a prediction interval for the true outcomes was also provided. The evaluation of potential outliers and/or influential studies in the context of the model was performed with the studentized residuals and Cook's distances. If a studentized residual larger than the $100 \times (1 - 0.05/(2 \times k))^{th}$ percentile of a standard normal distribution was found, the study was considered a potential outlier. If a Cook's distance larger than the median plus six times the interquartile range of the Cook's distances was found, the study was considered influential. Funnel plot asymmetry was checked through rank correlation and the regression tests. OpenMeta [Analyst] (http://www.cebm.brown.edu/open_meta/open_meta/open_meta, accessed on 1 June 2023) or other equivalent software for meta-analysis were employed, and the results were graphically illustrated and summarized with forest plots.

3. Results

3.1. Study Selection

The electronic search retrieved a total of 228 articles (205 articles from the electronic database search and 23 articles from the hand search) published up to June 2023. After the removal of duplicates, title and abstract analysis was performed on 211 articles. One hundred and seventy-eight articles were excluded following the screening of titles and abstracts. Full text analysis was performed on the remaining 33 articles, and 17 articles were further excluded. The final review included 16 articles [13–28], which all met the criteria for inclusion in the meta-analysis (Figure 1).

3.2. Population and Studies Characteristics

The study population consisted of 729 patients, with a mean age of 61.82 ± 5.56 years. Information on gender distribution was available for 14 out of 16 articles [13,15–26,28], accounting for a population of 696 patients, 420 males and 276 females.

In 12 studies [13–15,17,19,20,22–26,28], the AJCC/UICC classification was employed for tumor staging, while two studies did not report the classification system employed.

In 13 studies [13,15–17,20–28], ultrasonography was performed preoperatively. The frequencies employed ranged between a minimum of 5 and a maximum of 70 MHz (Table 1).

Table 1. Evidence table of the included studies.

Authors	Design	Patients	M:F	Mean Age	Staging Method	Tumor Location	T Stage (Patients No.)	Timing	Us Equipment	US Frequency	Correlation P-DOI/US-DOI
Kurokawa et al. 2005 [13]	Prospective study	28	18:10	59.4	UICC	Tongue	T1 (n = 11) T2 (n = 12) T3 (n = 3) T4 (n = 2) N0 (n = 20) N1 (n = 6) N2a (n = 1) N2b (n = 1)	Preoperative	Echo Camera SSD-1200CV; Aloka, Tokyo, Japan	7.5 MHz	0.976
Songra et al. 2006 [14]	Prospective study	14	NR	NR	AJCC	Tongue/floor of the mouth	T1 N0 M0 (n = 8) T2 N2a M0 (n = 2) T4 N3 M0 (n = 1) T2 N0 M0 (n = 2) T2 N1 M0 (n = 1)	Intraoperative	HDI 5000; Advanced Technologies Ltd., Seattle	5–10 MHz	0.648
Mark Taylor et al. 2010 [15]	Prospective study	21	12:9	65	AJCC/UICC	Tongue/floor of the mouth	T1 (n = 5) T2 (n = 6) T3 (n = 6) T4 (n = 4)	Preoperative	NR	10–12 MHz	0.981
Iida et al. 2018 [16]	Retrospective study	56	34:22	59	NR	Tongue	NR	Preoperative	Model UST-5713T/Intraoperative Electronic Linear Probe; Hitachi Aloka Medical, Ltd., Tokyo, Japan	16 MHz	0.867
Noorlag et al. 2020 [17]	Retrospective study	146	74:72	64	AJCC/UICC	Tongue	T1 (n = 84) T2 (n = 62)	Preoperative	EpiQ 5 with CL15-7 transducer; Philips Medical Systems, Best, The Netherlands	15	0.78
Yoon et al. 2020 [18]	Prospective study	20	13:07	60.35	NR	Tongue	NR	Intraoperative	L15-7io Philips Healthcare; Philips North America Corporation, Andover, MA, USA	7–15 MHz	0.95
Bulbul et al. 2021 [19]	Prospective study	23	15:8	59.1 ± 17.2	AJCC/UICC	Tongue	T1 (n = 13) T2 (n = 8) T3 (n = 2)	Intraoperative	L15-7io Philips Healthcare; Philips North America Corporation, Andover, MA, USA	7–15 MHz	0.9449

Table 1. Cont.

Authors	Design	Patients	M:F	Mean Age	Staging Method	Tumor Location	T Stage (Patients No.)	Timing	Us Equipment	US Frequency	Correlation P-DOI/US-DOI
Filauro et al. 2021 [20]	Retrospective study	49	27:22	65.6 ± 15.8	AJCC/UICC	Oral cavity (buccal mucosa, tongue, floor of the mouth)	T1 (n = 15) T2 (n = 21) T3 (n = 13)	Preoperative	L15-7io Philips Healthcare; Philips North America Corporation, Andover, MA, USA	7–15 MHz	0.76
Harada et al. 2021 [21]	Retrospective study	128	85:43	55.7	NR	Tongue	NR	Preoperative	HI VISION Avius, Hitachi Healthcare Systems, Japan	13	0.815
Izzetti et al. 2021 [22]	Retrospective study	10	4:6	68.7 ± 10.2	AJCC/UICC	Oral cavity	Tis (n = 2) T1 (n = 3) T2 (n = 4)	Preoperative	Vevo MD; VisualSonics, Toronto, ON, Canada	70	0.96
Rocchetti et al. 2021 [23]	Retrospective study	36	23:13	62.0 ± 16.1 (M) 71.2 ± 10.6 (F)	AJCC/UICC	Oral cavity	Tis (n = 3) T1 (n = 9) T2 (n = 20)	Preoperative	E-CUBE 15 EX US scanner; Alpinion Medical Systems, Seoul, Republic of Korea	8–17 MHz	0.907
Caprioli et al. 2022 [24]	Retrospective study	41	25:16	64.07 ± 17.67	AJCC/UICC	Tongue	T1s (n = 5) T1 (n = 21) T2 (n = 15)	Preoperative	NR	7–22 MHz	0.84
Nilsson et al. 2022 [25]	Prospective study	40	25:15	65 ± 14	AJCC/UICC	Tongue	T1 (n = 19) T2 (n = 10) T3 (n = 11)	Preoperative	8870 probe, BK Medical Flex Focus 500 US; Peabody, MA, USA	18 MHz	0.6
Takamura et al. 2022 [26]	Retrospective study	48	28:20	65.7	AJCC/UICC	Tongue	T1 (n = 28) T2 (n = 20)	Preoperative	EUP-O54J transducer, HI VISION Preirus; Hitachi, Tokyo, Japan	7–13 MHz	0.83
Au et al. 2023 [27]	Retrospective study	19	NR	NR	NR	Tongue	NR	Preoperative	NR	NR	0.910
Kumar et al. 2023 [28]	Prospective study	50	37:13	47.3 ± 11.7	AJCC/UICC	Tongue	T1 9 T2 32 T3 9	Preoperative	Aixplorer US system: SuperSonic Imagine, Aix-en-Provence, France	6–13 MHz	0.880

AJCC/UICC: American Joint Committee on Cancer/Union for International Cancer Control; NR: not reported; US: ultrasound.

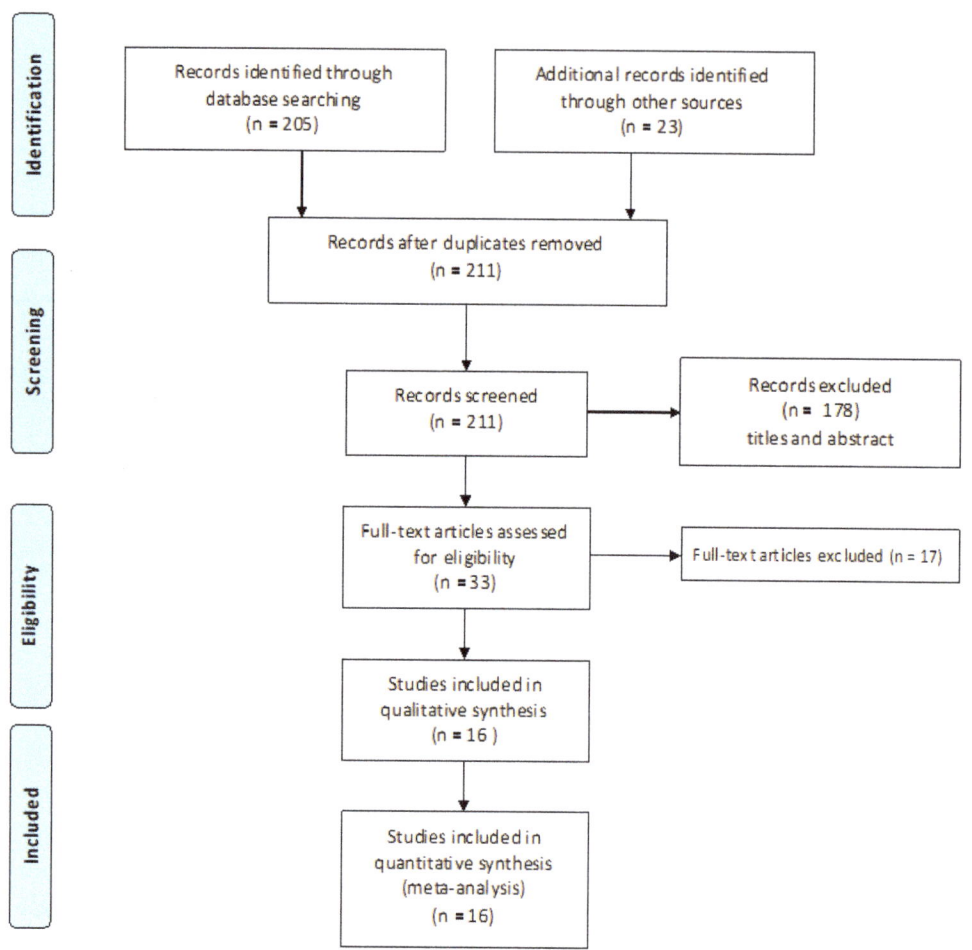

Figure 1. Study flowchart.

3.3. Synthesis of the Main Findings of the Included Studies

Kurokawa et al. [13] included 28 patients with OSCC of the tongue. The authors reported a correlation between DOI assessed with 7.5 MHz ultrasonography and T stage, tumor size, N stage, type of invasion, muscular invasion and deep invasive front grading. No correlation was found with growth type, differentiation, and Anneroth's malignancy. Ultrasound measurements correlated with histology. Other diagnostic techniques (computed tomography and magnetic resonance) tended to overestimate tumor dimensions.

Songra et al. [14] employed ultrasonography (frequency range 5–10 MHz) to assess deep margins intraoperatively half way through surgical resection. The authors reported good agreement between ultrasound and histology when applying a 5 mm threshold to indicate clear surgical margins. The technique was reported to have 83% sensitivity and 63% specificity.

In the study by Mark Taylor et al. [15], intraoral ultrasound (10–12 MHz) was performed in patients with biopsy proven squamous cell carcinoma of the tongue or floor of the mouth. The authors found that in cases of DOI < 5 mm, none of the patients presented positive lymph nodes, while in the presence of DOI ≥ 5 mm, 65% of the patients had nodal metastases. The authors concluded that preoperative ultrasonography was accurate in the assessment of tumor dimensions, and that in the presence of DOI ≥ 5 mm elective neck dissection is recommended.

Iida et al. [16] compared preoperative ultrasound measurement of DOI performed with a 16 MHz probe with histological DOI. The authors discriminated the accuracy of the technique depending on tumor size. In cases of superficial tumors, the comparison between ultrasonography and histology was 1 mm in 64.1% of cases and 2 mm in 92.3% of cases. In the presence of in situ OSCCs, the DOI ranged between 0.8 mm and 1.6 mm. Ultrasonography appeared reliable in tumors with DOI ≤ 5 mm, corresponding to T1 clinical staging according to the eighth edition of the AJCC, and was comparable to histology when analyzing superficial tongue carcinomas. The authors concluded that intraoral ultrasonography may constitute a diagnostic supplement especially in cases of superficial tumors where discordance between radiographic-derived and clinically derived values is encountered.

Noorlag et al. [17] analyzed a retrospective cohort of 209 patients with T1-T2 OSCC of the tongue, evaluated preoperatively with intraoral ultrasonography (15 MHz) and magnetic resonance (1.5–3.0 T). Ultrasonography showed a mean absolute difference with histology of 1.6 mm in smaller tumors and of 4.7 mm in larger tumors. Magnetic resonance showed a mean absolute difference with histology of 3.2 mm. The authors encountered an overall underestimation employing both diagnostic techniques compared to histological DOI. Among the presumable reasons for such a discrepancy, the authors listed (i) the timespan between imaging and surgery, which in some cases was more than four weeks; (ii) the pressure applied to the tumor during ultrasound scan; and (iii) tumor shrinkage following formalin fixation and/or slicing errors during specimen processing for histology. The conclusions reported a good correlation between magnetic resonance and intraoral ultrasonography measurements with histology. Ultrasonography showed higher accuracy in tumors with pathological DOI ≤ 10 mm (T1–T2 according to the eighth edition of the AJCC criteria) compared to magnetic resonance which tended to overestimate DOI, while in tumors >10 mm (T3) the accuracy of intraoral ultrasonography decreased.

Yoon et al. [18] performed tumor resection of OSCCs of the tongue under ultrasound guidance (7–15 MHz frequency) in 20 patients. Mean ultrasonographic DOI was 6.6 mm ± 3.4 mm and histopathologic DOI was 6.4 mm ± 4.4 mm, with a high correlation between the two measurements. Intraoperative application of ultrasonography resulted in an improvement in the achievement of clear resection margins and in the performance of elective neck dissection in the presence of DOI > 4 mm.

Bulbul et al. [19] included 23 patients with T1-T3 OSCC of the tongue and performed ultrasound (7–15 MHz)-guided tumor resection, and compared the surgical outcomes to a control group composed by 21 patients with T1-T3 OSCC surgically treated without ultrasound guidance. The mean closest margins for the ultrasound group were 6.3 mm ± 2.8 mm and 4.3 mm ± 2.7 mm for the control group. The mean deep margins for the ultrasound group were 8.5 mm ± 4.9 mm and 6.7 mm ± 3.8 mm for control group. Ultrasonographic guidance allowed for obtaining improved overall and deep margin clearance, 78% negative (≥5 mm) deep margins, and the absence of frankly positive deep margins.

Filauro et al. [20] performed a retrospective evaluation of 49 patients with T1-T3 OSCC who underwent intraoral ultrasound scan (7–15 MHz) and/or magnetic resonance imaging (1.5–3.0 T). The mean value of DOI was 7.0 mm with ultrasonography, 7.2 mm with magnetic resonance, and 7.3 mm with histology. Magnetic resonance provided a correct staging in 64% of cases, while intraoral ultrasound correctly staged all patients. For elective neck dissection, indicated in the presence of pathological DOI ≥ 4 mm, a 100% sensitivity was found for both the techniques, while 73% specificity for magnetic resonance and 47% specificity for ultrasonography were detected. The best cut-off for elective neck dissection was a radiological DOI ≥ 5 mm. Overall sensitivity was 92% for magnetic resonance and 87% for ultrasonography, while specificity was 93% for magnetic resonance and 76% for ultrasonography. While recognizing a good performance of ultrasonography compared to magnetic resonance, the authors recognized as limits to ultrasonography applicability the operator-dependency and the limited imaging capability for lesions close to bony structures or in the posterior half of the oral cavity.

Harada et al. [21] compared clinical DOI and radiological DOI assessed with ultrasound, MRI before biopsy, and MRI after biopsy. The authors performed a correction on pathological DOI values as a 10.3% shrinkage of the specimen after preparation was estimated. MRI before biopsy showed the highest concordance with clinical DOI, with a slight overestimation. Ultrasonography tended to underestimate clinical DOI. MRI after biopsy showed an overestimation of clinical DOI related to the inflammatory reaction of tongue muscles following bioptic sampling.

Izzetti et al. [22] assessed the correlation between ultrasonography performed at 70 MHz frequency and histology in a pilot sample of 10 patients affected by OSCC. A significant correlation was found between the two techniques. A 0.14 mm overestimation was registered for DOI values assessed through ultrasonography.

Rocchetti et al. [23] performed an ultrasonographic assessment of OSCC of the oral cavity using 8–17 MHz frequencies in 32 patients. The authors reported the following values for ultrasound assessment of tumor depth: 93.1% sensitivity, 100% specificity, 100% PPV, and 60% NPV. According to their results, ultrasonography appeared effective especially in the assessment of early-stage tumors.

Caprioli et al. [24] compared preoperative DOI assessed through MRI and ultrasonography (8–22 MHz frequency) with pathological DOI in 41 patients with tongue OSCC. While magnetic resonance tended to overestimate, ultrasonography showed a 92.31% sensitivity and 82.14% specificity in predicting a pathological DOI $\geq$ 4 mm, with a 100% specificity and a 94.7% sensitivity in discriminating an invasive cancer.

Nilsson et al. [25] enrolled 40 patients with biopsy-proven primary T1-T3 OSCC of the tongue and floor of the mouth and performed preoperative ultrasound employing an 18 MHz equipment. The authors compared DOI measurements obtained with ultrasound, magnetic resonance, computed tomography and histology. A DOI assessment was performed in all the patients employing ultrasonography, in 79% of patients with magnetic resonance and in 5% of patients with computed tomography. For magnetic resonance, motion artifacts and reduced tumor dimensions hindered DOI evaluation, while computed tomography was prone to artifacts. A comparison with histology revealed an error of 0.5 mm for ultrasonographic measurements, which further decreased to 0.1 mm in cases of T1-T2 tumors. A mean overestimation of 3.9 mm was reported for magnetic resonance, which appeared more reliable when assessing T3 tumors.

Takamura et al. [26] evaluated 48 patients with T1-T2 tongue OSCC (T1N0: 26 patients; T1N1: 17 patients, T2N0: 2 patients, and T2N1: 3 patients) and compared DOI as assessed with computed tomography, magnetic resonance (1.5 T), and ultrasonography (7–13 MHz). Computed tomography showed a mean difference of 2.7 mm between the histopathological DOI and radiological DOI, while for magnetic resonance the mean difference was around 2 mm. Ultrasonography DOI measurement differed by a mean of 0.2 mm, being the most accurate diagnostic imaging measurement method.

Au et al. [27] performed intraoral ultrasound assessment of biopsy-confirmed OSCC of the tongue in clinically nodal-negative patients treated with resection. In total, 19 patients were assessed with intraoral ultrasonography, and a strong correlation between ultrasonography and histology was found ($p < 0.001$), with a 90% sensitivity and 78% specificity.

Kumar et al. [28] performed intraoral ultrasonography (6–13 MHz) and contrast-enhanced magnetic resonance (1.5 T) in patients affected by T1-T3 biopsy-proven tongue OSCC. Ultrasonography was superior to magnetic resonance in T1 tumors with pathological DOI $\leq$ 5 mm compared to T2 tumors (DOI 5–10 mm).

3.4. Meta-Analysis

All 16 studies resulting from full text analysis were eligible for inclusion in the meta-analysis. The Fisher r-to-z transformed correlation coefficients range was 0.6931–2.3235, and all the estimates were positive. Based on the random-effects model, μ was 1.4041 (95% CI: 1.1783 to 1.6300), with the average outcome significantly differing from zero ($z = 12.1877$, $p < 0.0001$). The correlation coefficients appeared heterogeneous according to the Q-test ($Q(15) = 87.3755$, $p < 0.0001$, $tau^2 = 0.1740$, $I^2 = 87.5430\%$), with a 95% prediction interval between 0.5560 and 2.2523. However, the correlation coefficients of the included studies were in the same direction as the estimated average outcome. None of the studies had a value larger than ± 2.9552 after studentized residuals analysis, thus revealing the absence of outliers. According to the Cook's distances, none of the studies could be considered to be overly influential. The regression test indicated funnel plot asymmetry ($p = 0.0415$) but not the rank correlation test ($p = 0.0517$). (Figure 2).

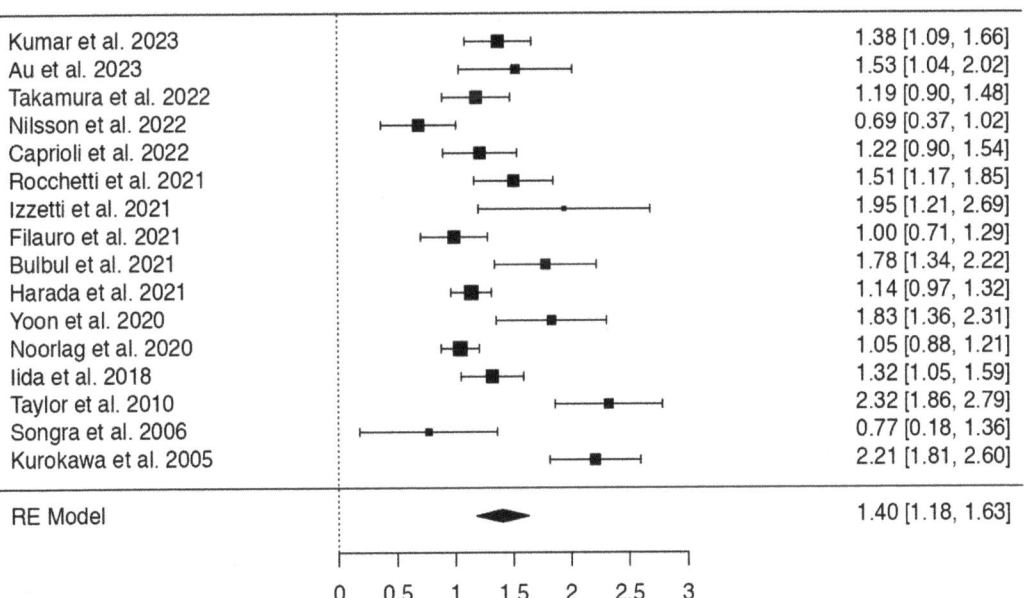

Figure 2. Forest plot of the meta-analysis.

3.5. Risk of Bias Assessment

All 16 studies showed a moderate/low risk of bias. Four studies showed a high risk of bias in the selection of participants, as the classification criteria employed for OSCC diagnosis were not reported (Figure 3).

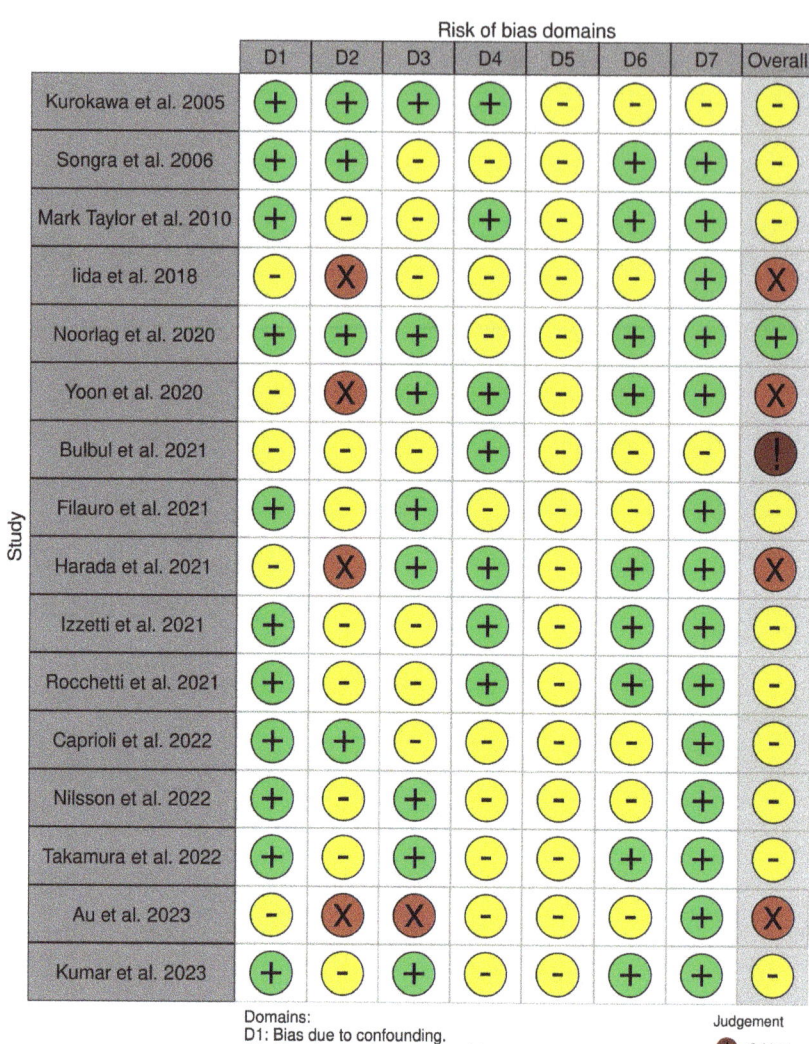

Figure 3. Risk of bias assessment of the 16 articles included in the review [13–28]. Table generated with *robvis* tool [29].

4. Discussion

The present results support the application of ultrasonography as a reliable tool in the assessment of DOI. Although the body of evidence is limited and the available literature is inhomogeneous in terms of frequencies and protocols employed, an overall consistency in the reporting is observed, suggesting a correlation between ultrasonographic DOI assessment and histology.

The role of preoperative DOI assessment has been extensively investigated in the literature, and its validation as a prognosticator for OSCC is represented by the inclusion in the eighth edition of the AJCC staging as a T-category modifier. Importantly, DOI appears extremely valuable in the presence of early OSCC, improving prognostication. Murthy et al. reported that increasing DOI is associated with poorer prognosis in T1-T2 OSCC, although a plateau in estimated survival rates is observed for tumor DOI > 5 mm [30]. Moreover, 5 mm DOI was reported to be a cut-off for the presence of occult nodal metastases in T2 patients [30]. From this perspective, DOI is an independent predictor of nodal metastases, and its inclusion in the staging system improved the decision-making of elective neck dissection, especially in patients with early OSCC [31].

The application of the eighth AJCC has been reported to result in an upstaging of patients with early OSCC compared to the seventh edition, improving the discrimination among pT1, pT2, and pT3 for disease-free survival and five-year overall survival [31]. However, Tsai et al. described a more favorable prognosis for pT1N1 than pN2-3N1 in stage III OSCC, and highlighted the need for a re-classification and a down-staging patients with pT1N1 disease [32]. Similarly, Kang et al. suggested a downstaging of pT4bN0-2 and pT1-2N3b to pStage IVA due to their less adverse prognosis [33]. Berdugo et al. suggested the incorporation of tumor size along with DOI for pT staging, describing tumor dimensions as a robust prognosticator limitedly dependent on histological variables [34]. Conversely, Newman et al. proposed a distinction between two prognostic groups in the pT3N0M0 stage depending on the DOI, with treatment escalation for deeper tumors [35]. As deeper DOI is a predictor of poorer relapse-free and overall survival, it has also been hypothesized to subdivide stage III OSCC based on DOI cut-off [36]. Undoubtedly, the eighth edition of the TNM clinical staging system has improved the ability to discriminate and prognosticate OSCC, by identifying patients with higher mortality rated through the application of clinical DOI and extranodal extension [2].

Ultrasonography has seen an increasing application in several medical fields, due to its ability to provide diagnostic information without the application of ionizing radiations, at a relatively lower cost compared to other diagnostic techniques [37–42]. Ultrasonography has been reported to be extremely high-performing in the preoperative assessment of OSCC, as it is estimated to have a 91–93% sensitivity [43]. In particular, ultrasonography finds indication in the presence of small tumors, which are not detectable through other diagnostic imaging techniques such as computed tomography and magnetic resonance [44]. The results of the present study confirm the good performance of ultrasonography in assessing DOI, and the available body of literature supports its application for the preoperative and/or intraoperative evaluation of OSCC.

The present study has some limitations. First, the variability of frequencies employed and ultrasound acquisition protocols may hinder comparison between studies, and thus the drawing of firm conclusions. However, it could be observed that the current literature consistently reports the use of linear probes, although the variability in the frequencies employed may hinder the recommendation of a specific ultrasound frequency. Importantly, although some differences were detected in terms of the timing of ultrasonographic scan, it could be hypothesized that preoperative ultrasonography may prove beneficial for surgical planning. Nevertheless, the evidence on the intraoperative ultrasound acquisition supports a role of this technique in tumor resection with clear margins. Secondly, although the definition for DOI was cautiously screened in order to discriminate studies reporting on other parameters (e.g., tumor thickness), great variability is encountered in the literature, hindering further assumptions regarding the measurement of DOI depending on the ultrasound frequencies employed. Finally, some of the included studies reported the application of ultrasonography to sites other than tongue, thus potentially representing a confounding factor. Nevertheless, our results support a role for intraoral ultrasonography in evaluating DOI.

5. Conclusions

Ultrasonographic assessment of DOI is a reliable tool in the evaluation of OSCC and the studies present in the literature consistently report high correlation coefficients with histopathology. Further studies aimed at improving the definition of acquisition protocols and the frequencies to be used are needed.

Author Contributions: Conceptualization, R.I., M.N. and S.G.; methodology, S.G.; software, S.G.; validation, M.N., R.I. and F.G.; formal analysis, M.N., R.I. and S.G.; investigation, M.N., R.I. and S.G.; resources, F.G.; data curation, S.G.; writing—original draft preparation, M.N., R.I. and S.G.; writing—review and editing, R.I. and F.G.; visualization, M.N., R.I. and S.G.; supervision, F.G.; project administration, F.G.; funding acquisition, F.G. All authors have read and agreed to the published version of the manuscript.

Funding: This research received no external funding.

Institutional Review Board Statement: Not applicable.

Informed Consent Statement: Not applicable.

Data Availability Statement: No new data generated.

Conflicts of Interest: The authors declare no conflict of interest.

References

1. Lee, M.K.; Choi, Y. Correlation between radiologic depth of invasion and pathologic depth of invasion in oral cavity squamous cell carcinoma: A systematic review and meta-analysis. *Oral Oncol.* **2023**, *136*, 106249. [CrossRef] [PubMed]
2. Yokota, Y.; Hasegawa, T.; Yamakawa, N.; Rin, S.; Otsuru, M.; Yamada, S.I.; Hirai, E.; Ashikaga, Y.; Yamamoto, K.; Ueda, M.; et al. Comparison of the 8th edition of TNM staging of oral cancer with the 7th edition and its prognostic significance using clinical depth of invasion and extranodal extension. *Oral Oncol.* **2023**, *145*, 106519. [CrossRef] [PubMed]
3. Park, K.S.; Choi, Y.; Kim, J.; Ahn, K.J.; Kim, B.S.; Lee, Y.S.; Sun, D.I.; Kim, M.S. Prognostic value of MRI-measured tumor thickness in patients with tongue squamous cell carcinoma. *Sci. Rep.* **2021**, *11*, 11333. [CrossRef] [PubMed]
4. Majumdar, K.S.; Kaul, P.; Kailey, V.S.; Maharaj, D.D.; Thaduri, A.; Ilahi, I.; Panuganti, A.; Usmani, S.A.; Singh, A.; Poonia, D.R.; et al. Radiological tumor thickness as a clinical predictor of pathological depth of invasion in oral squamous cell carcinoma: A retrospective analysis. *Eur. Arch. Otorhinolaryngol.* **2023**, *280*, 1417–1423. [CrossRef] [PubMed]
5. Waech, T.; Pazahr, S.; Guarda, V.; Rupp, N.J.; Broglie, M.A.; Morand, G.B. Measurement variations of MRI and CT in the assessment of tumor depth of invasion in oral cancer: A retrospective study. *Eur. J. Radiol.* **2021**, *135*, 109480. [CrossRef]
6. Li, M.; Yuan, Z.; Tang, Z. The accuracy of magnetic resonance imaging to measure the depth of invasion in oral tongue cancer: A systematic review and meta-analysis. *Int. J. Oral Maxillofac. Surg.* **2022**, *51*, 431–440. [CrossRef]
7. Tarabichi, O.; Bulbul, M.G.; Kanumuri, V.V.; Faquin, W.C.; Juliano, A.F.; Cunnane, M.E.; Varvares, M.A. Utility of intraoral ultrasound in managing oral tongue squamous cell carcinoma: Systematic review. *Laryngoscope* **2019**, *129*, 662–670. [CrossRef] [PubMed]
8. Liberati, A.; Altman, D.G.; Tetzlaff, J.; Mulrow, C.; Gøtzsche, P.C.; Ioannidis, J.P.; Clarke, M.; Devereaux, P.J.; Kleijnen, J.; Moher, D. The PRISMA statement for reporting systematic reviews and meta-analyses of studies that evaluate healthcare interventions: Explanation and elaboration. *BMJ* **2009**, *339*, b2700. [CrossRef] [PubMed]
9. Moher, D.; Liberati, A.; Tetzlaff, J.; Altman, D.G.; PRISMA Group. Preferred reporting items for systematic reviews and meta-analyses: The PRISMA statement. *PLoS Med.* **2009**, *6*, e1000097. [CrossRef] [PubMed]
10. Hutton, B.; Salanti, G.; Caldwell, D.M.; Chaimani, A.; Schmid, C.H.; Cameron, C.; Ioannidis, J.P.; Straus, S.; Thorlund, K.; Jansen, J.P.; et al. The PRISMA extension statement for reporting of systematic reviews incorporating network meta-analyses of health care interventions: Checklist and explanations. *Ann. Intern. Med.* **2015**, *162*, 777–784. [CrossRef]
11. Sterne, J.A.; Hernán, M.A.; Reeves, B.C.; Savović, J.; Berkman, N.D.; Viswanathan, M.; Henry, D.; Altman, D.G.; Ansari, M.T.; Boutron, I.; et al. ROBINS-I: A tool for assessing risk of bias in non-randomised studies of interventions. *BMJ* **2016**, *355*, i4919. [CrossRef] [PubMed]
12. Viechtbauer, W. Conducting meta-analyses in R with the metafor package. *J. Stat. Soft.* **2010**, *36*, 1–48. [CrossRef]
13. Kurokawa, H.; Hirashima, S.; Morimoto, Y.; Yamashita, Y.; Tominaga, K.; Takamori, K.; Igawa, K.; Takahashi, T.; Fukuda, J.; Sakoda, S. Preoperative Ultrasound Assessment of Tumour Thickness in Tongue Carcinomas. *Asian J. Oral Maxillofac. Surg.* **2005**, *117*, 173–178. [CrossRef]
14. Songra, A.K.; Ng, S.Y.; Farthing, P.; Hutchison, I.L.; Bradley, P.F. Observation of tumour thickness and resection margin at surgical excision of primary oral squamous cell carcinoma—Assessment by ultrasound. *Int. J. Oral Maxillofac. Surg.* **2006**, *35*, 324–331. [CrossRef]
15. Mark Taylor, S.; Drover, C.; Maceachern, R.; Bullock, M.; Hart, R.; Psooy, B.; Trites, J. Is preoperative ultrasonography accurate in measuring tumor thickness and predicting the incidence of cervical metastasis in oral cancer? *Oral Oncol.* **2010**, *46*, 38–41. [CrossRef] [PubMed]
16. Iida, Y.; Kamijo, T.; Kusafuka, K.; Omae, K.; Nishiya, Y.; Hamaguchi, N.; Morita, K.; Onitsuka, T. Depth of invasion in superficial oral tongue carcinoma quantified using intraoral ultrasonography. *Laryngoscope* **2018**, *128*, 2778–2782. [CrossRef]

17. Noorlag, R.; Klein Nulent, T.J.W.; Delwel, V.E.J.; Pameijer, F.A.; Willems, S.M.; de Bree, R.; van Es, R.J.J. Assessment of tumour depth in early tongue cancer: Accuracy of MRI and intraoral ultrasound. *Oral Oncol.* **2020**, *110*, 104895. [CrossRef]
18. Yoon, B.C.; Bulbul, M.D.; Sadow, P.M.; Faquin, W.C.; Curtin, H.D.; Varvares, M.A.; Juliano, A.F. Comparison of Intraoperative Sonography and Histopathologic Evaluation of Tumor Thickness and Depth of Invasion in Oral Tongue Cancer: A Pilot Study. *AJNR Am. J. Neuroradiol.* **2020**, *41*, 1245–1250. [CrossRef]
19. Bulbul, M.G.; Tarabichi, O.; Parikh, A.S.; Yoon, B.C.; Juliano, A.; Sadow, P.M.; Faquin, W.; Gropler, M.; Walker, R.; Puram, S.V.; et al. The utility of intra-oral ultrasound in improving deep margin clearance of oral tongue cancer resections. *Oral Oncol.* **2021**, *122*, 105512. [CrossRef]
20. Filauro, M.; Missale, F.; Marchi, F.; Iandelli, A.; Carobbio, A.L.C.; Mazzola, F.; Parrinello, G.; Barabino, E.; Cittadini, G.; Farina, D.; et al. Intraoral ultrasonography in the assessment of DOI in oral cavity squamous cell carcinoma: A comparison with magnetic resonance and histopathology. *Eur. Arch. Otorhinolaryngol.* **2021**, *278*, 2943–2952. [CrossRef]
21. Harada, H.; Tomioka, H.; Hirai, H.; Kuroshima, T.; Oikawa, Y.; Nojima, H.; Sakamoto, J.; Kurabayashi, T.; Kayamori, K.; Ikeda, T. MRI before biopsy correlates with depth of invasion corrected for shrinkage rate of the histopathological specimen in tongue carcinoma. *Sci. Rep.* **2021**, *11*, 20992. [CrossRef] [PubMed]
22. Izzetti, R.; Nisi, M.; Gennai, S.; Oranges, T.; Crocetti, L.; Caramella, D.; Graziani, F. Evaluation of Depth of Invasion in Oral Squamous Cell Carcinoma with Ultra-High Frequency Ultrasound: A Preliminary Study. *Appl. Sci.* **2021**, *11*, 7647. [CrossRef]
23. Rocchetti, F.; Tenore, G.; Montori, A.; Cassoni, A.; Cantisani, V.; Di Segni, M.; Di Gioia, C.R.T.; Carletti, R.; Valentini, V.; Polimeni, A.; et al. Preoperative evaluation of tumor depth of invasion in oral squamous cell carcinoma with intraoral ultrasonography: A retrospective study. *Oral Surg. Oral Med. Oral Pathol. Oral Radiol.* **2021**, *131*, 130–138. [CrossRef] [PubMed]
24. Caprioli, S.; Casaleggio, A.; Tagliafico, A.S.; Conforti, C.; Borda, F.; Fiannacca, M.; Filauro, M.; Iandelli, A.; Marchi, F.; Parrinello, G.; et al. High-Frequency Intraoral Ultrasound for Preoperative Assessment of Depth of Invasion for Early Tongue Squamous Cell Carcinoma: Radiological-Pathological Correlations. *Int. J. Environ. Res. Public Health* **2022**, *19*, 14900. [CrossRef]
25. Nilsson, O.; Knutsson, J.; Landström, F.J.; Magnuson, A.; von Beckerath, M. Ultrasound accurately assesses depth of invasion in T1-T2 oral tongue cancer. *Laryngoscope Investig. Otolaryngol.* **2022**, *7*, 1448–1455. [CrossRef]
26. Takamura, M.; Kobayashi, T.; Nikkuni, Y.; Katsura, K.; Yamazaki, M.; Maruyama, S.; Tanuma, J.I.; Hayashi, T. A comparative study between CT, MRI, and intraoral US for the evaluation of the depth of invasion in early stage (T1/T2) tongue squamous cell carcinoma. *Oral Radiol.* **2022**, *38*, 114–125. [CrossRef]
27. Au, V.H.; Miller, L.E.; Deschler, D.G.; Lin, D.T.; Richmon, J.D.; Varvares, M.A. Comparison of Preoperative DOI Estimation in Oral Tongue Cancer with cN0 Disease. *Otolaryngol. Head Neck Surg.* **2023**. [CrossRef]
28. Kumar, R.; Sherif, M.P.; Manchanda, S.; Barwad, A.; Sagar, P.; Khan, M.A.; Bhalla, A.S.; Singh, C.A.; Kumar, R. Depth of Invasion in Carcinoma Tongue: Evaluation of Clinical and Imaging Techniques. *Laryngoscope* **2023**. [CrossRef]
29. McGuinness, L.A.; Higgins, J.P.T. Risk-of-bias VISualization (robvis): An R package and Shiny web app for visualizing risk-of-bias assessments. *Res. Synth. Methods* **2021**, *12*, 55–61. [CrossRef]
30. Murthy, S.; Low, T.H.; Subramaniam, N.; Balasubramanian, D.; Sivakumaran, V.; Anand, A.; Vijayan, S.N.; Nambiar, A.; Thankappan, K.; Iyer, S. Validation of the eighth edition AJCC staging system in early T1 to T2 oral squamous cell carcinoma. *J. Surg. Oncol.* **2019**, *119*, 449–454. [CrossRef]
31. Matos, L.L.; Dedivitis, R.A.; Kulcsar, M.A.V.; de Mello, E.S.; Alves, V.A.F.; Cernea, C.R. External validation of the AJCC Cancer Staging Manual, 8th edition, in an independent cohort of oral cancer patients. *Oral Oncol.* **2017**, *71*, 47–53. [CrossRef] [PubMed]
32. Tsai, M.H.; Chuang, H.C.; Lin, Y.T.; Huang, T.L.; Fang, F.M.; Lu, H.; Chien, C.Y. Prognostic stratification of patients with AJCC 2018 pN1 disease in stage III oral squamous cell carcinoma. *J. Otolaryngol. Head Neck Surg.* **2022**, *51*, 18. [CrossRef] [PubMed]
33. Kang, C.J.; Tsai, C.Y.; Lee, L.Y.; Lin, C.Y.; Yang, L.Y.; Cheng, N.M.; Hsueh, C.; Fan, K.H.; Wang, H.M.; Hsieh, C.H.; et al. Prognostic stratification of patients with AJCC 2018 pStage IVB oral cavity cancer: Should pT4b and pN3 disease be reclassified? *Oral Oncol.* **2021**, *119*, 105371. [CrossRef] [PubMed]
34. Berdugo, J.; Thompson, L.D.R.; Purgina, B.; Sturgis, C.D.; Tuluc, M.; Seethala, R.; Chiosea, S.I. Measuring Depth of Invasion in Early Squamous Cell Carcinoma of the Oral Tongue: Positive Deep Margin, Extratumoral Perineural Invasion, and Other Challenges. *Head Neck Pathol.* **2019**, *13*, 154–161. [CrossRef]
35. Newman, M.; Dziegielewski, P.T.; Nguyen, N.T.A.; Seikaly, H.S.; Xie, M.; O'Connell, D.A.; Harris, J.R.; Biron, V.L.; Gupta, M.K.; Archibald, S.D.; et al. Relationship of depth of invasion to survival outcomes and patterns of recurrence for T3 oral tongue squamous cell carcinoma. *Oral Oncol.* **2021**, *116*, 105195. [CrossRef]
36. Tandon, S.; Ahlawat, P.; Pasricha, S.; Purohit, S.; Simson, D.K.; Dobriyal, K.; Umesh, P.; Mishra, M.; Kumar, L.; Karimi, A.M.; et al. Depth of Invasion as an Independent Predictor of Survival in Patients of Stage III Squamous Cell Carcinoma of the Oral Tongue. *Laryngoscope* **2022**, *132*, 1594–1599. [CrossRef]
37. Izzetti, R.; Fantoni, G.; Gelli, F.; Faggioni, L.; Vitali, S.; Gabriele, M.; Caramella, D. Feasibility of intraoral ultrasonography in the diagnosis of oral soft tissue lesions: A preclinical assessment on an ex vivo specimen. *Radiol. Med.* **2018**, *123*, 135–142. [CrossRef]
38. Aringhieri, G.; Izzetti, R.; Vitali, S.; Ferro, F.; Gabriele, M.; Baldini, C.; Caramella, D. Ultra-high frequency ultrasound (UHFUS) applications in Sjogren syndrome: Narrative review and current concepts. *Gland Surg.* **2020**, *9*, 2248–2259. [CrossRef]
39. Izzetti, R.; Vitali, S.; Aringhieri, G.; Caramella, D.; Nisi, M.; Oranges, T.; Dini, V.; Graziani, F.; Gabriele, M. The efficacy of Ultra-High Frequency Ultrasonography in the diagnosis of intraoral lesions. *Oral Surg. Oral Med. Oral Pathol. Oral Radiol.* **2020**, *129*, 401–410. [CrossRef]

40. Oranges, T.; Janowska, A.; Vitali, S.; Loggini, B.; Izzetti, R.; Romanelli, M.; Dini, V. Dermatoscopic and ultra-high frequency ultrasound evaluation in cutaneous postradiation angiosarcoma. *J. Eur. Acad. Dermatol. Venereol.* **2020**, *34*, e741. [CrossRef]
41. Izzetti, R.; Ferro, F.; Vitali, S.; Nisi, M.; Fonzetti, S.; Oranges, T.; Donati, V.; Caramella, D.; Baldini, C.; Gabriele, M. Ultra-high frequency ultrasonography (UHFUS)-guided minor salivary gland biopsy: A promising procedure to optimize labial salivary gland biopsy in Sjögren's syndrome. *J. Oral Pathol. Med.* **2021**, *50*, 485–491. [CrossRef] [PubMed]
42. Izzetti, R.; Vitali, S.; Aringhieri, G.; Nisi, M.; Oranges, T.; Dini, V.; Ferro, F.; Baldini, C.; Romanelli, M.; Caramella, D.; et al. Ultra-High Frequency Ultrasound, A Promising Diagnostic Technique: Review of the Literature and Single-Center Experience. *Can. Assoc. Radiol. J.* **2021**, *72*, 418–431. [CrossRef] [PubMed]
43. Izzetti, R.; Nisi, M.; Aringhieri, G.; Vitali, S.; Oranges, T.; Romanelli, M.; Caramella, D.; Graziani, F.; Gabriele, M. Ultra-high frequency ultrasound in the differential diagnosis of oral pemphigus and pemphigoid: An explorative study. *Skin Res. Technol.* **2021**, *27*, 682–691. [CrossRef] [PubMed]
44. Marcello Scotti, F.; Stuepp, R.T.; Leonardi Dutra-Horstmann, K.; Modolo, F.; Gusmão Paraiso Cavalcanti, M. Accuracy of MRI, CT, and Ultrasound imaging on thickness and depth of oral primary carcinomas invasion: A systematic review. *Dentomaxillofac. Radiol.* **2022**, *51*, 20210291. [CrossRef]

Disclaimer/Publisher's Note: The statements, opinions and data contained in all publications are solely those of the individual author(s) and contributor(s) and not of MDPI and/or the editor(s). MDPI and/or the editor(s) disclaim responsibility for any injury to people or property resulting from any ideas, methods, instructions or products referred to in the content.

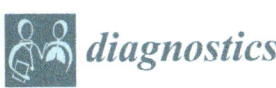

Article

The Role of Ultra-High-Frequency Ultrasound in Pyoderma Gangrenosum: New Insights in Pathophysiology and Diagnosis

Giammarco Granieri [1], Alessandra Michelucci [1,*], Flavia Manzo Margiotta [1], Bianca Cei [1], Saverio Vitali [2], Marco Romanelli [1] and Valentina Dini [1]

1. Department of Dermatology, University of Pisa, 56126 Pisa, Italy; giammarcogranieri@gmail.com (G.G.); manzomargiottaflavia@gmail.com (F.M.M.); ceibianca95@gmail.com (B.C.); marco.romanelli@unipi.it (M.R.); valentina.dini@unipi.it (V.D.)
2. Diagnostic and Interventional Radiology, University Hospital of Pisa, 56126 Pisa, Italy; vitalisaverio@gmail.com
* Correspondence: alessandra.michelucci@gmail.com

Abstract: Pyoderma gangrenosum (PG) is a neutrophilic dermatological disease, whose pathogenesis is still poorly clarified. Because of the lack of validated criteria for diagnosis and response, PG treatment is still challenging and should be differentiated in the inflammatory and non-inflammatory phases. Our study aimed to provide a new semi-quantitative approach for PG diagnosis and monitoring, identifying ultra-high-frequency ultrasound (UHFUS) early biomarkers associated with the transition between the two phases. We enrolled 13 patients affected by painful PG lesions evaluated during the inflammatory phase (T0) and during the non-inflammatory phase (T1): pain was measured by the Visual Analogue Scale (VAS); clinical features were recorded through digital photography; epidermis and dermis ultrasound (US) characteristics were evaluated by UHFUS examination with a 70 MHz probe (Vevo MD® FUJIFILM VisualSonics). In T1 UHFUS examination, the presence of hyperechoic oval structures was lower compared to T0 (p value < 0.05). An hyperechogenic structure within the oval structure, suggestive of a hair tract, was evident in T0 and absent in T1 (p value < 0.05). In T0, blood vessels appear as U-shaped and V-shaped anechoic structures with a predominance of U-shaped vessels (p value < 0.05) compared to the more regular distribution found in T1. Finding early biomarkers of the transition from the inflammatory to the non-inflammatory phase could provide new insight in terms of therapeutic decision making and response monitoring. The differences found by this study suggest a potential use of UHFUS for the development of an objective standardized staging method. Further investigations will be necessary to confirm our preliminary results, thus providing a turning point in PG early detection, differential diagnosis and treatment monitoring.

Keywords: pyoderma gangrenosum; ultra-high-frequency ultrasound; UHFUS; PG

1. Introduction

Pyoderma gangrenosum (PG) is a neutrophilic dermatosis of unknown etiology and uncertain epidemiology due to its challenging diagnosis. Its estimated prevalence is approximately 58 cases per million people, with an incidence of approximately 6 cases per million [1,2].

The average age of onset is 59 years with a higher prevalence in women, even if some studies suggest that the higher incidence occurs between 20 and 50 years old, without gender differences [2,3]. The mortality rate associated with PG ranges from 16% to 27% [4].

Furthermore, approximately 50% of PG patients are affected by another immune disease, although some studies report a slightly lower frequency [5]. Notably, PG is the second most common cutaneous manifestation of inflammatory bowel disease (IBD) [4].

The epidemiology of PG varies depending on the clinical phenotypes, which includes ulcerative, pustular, bullous and vegetative forms. Post-surgical PG is considered a specific entity that can represent a climax of pathergy phenomenon. The ulcerative phenotype is the most prevalent form, primarily affecting the lower limbs. PG is frequently associated with IBD, rheumatoid arthritis (RA), seronegative arthritis, monoclonal gammopathy, and hematological malignancies [5–7].

Ulcerative PG is characterized by rapidly expanding painful ulcers, often exhibiting a distinctive lilac ring at the edge [4].

All phenotypes of PG present an inflammatory phase characterized by high levels of pain. Therefore, the primary step of therapy is to block the inflammatory process, with immunosuppressive/immunomodulatory drugs and appropriate wound care, based on PG TIME [5,8]. Following the proper treatment, this phase moved toward a non-inflammatory phase that allows wound re-epithelialization [9–11].

Because of the chronic and relapsing course of PG, finding early biomarkers of this transition could be useful in terms of therapeutic decision making and response monitoring [5].

Currently, PG remains a diagnosis of exclusion as there are no validated and specific clinical, instrumental, or serological markers. Histological examination is non-specific and can vary depending on the sample site and stage of the lesion [12].

As a result, diagnostic tools, such as the PARACELSUS score, have been proposed, incorporating major, minor and additional criteria based on clinical, histological and therapeutic features of the ulcer [5,13]. Only one study is in the literature regarding the use of UltraSonography (US) with a linear probe up to 18 MHz in PG. This examination performed at the level of a painful nodule from PG showed a well-defined hypoechogenic structure at the subepidermal level, which continued with a hypoechogenic, heterogeneous, irregular area that disposed in sections reaching a destructured hypodermis. Doppler color modality showed increased local vascularity. After one week of treatment, a reduction in local vascularity and lesion dimensions was identified. There are no applications of ultra-high-frequency ultrasound (UHFUS) in PG lesions in the literature [14].

As technology continues to advance and research progresses, UHFUS is poised to become an indispensable tool in dermatology, revolutionizing the way we understand and address various skin conditions. Furthermore, the advancement in imaging techniques, specifically UHFUS, could offer distinct advantages over conventional diagnostic methods, as it is a non-invasive procedure that delivers a spatial resolution in the order of 30 μm. This level of resolution allows for the visualization of skin structures with unprecedented clarity, comparable to what is achievable through histological examination. UHFUS provides clinicians and researchers with a powerful tool to delve deep into the skin's microanatomy, revealing intricate details that were previously inaccessible without invasive procedures. The technique captures comprehensive images of various skin components, such as the dermo-epidermal junction, hair follicles, pilo-erector muscles, and blood vessels [15–21]. The distinct patterns observed through UHFUS imaging could assist in the early detection of PG, enabling timely intervention and management. Moreover, UHFUS serves as an essential tool in monitoring the progression of PG and evaluating the efficacy of treatment. By conducting longitudinal UHFUS assessments, clinicians could track changes in the affected skin over time, observing how the lesions evolve and respond to therapeutic interventions. This real-time feedback enhances the precision of treatment plans, as adjustments can be made based on objective imaging data, leading to more personalized and effective patient care.

The non-invasive nature of UHFUS also addresses concerns related to the risk of pathergy phenomenon often associated with invasive procedures such as skin biopsies. This reduction in invasiveness not only ensures patient comfort and safety but also encourages more frequent monitoring, facilitating a proactive approach to PG management.

Despite its tremendous potential, UHFUS is still a developing field, and further research is warranted to fully understand its capabilities in PG diagnosis and management. Collaborative efforts between dermatologists, imaging specialists, and researchers will be essential to optimize UHFUS protocols and establish standardized criteria for PG diagnosis based on imaging findings.

Its non-invasive nature, coupled with remarkable spatial resolution, could provide valuable insights for accurate diagnosis, treatment planning, and monitoring of PG.

The aim of this study was to identify UHFUS biomarkers associated with the inflammatory and non-inflammatory phases of different phenotypes of PG.

2. Materials and Methods

We enrolled 13 patients affected by painful PG lesions (Visual Analogue Scale (VAS) > 8): 11/13 presented an ulcerative phenotype, 2/13 had a pustular phenotype and 5/13 showed multiple PG lesions in different body areas. PG diagnosis was performed by a PARACELSUS score ≥ 10 and a skin biopsy with histological findings revealing intense neutrophilic infiltrate [13].

All patients were evaluated during the inflammatory phase (T0) and during the non-inflammatory phase (T1). T0 is defined by VAS > 7 and rapid growth and development of new lesions. In ulcerative PG, this phase was also characterized by the presence of a lilac ring, severe exudate and necrosis on the wound bed. In the pustular phenotype, the occurrence of new pustular satellite lesions and the increase in perilesional skin erythema suggested the presence of the inflammatory phase.

T1 was defined by VAS < 2, the absence of a lilac ring, wound bed necrosis and new satellite lesions for more than 4 weeks.

PG management was performed with a combination of local and systemic therapy, according to evidence and expert opinions presented in the literature [8,22,23].

A comprehensive patient's assessment was performed at T0 and T1. The clinical investigation was performed by a dermatologist expert in pyoderma gangrenosum which collected a photographic record of the patient and assessed clinical disease parameters such as pain, measured with VAS. UHFUS investigation was performed by a dermatologist expert in UHFUS blinded from the clinical diagnosis by three UHFUS clips with a 70 MHz linear probe (Vevo MD® FUJIFILM VisualSonics, Toronto, Ontario, Canada), in B-MODE. The use of UHFUS with a 70 MHz probe allows to examine the more superficial cutaneous and adnexal features with a spatial resolution in the order of 30 μm (Figure 1). A correlation between digital photograph and US clip was performed: two regions of interest (ROI) at the wound bed and edge were provided for the ulcerative phenotype, while one ROI was provided for the pustular phenotype. The probe was placed perpendicular to the lesion and a large amount of gel was used to maintain the adequate distance from the skin surface. The US parameters (such as gains, depth, time gain control, focus) were optimized during the examinations. A qualitative-quantitative analysis of the US features was performed by 2 dermatologists experienced in UHFUS imaging.

The UHFUS characteristics evaluated were:

Epidermis and dermis US morphology

Vessel's morphology

Dermal oedema as dermal hypoechogenicity, classified in three degrees (mild, moderate, severe)

Aliasing as the presence of image background noise, classified in three degrees (mild, moderate, severe).

Categorical data were described with absolute and relative (%) frequency, continuous data were summarized with mean and standard deviation. Fisher test was performed to compare UHFUS results obtained by the population evaluated in T0 and T1. Significance was set at <0.05 and all analyses were carried out by SPSS v. 28 technology.

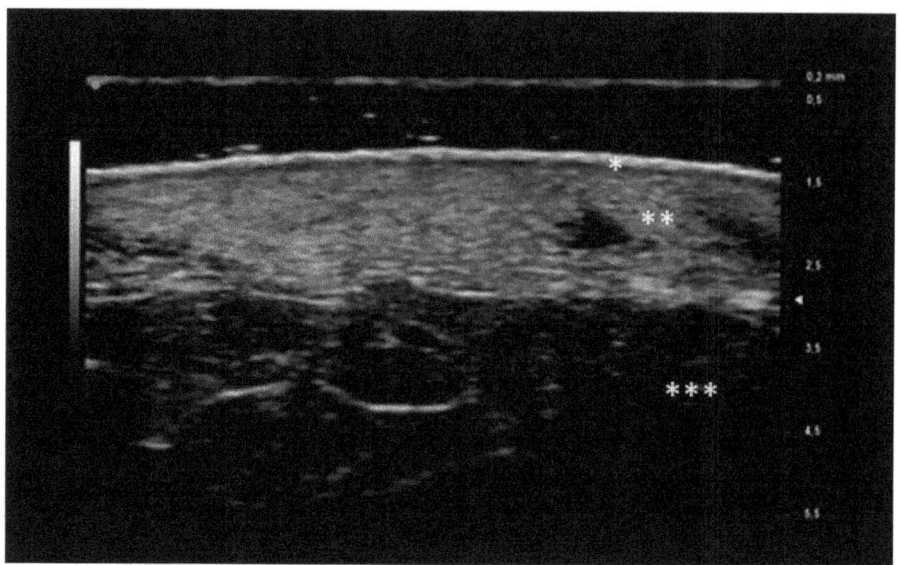

Figure 1. UHFUS features of healthy skin: epidermis (*), dermis (**) and hypodermis (***).

3. Results

Our population consisted of 13 patients (11 females and 2 males) with a mean age of 60.38 (17.4) years, a mean disease duration of 5 years and a mean BMI of 30.55 (5.7). The clinical and anamnestic features of the population are reported in Table 1, while the results obtained by UHFUS examination are presented in Table 2. The mean time needed to switch from the T0 phase to the T1 phase was 2 months.

Table 1. Characteristics of the population ($n = 13$). Statistics: frequency (%).

Characteristics		Statistics
Onset	Confluent pustules	2 (15.4)
	Non-confluent pustules	3 (23.1)
	Nodule	5 (38.5)
	Blister	3 (23.1)
	Trauma	2 (15.4)
Current phenotype	Ulcerative	11 (84.6)
	Pustular	2 (15.4)
Location	Face	2 (15.4)
	Lower limbs	11 (84.6)
	Upper limbs	1 (7.7)
	Back	4 (30.8)
Family history	Hematological malignancies	1 (7.7)
	Solid tumors	7 (54.0)
	Rheumatoid arthritis	2 (15.4)
	Hypertension	6 (46.2)
	Diabetes	6 (46.2)

Table 1. Cont.

Characteristics		Statistics
	Acne/hidradenitis suppurativa/pilonidal cyst	4 (30.8)
	Psoriasis	4 (30.8)
Comorbidities	Hematological malignancies	2 (15.4)
	Solid tumors	1 (7.7)
	Cardiovascular disease	7 (54.0)
	Diabetes	1 (7.7)
	IBD	1 (7.7)
	Acne/Hidradenitis suppurativa	8 (61.4)
	Psoriasis	3 (23.1)

Table 2. Ultra-High Frequency UltraSound (UHFUS) features of the population ($n = 13$). Statistics: frequency (%).

UHFUS Parameter		T0	T1	p-Value
Hyperechoic oval structures		12 (92.3)	4 (30.8)	0.001
Hair tract		7 (53.8)	0 (0)	0.005
V-shaped vessels		6 (46.2)	7 (53.8)	0.695
U-shaped vessels		12 (92.3)	5 (38.5)	0.004
Dermal hypercogenicity		0 (0)	2 (15.4)	0.8634
Dermal hypoechonicity	Mild	5 (38.5)	10 (69.2)	0.8634
	Moderate	6 (46.2)	1 (7.7)	
	severe	2 (15.4)	0 (0)	
Aliasing	Mild	3 (23.1)	9 (69.2)	0.636
	Moderate	6 (46.2)	1 (7.7)	
	Severe	5 (38.5)	0 (0)	

Oval hyperechoic structures were identified in the reticular and papillary dermis during the initial T0 UHFUS examination. These structures were surrounded by a consistent, homogeneous hypoechoic background. Notably, this peculiar arrangement was observed in both the pustular and ulcerative phenotypes, indicating a common underlying feature.

As the examination progressed towards the inflamed edge, these oval structures exhibited a noticeable increase in prevalence, reinforcing their association with the inflammatory process.

A statistically significant decrease in the presence of these hyperechoic oval structures was observed during the subsequent T1 UHFUS examination. This reduction in prevalence (p value < 0.05) underscores the dynamic nature of these structures and their potential correlation with the progression of the inflammatory response (Figure 2).

Additionally, a distinct finding emerged during the T0 UHFUS examination—an internal hyperechogenic structure within the oval entities. This internal structure, suggestive of a hair tract, was consistently identified during the initial examination (T0) but was notably absent in the follow-up examination (T1) (p value < 0.05) (Figure 3).

During the initial T0 examination, blood vessels appeared as U-shaped and V-shaped anechoic structures within the observed lesion. Notably, these vessels exhibited a distinct orientation, with their concavity consistently facing the center of the lesion. Moreover, a statistically significant predominance of U-shaped vessels was detected in T0 (p value < 0.05).

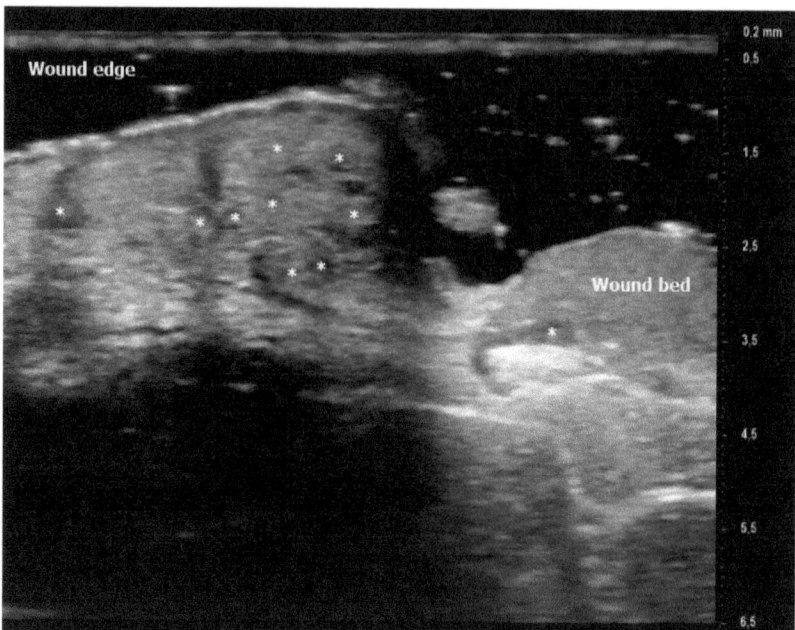

Figure 2. Pyoderma Gangrenosum (PG) Ultra-High Frequency UltraSound (UHFUS) features during the inflammatory phase (T0): oval hyperechoic structures (*) surrounded by hypoechoic borders predominantly located at the ulcer edge.

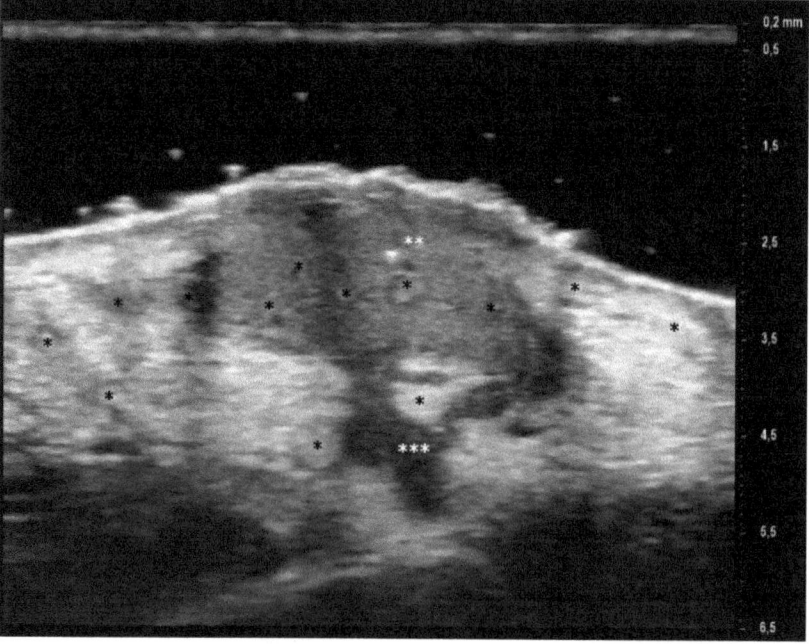

Figure 3. PG pustular lesion: hyperecoic oval structures (*), hair tract (**), hypoechoic U-shaped and V-shaped vessels (***).

Transitioning to the subsequent T1 examination, the blood vessels appeared to adopt a more regular distribution within the lesion. This shift was accompanied by a decline in both U-shaped and V-shaped vessels, indicative of an evolving vascular pattern over the course of progression.

The phenomenon of aliasing, characterized by the distortion of signals in ultrasound imaging, was notably pronounced (moderate to severe) during the initial assessment at T0. As the examination progressed to the subsequent time point, T1, a discernible improvement was observed in the degree of aliasing.

4. Discussion

Pyoderma gangrenosum is a dermatological disease with a great socio-economic burden on patients' quality of life. Its chronic and relapsing nature necessitates the need for an early recognition and prompt management of a new disease flare. Goldust et al. assessed that the main research gap in the PG field is related to the identification of diagnostic biomarkers and standardized staging methods [24–27].

The substantial therapeutic differences between inflammatory and non-inflammatory phases require imaging tools and quantitative parameters to guide and support treatment choice. Moreover, recognition of early inflammatory signs would be crucial to avoid the pathergy phenomenon occurrence.

The distinction between the inflammatory and non-inflammatory phases of PG is essential for the choice of the correct therapeutic approach, either topical or systemic. Surgical debridement, as well as other traumatic treatments, can be carried out only during the non-inflammatory phase, because of the pathergy phenomenon. On the other hand, the choice of frequency and dose administration of immunosuppressive and immunomodulatory drugs is guided by the disease phase. During the active and acute phases of the disease, a more aggressive treatment approach may be necessary. Higher doses and more frequent administrations of immunosuppressive drugs may be prescribed to quickly suppress the overactive immune response and control the progression of the condition. Close monitoring by medical professionals is essential during this phase to assess the response to treatment and to ensure the patient's safety. Conversely, during the remission or maintenance phase of the disease, the treatment strategy may shift towards a more conservative approach. Lower doses or less frequent administrations of immunosuppressive drugs might be prescribed to maintain the disease in a controlled state and prevent flare-ups. The objective in this phase is to find a balance between regulating the immune system and avoiding excessive risks linked to prolonged immunosuppression. To date, the assessment of the inflammatory phase in PG is performed exclusively by clinical examination of the lesions: an intensified pain experienced by the patient, an increase in the number of lesions, and the presence of lilac ring are clinical parameters suggestive of a transition to the inflammatory phase. The presence of comorbidities or wound superinfections may mask or mimic an inflammatory phase, thus making its detection more difficult.

It is therefore a current challenge to identify early and more objective biomarkers, detectable even before clinical parameters, suggestive of the transition from the inflammatory phase to the non-inflammatory one, to guide therapeutic choice.

In our population, the mean age of PG onset was 55 years old, with a higher prevalence in women (M/F ratio of 0.18) in agreement with evidence presented in the literature [2]. The most frequently involved site was the lower limbs (84.6%), and the most observed comorbidities were HS (61.4%), hematologic malignancies (15.4%) and IBD (7.7%) as Maverakis et al. had already reported [5]. Moreover, in our population PG was often associated with psoriasis: 30.8% of patients presented a positive family history while 23.1% were affected by psoriasis. These results could be explained by the common proinflammatory pathways shared between the two diseases [4].

In this study, for the first time in the literature, clinical parameters were correlated with UHFUS findings obtained with a 70 MHz probe. Only one case report described the use of US (18 MHz) in PG, revealing the presence of heterogeneous and irregular hypoechogenic dermis that changes after systemic corticosteroid therapy with an increased dermal echogenicity [14].

The results obtained by our investigation revealed some UHFUS differences between the inflammatory and non-inflammatory phases. At T0, oval hyperechoic structures, that statistically significantly decreased in T1, were identified in the papillary and reticular dermis (p-value < 0.05) (Figures 4 and 5).

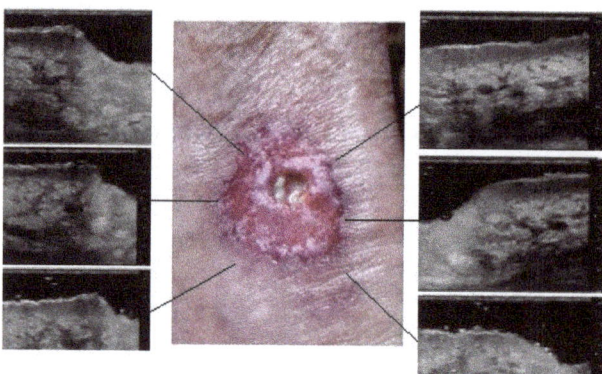

Figure 4. Patient affected by ulcerative Pyoderma Gangrenosum (PG) of the calf during the inflammatory phase: clinical aspect of the wound and its Ultra-High Frequency UltraSound (UHFUS) correlates.

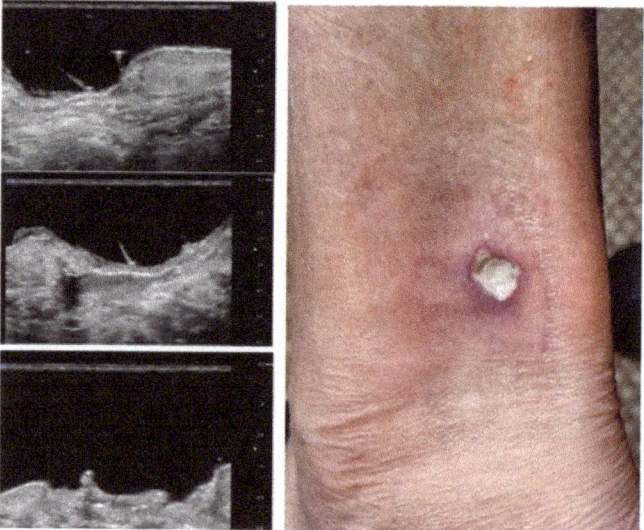

Figure 5. Patient affected by ulcerative Pyoderma Gangrenosum (PG) of the calf during the non-inflammatory phase: clinical aspect of the wound and its Ultra-High Frequency UltraSound (UHFUS) correlates.

These US findings spared the epidermis and were well demarcated from the surrounding dermis, thus suggesting a hypothesis of "dermal destruction" that we called "tsunami sign" because of the presence of a US image resembling a wave breaking towards the center of the lesion (Figure 6). In T0, hyperechoic oval structures were mainly located at the level of the lesion edges, near V-shaped and U-shaped blood vessels, where the inflammatory response presented a higher activity. Particularly, in T0 an increased expression of U-shaped vessels compared to V-shaped vessels was detectable. In contrast, T1 was characterized by a more uniform vascularization with a significant reduction in U-shaped vessels (p-value < 0.05). These UHFUS findings could be explained by the increased dermal oedema in T0, which resulted in surrounding connective tissue compression and morphological blood vessels changes.

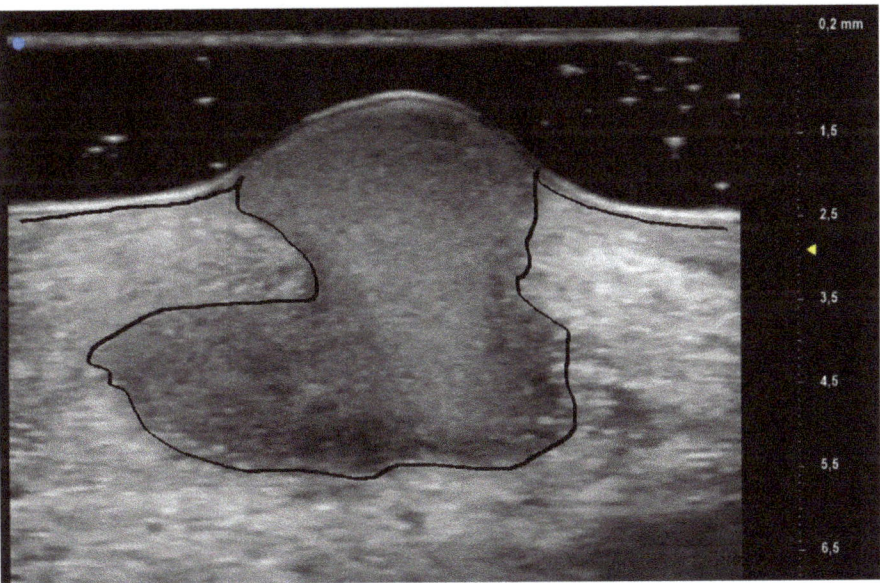

Figure 6. Early PG lesion: the purulent material (included by the black line) is well demarcated and undermined from the surrounding dermis giving a wave-like appearance, the so-called "tsunami sign".

In addition, we identified an augmented echogenicity of the dermis in T0 compared to T1, probably due to increased dermal oedema during the inflammatory phase.

On T0 B-MODE examination we also noticed an enhancement of background noise (called "aliasing") in proximity of V-shaped and U-shaped vessels and oval formations. While the vascular signal in C-MODE could be non-specific, the B-MODE signal allowed us to identify a background noise related to increased reflection phenomena, caused by the presence of corpuscular elements, that, due to vasodilation and stasis, are piled in the blood vessels. The aliasing signal was more easily detectable at the wound edges, probably because of the increased vasodilatation responsible for the lilac ring formation, and it was reduced in T1.

The UHFUS characteristics found in T0 decreased in number and density in T1, but did not disappear. This result could be explained by two theories. First, the permanence of some UHFUS features could be suggestive of a new potential inflammatory flair, thus justifying the need for immunomodulatory maintenance therapy even in the non-inflammatory phase. In addition, the persistence of oval formations/micro-abscesses and V-shaped vessels in the non-inflammatory phase promoted the hypothesis that these UHFUS patterns were pathognomonic signs of PG.

Moreover, the presence of similar UHFUS findings between the pustular and ulcerative phenotypes in T0, suggested the idea, not yet confirmed in the literature, that the pustular phenotype was an early stage of the ulcerative one, in agreement with the assumption of Powell et al. this hypothesis could be supported by our population's anamnestic data that reveal a clinical onset with confluent or non-confluent pustules in 5 patients. (Figure 7) [12].

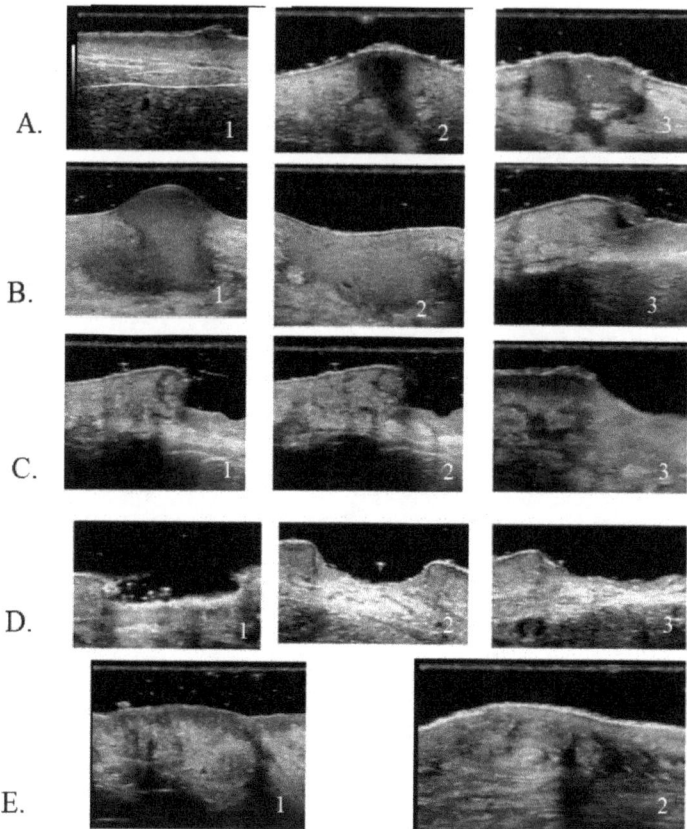

Figure 7. UHFUS PG features: early PG pustule with hair tract (**A1-2-3**); undermined purulent material with the "tsunami sign" formation (**B1-2-3**); PG evolution toward ulceration (**C1-2-3**); PG lesion during non-inflammatory phase (**D1-2-3**); healed PG lesion (**E1-2**).

UHFUS examination showed the presence of a hair track within the oval hyperechoic structures in T0 and their disappearance in T1 (p-value < 0.05). This finding, as well as the increased U-shaped and V-shaped vessels in T0, could also support the idea that the pilosebaceous unit could play a pivotal role in PG pathogenesis.

Wang et al. demonstrated that healed PG scars presented a complete loss of the pilosebaceous unit. Perilesional ulcer skin biopsy revealed a predominance of lymphocytes T polyclonal against dermal and follicular antigens. Moreover, early PG papules revealed higher expression of genes coding for chemokines that attract lymphocytes T, thus causing perivascular and peri pilosebaceous T cell infiltrates [28,29].

In addition, Marzano et al. identified increased activation of adaptive immunity toward hair follicle Ag, as histological analysis performed at the ulcer edge demonstrated the presence of clonally expanded T cells, which could indicate an antigen-driven phenomenon [5].

Hurwitz et al. conducted a comparative study between the different stages of PG: nine skin biopsies were performed on evolving, active, regressing or resolved PG lesions.

The early papule-pustules presented deep folliculitis involving the pilosebaceous unit, with neutrophils located in and surrounding the infundibulum that showed signs of rupture or perforation.

Ulcerated and inflamed lesions were characterized by a massive papillary dermal edema with epidermal neutrophilic abscesses that contributed to the peripheral violaceous undermined edges.

The healing phase presented infiltrates of lymphocytes and histiocytes, while completely healed lesions showed marked signs of fibroplasia [30].

However, a skin biopsy is an invasive exam that depends on the sample site and the lesion's stage. UHFUS (70 MHz) with a spatial resolution in the order of 30 microns permitted us to perform a kind of in vivo histological examination. This non-invasive and repeatable exam allowed real-time monitoring of PG lesions, and finding a correlation between UHFUS morphological structures and histological features would represent a breakthrough in PG diagnosis and treatment monitoring.

The histological findings reported by Hurwitz et al. were comparable with UHFUS ones: the "hair tract" as a sign of pilosebaceous unit involvement; the "dermal hypoecogenity" as a mark of oedema; the "oval hyperechogenic structure" as neutrophilic microabscesses and the "increasing in dermal echogenicity" as increased fibroplasia in the healing phase.

Moreover, our study provides new insight into PG pathogenesis comprehension: dermal abscesses and their subsequent ulceration could derive from an immune response directed toward exposed follicular antigens [29].

5. Conclusions

Our study aimed to provide a new semi-quantitative approach for PG diagnosis and monitoring.

The use of US, particularly UHFUS examination, has demonstrated its potential to revolutionize the field of dermatology by providing valuable insights into the development of an objective and standardized staging method for various skin disorders [31–34]. In this context, our study represents the first experience with UHFUS in patients affected by PG lesions presented in the literature. Notably, one of the significant advantages of UHFUS examination is its ability to facilitate early diagnosis without the associated risks of pathergy phenomenon induced by invasive procedures such as skin biopsies. From the preliminary results obtained with this study, the use of UHFUS examination has shown promising potential in standardizing staging methods and enabling early diagnosis of various skin conditions, including PG.

However, there are some limitations in our study that need to be analyzed and overcome with further investigations in order to understand the full potential of UHFUS as an invaluable tool in PG diagnosis and patient care.

The foremost limitation lies in the small sample size, which might have impacted the generalizability of the findings. In future studies, it will be necessary to include larger and more different patient cohorts to ensure more comprehensive results. Moreover, it would be interesting to perform a quantitative assessment of the vascular signal for a better US characterization of the lesions.

Additionally, the variation in treatments received by the patients in this study poses another challenge. Different treatment approaches might have influenced the presentation of the pustules or ulcerative lesions, which could potentially confound the interpretation of the UHFUS results. To overcome this limitation, future investigations should include patients with more uniform treatment plans, allowing for a more focused evaluation of the imaging biomarkers.

To enhance the applicability of UHFUS in diagnosing PG and distinguish it from other chronic wounds, further research should include a broader spectrum of pustules or ulcerative lesions. By expanding the scope of investigation, we can identify specific imaging biomarkers that are uniquely associated with PG and aid in its differential diagnosis.

Lastly, while our study proposed a hypothesis regarding the pathogenesis of PG, it is crucial to validate this hypothesis through histological correlation. Histological examination of tissue samples from PG patients can provide valuable insights into the underlying mechanisms and confirm the accuracy of UHFUS findings.

Author Contributions: Conceptualization, V.D. and M.R.; methodology, V.D. and M.R.; validation, V.D., M.R. and S.V.; formal analysis, A.M. and B.C.; investigation, G.G., A.M. and B.C.; data curation, G.G., F.M.M. and B.C.; writing—original draft preparation, A.M. and B.C.; writing—review and editing, G.G., A.M. and F.M.M.; visualization, V.D. and M.R.; supervision, V.D. and M.R.; project administration, V.D. All authors have read and agreed to the published version of the manuscript.

Funding: This research received no external funding.

Institutional Review Board Statement: All patients in this manuscript have given written informed consent for participation in this study and the use of their de-identified, anonymized, aggregated data and their case details (including photographs) for publication. This study was conducted in accordance with the Declaration of Helsinki, and approved by the Institutional Review Board (or Ethics Committee) of UO Dermatology, AOUP, Pisa (SUS1-AD ASTRA, 8 July 2019).

Informed Consent Statement: Informed consent was obtained from all subjects involved in the study.

Data Availability Statement: The authors confirm that the data supporting the findings of this study are available from the corresponding author on request.

Conflicts of Interest: The authors declare no conflict of interest.

References

1. Xu, A.; Balgobind, A.; Strunk, A.; Garg, A.; Alloo, A. Prevalence estimates for pyoderma gangrenosum in the United States: An age- and sex-adjusted population analysis. *J. Am. Acad. Dermatol.* **2020**, *83*, 425–429. [CrossRef] [PubMed]
2. Langan, S.M.; Groves, R.W.; Card, T.R.; Gulliford, M.C. Incidence, mortality, and disease associations of pyoderma gangrenosum in the United Kingdom: A retrospective cohort study. *J. Investig. Dermatol.* **2012**, *132*, 2166–2170. [CrossRef] [PubMed]
3. Marzano, A.V.; Borghi, A.; Wallach, D.; Cugno, M. A Comprehensive Review of Neutrophilic Diseases. *Clin. Rev. Allergy Immunol.* **2018**, *54*, 114–130. [CrossRef] [PubMed]
4. Alavi, A.; French, L.E.; Davis, M.D.; Brassard, A.; Kirsner, R.S. Pyoderma Gangrenosum: An Update on Pathophysiology, Diagnosis and Treatment. *Am. J. Clin. Dermatol.* **2017**, *18*, 355–372. [CrossRef]
5. Maverakis, E.; Marzano, A.V.; Le, S.T.; Callen, J.P.; Brüggen, M.C.; Guenova, E.; Dissemond, J.; Shinkai, K.; Langan, S.M. Pyoderma gangrenosum. *Nat. Rev. Dis. Primers* **2020**, *6*, 81. [CrossRef]
6. Dhooghe, N.; Oieni, S.; Peeters, P.; D'Arpa, S.; Roche, N. Post Surgical Pyoderma Gangrenosum in flap surgery: Diagnostic clues and treatment recommendations. *Acta Chir. Belg.* **2017**, *117*, 69–76. [CrossRef] [PubMed]
7. Bevilacqua, M.; Granieri, G.; Fidanzi, C.; Salvia, G.; Margiotta, F.M.; Michelucci, A.; Romanelli, M.; Dini, V. Pyoderma gangrenosum in a patient with Dubowitz syndrome: A new comorbidity? *Wounds* **2023**, *35*, E123–E125. [CrossRef] [PubMed]
8. Janowska, A.; Oranges, T.; Fissi, A.; Davini, G.; Romanelli, M.; Dini, V. PG-TIME: A practical approach to the clinical management of pyoderma gangrenosum. *Dermatol. Ther.* **2020**, *33*, e13412. [CrossRef]
9. Molinelli, E.; Brisigotti, V.; Paolinelli, M.; Offidani, A. Novel Therapeutic Approaches and Targets for the Treatment of Neutrophilic Dermatoses, Management of Patients with Neutrophilic Dermatoses and Future Directions in the Era of Biologic Treatment. *Curr. Pharm. Biotechnol.* **2021**, *22*, 46–58. [CrossRef]
10. Maronese, C.A.; Pimentel, M.A.; Li, M.M.; Genovese, G.; Ortega-Loayza, A.G.; Marzano, A.V. Pyoderma Gangrenosum: An Updated Literature Review on Established and Emerging Pharmacological Treatments. *Am. J. Clin. Dermatol.* **2022**, *23*, 615–634. [CrossRef]
11. Patel, F.; Fitzmaurice, S.; Duong, C.; He, Y.; Fergus, J.; Raychaudhuri, S.P.; Garcia, M.S.; Maverakis, E. Effective strategies for the management of pyoderma gangrenosum: A comprehensive review. *Acta Derm. Venereol.* **2015**, *95*, 525–531. [CrossRef]
12. Powell, F.C.; Su, W.P.; Perry, H.O. Pyoderma gangrenosum: Classification and management. *J. Am. Acad. Dermatol.* **1996**, *34*, 395–409; quiz 410–412. [CrossRef]
13. Jockenhöfer, F.; Wollina, U.; Salva, K.A.; Benson, S.; Dissemond, J. The PARACELSUS score: A novel diagnostic tool for pyoderma gangrenosum. *Br. J. Dermatol.* **2019**, *180*, 615–620. [CrossRef]
14. Pousa-Martínez, M.; Sánchez-Aguilar, D.; Aliste, C.; Vázquez-Veiga, H. Usefulness of ultrasound in the diagnosis and follow-up of pyoderma gangrenosum. *Actas Dermosifiliogr.* **2017**, *108*, 962–964. [CrossRef] [PubMed]
15. Russo, A.; Reginelli, A.; Lacasella, G.V.; Grassi, E.; Karaboue, M.A.A.; Quarto, T.; Busetto, G.M.; Aliprandi, A.; Grassi, R.; Berritto, D. Clinical Application of Ultra-High-Frequency Ultrasound. *J. Pers. Med.* **2022**, *12*, 1733. [CrossRef]
16. Granieri, G.; Oranges, T.; Morganti, R.; Janowska, A.; Romanelli, M.; Manni, E.; Dini, V. Ultra-high frequency ultrasound detection of the dermo-epidermal junction: Its potential role in dermatology. *Exp. Dermatol.* **2022**, *31*, 1863–1871. [CrossRef]
17. Almuhanna, N.; Wortsman, X.; Wohlmuth-Wieser, I.; Kinoshita-Ise, M.; Alhusayen, R. Overview of Ultrasound Imaging Applications in Dermatology. *J. Cutan. Med. Surg.* **2021**, *25*, 521–529. [CrossRef] [PubMed]

18. Albano, D.; Aringhieri, G.; Messina, C.; De Flaviis, L.; Sconfienza, L.M. High-Frequency and Ultra-High Frequency Ultrasound: Musculoskeletal Imaging up to 70 MHz. *Semin. Musculoskelet. Radiol.* **2020**, *24*, 125–134. [CrossRef]
19. Wortsman, X.; Carreño, L.; Ferreira-Wortsman, C.; Poniachik, R.; Pizarro, K.; Morales, C.; Calderon, P.; Castro, A. Ultrasound Characteristics of the Hair Follicles and Tracts, Sebaceous Glands, Montgomery Glands, Apocrine Glands, and Arrector Pili Muscles. *J. Ultrasound Med.* **2019**, *38*, 1995–2004. [CrossRef] [PubMed]
20. Oranges, T.; Vitali, S.; Benincasa, B.; Izzetti, R.; Lencioni, R.; Caramella, D.; Romanelli, M.; Dini, V. Advanced evaluation of hidradenitis suppurativa with ultra-high frequency ultrasound: A promising tool for the diagnosis and monitoring of disease progression. *Skin Res. Technol.* **2020**, *26*, 513–519. [CrossRef]
21. Wortsman, X. Top applications of dermatologic ultrasonography that can modify management. *Ultrasonography* **2023**, *42*, 183–202. [CrossRef] [PubMed]
22. McKenzie, F.; Cash, D.; Gupta, A.; Cummings, L.W.; Ortega-Loayza, A.G. Biologic and small-molecule medications in the management of pyoderma gangrenosum. *J. Dermatol. Treat.* **2019**, *30*, 264–276. [CrossRef] [PubMed]
23. Salvia, G.; Michelucci, A.; Granieri, G.; Manzo Margiotta, F.; Bevilacqua, M.; Fidanzi, C.; Panduri, S.; Romanelli, M.; Dini, V. An Integrated Systemic and Local Wound Management in Recalcitrant Pyoderma Gangrenosum. *Int. J. Low Extrem. Wounds* **2023**. [CrossRef] [PubMed]
24. Goldust, M.; Hagstrom, E.L.; Rathod, D.; Ortega-Loayza, A.G. Diagnosis and novel clinical treatment strategies for pyoderma gangrenosum. *Expert Rev. Clin. Pharmacol.* **2020**, *13*, 157–161. [CrossRef] [PubMed]
25. George, C.; Deroide, F.; Rustin, M. Pyoderma gangrenosum—A guide to diagnosis and management. *Clin. Med.* **2019**, *19*, 224–228. [CrossRef]
26. Yang, L.; Yang, Q.W.; Fu, Y.J. Research advances on the pathogenesis and diagnosis of pyoderma gangrenosum. *Zhonghua Shao Shang Za Zhi* **2022**, *38*, 569–573. (In Chinese) [CrossRef]
27. Chen, B.; Li, W.; Qu, B. Practical aspects of the diagnosis and management of pyoderma gangrenosum. *Front. Med.* **2023**, *10*, 1134939. [CrossRef]
28. Ackerman, A.B. An algorithmic method for histologic diagnosis of inflammatory and neoplastic skin diseases by analysis of their patterns. *Am. J. Dermatopathol.* **1985**, *7*, 105–107. [CrossRef] [PubMed]
29. Wang, E.A.; Steel, A.; Luxardi, G.; Mitra, A.; Patel, F.; Cheng, M.Y.; Wilken, R.; Kao, J.; de Ga, K.; Sultani, H.; et al. Classic Ulcerative Pyoderma Gangrenosum Is a T Cell-Mediated Disease Targeting Follicular Adnexal Structures: A Hypothesis Based on Molecular and Clinicopathologic Studies. *Front. Immunol.* **2018**, *8*, 1980. [CrossRef]
30. Hurwitz, R.M.; Haseman, J.H. The evolution of pyoderma gangrenosum. A clinicopathologic correlation. *Am. J. Dermatopathol.* **1993**, *15*, 28–33. [CrossRef]
31. Krajewska-Włodarczyk, M.; Owczarczyk-Saczonek, A. Usefulness of Ultrasound Examination in the Assessment of the Nail Apparatus in Psoriasis. *Int. J. Environ. Res. Public Health* **2022**, *19*, 5611. [CrossRef] [PubMed]
32. Wortsman, X. Top Advances in Dermatologic Ultrasound. *J. Ultrasound Med.* **2023**, *42*, 521–545. [CrossRef] [PubMed]
33. Zhang, Y.Q.; Wang, L.F.; Ni, N.; Li, X.L.; Zhu, A.Q.; Guo, L.H.; Wang, Q.; Xu, H.X. The Value of Ultra-High-Frequency Ultrasound for the Differentiation between Superficial Basal Cell Carcinoma and Bowen's Disease. *Dermatology* **2023**, *239*, 572–583. [CrossRef] [PubMed]
34. Mendes-Bastos, P.; Martorell, A.; Bettoli, V.; Matos, A.P.; Muscianisi, E.; Wortsman, X. The use of ultrasound and magnetic resonance imaging in the management of hidradenitis suppurativa: A narrative review. *Br. J. Dermatol.* **2023**, *188*, 591–600. [CrossRef] [PubMed]

Disclaimer/Publisher's Note: The statements, opinions and data contained in all publications are solely those of the individual author(s) and contributor(s) and not of MDPI and/or the editor(s). MDPI and/or the editor(s) disclaim responsibility for any injury to people or property resulting from any ideas, methods, instructions or products referred to in the content.

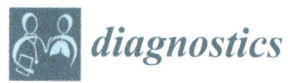

Brief Report

UHFUS: A Valuable Tool in Evaluating Exocrine Gland Abnormalities in Sjögren's Disease

Giovanni Fulvio [1,2,*], Rossana Izzetti [3], Giacomo Aringhieri [4], Valentina Donati [5], Francesco Ferro [1], Giovanna Gabbriellini [6], Marta Mosca [1] and Chiara Baldini [1]

1. Rheumatology Unit, Department of Clinical and Experimental Medicine, University of Pisa, 56126 Pisa, Italy
2. Department of Clinical and Translational Science, University of Pisa, 56126 Pisa, Italy
3. Unit of Dentistry and Oral Surgery, Department of Surgical, Medical and Molecular Pathology and Critical Care Medicine, University of Pisa, 56126 Pisa, Italy
4. Academic Radiology, Department of Clinical and Translational Research, University of Pisa, 56126 Pisa, Italy
5. Unit of Pathological Anatomy 2, Department of Laboratory Medicine, University of Pisa, 56126 Pisa, Italy
6. Ophthalmology, Department of Surgical, Medical and Molecular Pathology and Critical Care Medicine, University of Pisa, 56126 Pisa, Italy
* Correspondence: giovanni.fulvio92@gmail.com

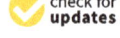

Citation: Fulvio, G.; Izzetti, R.; Aringhieri, G.; Donati, V.; Ferro, F.; Gabbriellini, G.; Mosca, M.; Baldini, C. UHFUS: A Valuable Tool in Evaluating Exocrine Gland Abnormalities in Sjögren's Disease. *Diagnostics* **2023**, *13*, 2771. https://doi.org/10.3390/diagnostics13172771

Academic Editor: Mara Carsote

Received: 15 July 2023
Revised: 22 August 2023
Accepted: 25 August 2023
Published: 26 August 2023

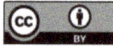

Copyright: © 2023 by the authors. Licensee MDPI, Basel, Switzerland. This article is an open access article distributed under the terms and conditions of the Creative Commons Attribution (CC BY) license (https://creativecommons.org/licenses/by/4.0/).

Abstract: Sjögren's Disease (SjD) is a chronic autoimmune disorder that affects the salivary and lacrimal glands, leading to xerostomia and xerophthalmia. Ultrasonography of Major Salivary Glands (SGUS) is a well-established tool for the identification of the salivary glands' abnormalities in SjD. Recently, a growing interest has arisen in the assessment of the other exocrine glands with ultrasonography: lacrimal glands (LGUS) and labial salivary glands (LSGUS). The objective of this study is to explore the practical applications of ultra-high frequency ultrasound (UHFUS) in the assessment of lacrimal glands and labial salivary glands. Indeed, UHFUS, with its improved spatial resolution compared to conventional ultrasonography, allows for the evaluation of microscopic structures and has been successfully applied in various medical fields. In lacrimal glands, conventional high-frequency ultrasound (HFUS) can detect characteristic inflammatory changes, atrophic alterations, blood flow patterns, and neoplastic lesions associated with SjD. However, sometimes it is challenging to identify lacrimal glands characteristics, thus making UHFUS a promising tool. Regarding labial salivary glands, limited research is available with conventional HFUS, but UHFUS proves to be a good tool to evaluate glandular inhomogeneity and to guide labial salivary glands biopsy. The comprehensive understanding of organ involvement facilitated by UHFUS may significantly improve the management of SjD patients.

Keywords: ultra-high frequency ultrasound; Sjögren's disease (SjD); exocrine glands; lacrimal glands; labial salivary glands; minor salivary glands; major salivary glands; major salivary glands ultrasonography

1. Introduction

Sjögren's Disease (SjD) is a chronic autoimmune disorder characterized by inflammation and dysfunction of the exocrine glands, particularly the salivary and lacrimal glands. These glands are responsible for producing saliva and tears, respectively, and their impairment in SjD leads to dryness of the mouth and eyes, known as xerostomia and xerophthalmia, respectively [1]. A valuable tool in evaluating exocrine gland abnormalities is ultrasonography of the major salivary glands (SGUS), largely employed for clinical and research purposes since it allows for the assessment of gland size, morphology, stiffness, and vascularity [2–4]. In SjD, SGUS can detect characteristic elementary findings such as hypoechoic areas, dilated ducts, and changes in blood flow patterns [5–7]. By ultrasonography, clinicians may identify the disease phenotype, disease activity, glandular damage, and prognostic information [8–10]. In addition, SGUS plays an important role in the detection of major salivary gland lymphoma, a possible complication of SjD [11]. In recent years, great interest has arisen in the application of ultrasonography for the diagnosis and phenotypic stratification of SjD, expanding beyond the conventional ultrasonography of major salivary glands to the ultrasonography of the other exocrine glands: lacrimal glands (LGUS) and labial salivary glands (LSGUS). Particularly, from this perspective, great potential has been seen in ultra-high frequency ultrasound (UHFUS). This study aims to provide insights into the practical applications and role of ultra-high frequency ultrasound in evaluating lacrimal glands and labial salivary glands.

2. Ultra-High Frequency Ultrasound

Ultra-high frequency ultrasound is a diagnostic technique that uses ultrasound frequencies higher than 30 MHz, providing improved spatial resolution compared to conventional ultrasonography. It was first introduced in the preclinical setting in the mid-90s and in the clinical setting at the beginning of the 2000s. UHFUS allows for the evaluation of anatomical structures with submillimeter resolution, making it useful in dermatology, angiology, intraoral pathology, pediatric imaging, peripheral nerve evaluation, and musculoskeletal disorders. It offers the ability to assess microscopic structures such as cutaneous and vessel layers, nerve anatomy, and lymph node structures, which are not easily visualized with conventional high-frequency ultrasound (HFUS). UHFUS has the potential to aid in the diagnosis, surgical planning, follow-up of different pathologies, and assessment of histoanatomy. However, it has a lower penetration depth compared to HFUS, and its use requires a deeper understanding of microscopic anatomy for accurate differential diagnosis. The safety of UHFUS has been studied in preclinical research, showing no significant adverse effects, but the increased frequency does raise concerns about thermal and mechanical energy deposition in human tissues. To ensure patient safety, UHFUS equipment includes real-time thermal and mechanical indices to monitor risks during the examination. Moreover, UHFUS equipment is designed to automatically adjust its output to ensure that mechanical and thermal limits are not exceeded for all imaging modalities. Overall, UHFUS offers versatility, cost-effectiveness, and non-invasiveness, making it a promising imaging modality that is continually evolving and expanding its applications in clinical practice [12–14].

3. Anatomy of Lacrimal Glands and Labial Salivary Glands

The lacrimal gland is anatomically divided into two distinct lobes: the orbital lobe and the palpebral lobe. The orbital lobe is larger, comprising approximately 76.6% of the entire gland's weight, while the palpebral lobe accounts for the remaining 23.4%. Lacrimal gland dimensions may vary among individuals: the long axis of the orbital lobe ranges from 20 to 25 mm, its short axis from 10 to 14 mm, and its thickness from 3 to 6 mm. Instead, the long axis of the palpebral lobe ranges from 9 to 15 mm, its short axis is approximately 8 mm, and its thickness is 2 mm. The lacrimal gland's total dimensions include a long axis of 15–20 mm, a short axis of 10–12 mm, and a thickness of 5 mm. The space between the orbital wall and the globe accommodates the orbital lobe. The palpebral lobe extends anteriorly beyond the superior orbital margin, allowing its inferior surface to contact the lateral portion of the superior fornix where its ducts open. In terms of anatomical relationships, the orbital lobe is above the elevator palpebrae superioris aponeurosis, while the palpebral lobe lies beneath it. Overall, the lacrimal gland is a bilobed serous gland situated in the superolateral aspect of the orbit, with the orbital lobe being larger and situated in the lacrimal fossa, while the palpebral lobe lies below. The lacrimal gland's relationship with the elevator palpebrae superioris aponeurosis changes depending on eyelid movement. When the eyelids are closed, the narrower and more proximal region of the elevator palpebrae aponeurosis lies between the orbital lobe above and the palpebral lobe below that, in this position, is well detectable with ultrasonography. Conversely, during eyelid retraction, the wider anterior part of the aponeurosis moves up and back, displacing the gland in the supratemporal region of the orbit. It is worth noting that the size of the lacrimal gland might vary in individuals, particularly in older individuals, where atrophy can lead to a smaller footprint on the globe, thus making it challenging to identify with ultrasonography [15–17].

There are more than 1000 minor salivary glands that can be found in various anatomical regions, including the sinonasal cavity, oral cavity, pharynx, larynx, trachea, lungs, and middle ear cavity, although they are most densely concentrated in specific areas such as the buccal mucosa (inner lining of the cheeks), labial mucosa (inner lining of the lips), lingual mucosa (underside of the tongue), soft and hard palate (roof of the mouth), and floor of the mouth. The labial salivary glands are located between the mucosal epithelium of the lips and the orbicularis oris muscle and are differently distributed between the two lips: in the upper lip glands they are densely situated between the corners of the mouth, conversely, in the inferior lip they are densely situated outside the corners [18].

4. Ultra-High Frequency Ultrasound Scanning Technique

In our centre, Ultra-high frequency ultrasound is currently performed with Vevo MD (Visual Sonics, Toronto, ON, Canada). Regarding lacrimal glands, a linear scanner UHF48 (20–46 MHz, axial resolution 50 μm) is employed and gel is applied on the probe to allow the transmission of ultrasound. The subjects undergoing the examination are positioned in a supine (lying face up) position with their eyelids closed. The first scan is obtained placing the probe perpendicular to the skin in the upper outer space between the ocular globe and the orbit (Figure 1). Unlike HFUS, the small size of the probe allows for another scan: tilting the transducer obliquely and pointing upwards and outwards, a greater view of the gland may be achieved (Figure 2c,d). B-mode, Doppler mode, and Spectral Doppler of the lacrimal artery are acquired [19].

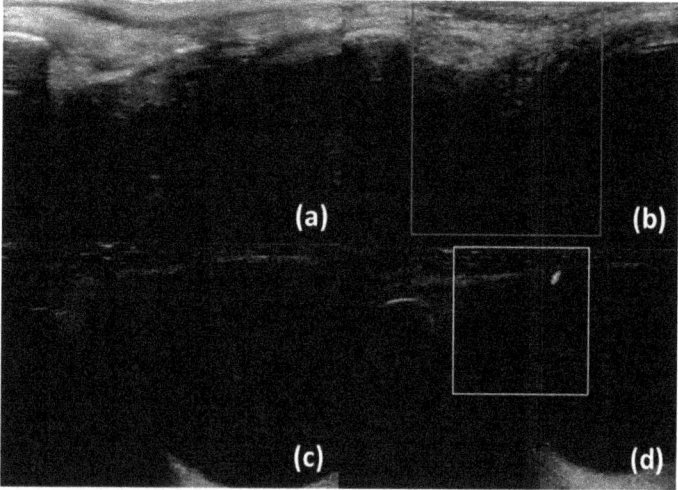

Figure 1. Normal lacrimal glands with a branch of the lacrimal artery. UHFUS (**a**,**b**) and HFUS (**c**,**d**); B-scale (**a**,**c**) and Colour Doppler (**b**,**d**).

Regarding labial salivary glands, subjects are examined with a linear scanner UHF70 (29–71 MHz, axial resolution 30 μm) in a supine position with their neck slightly extended, the mouth subtly open, and the lower lip gently stretched. First, the transducer is adequately cleaned and disinfected. Subsequently, the gel is placed on the probe, which is enveloped with a disposable probe cover, to avoid cross-infection during an intraoral UHFUS scan. Finally, the labial mucosa (intraoral part of the lip) is scanned in successive order: the central compartment, the right compartment, and the left compartment. B-mode, Doppler mode, and Spectral Doppler of lip small vessels are acquired (Figures 3 and 4) [20].

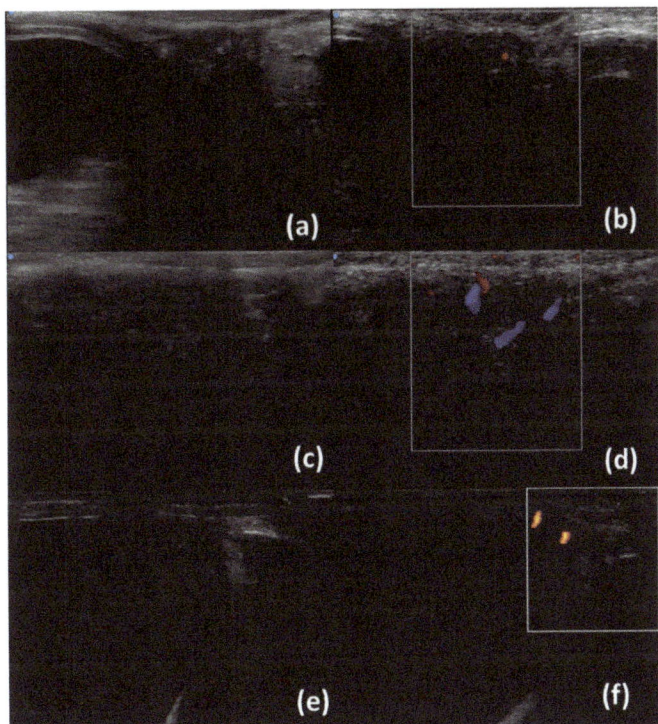

Figure 2. Lacrimal glands with inhomogeneity. UHFUS (**a–d**) and HFUS (**c,d**); B-scale (**a,c,f**) and Colour Doppler (**b,d,e**). Scans in figures (**c,d**) were obtained by tilting the probe upwards and outwards.

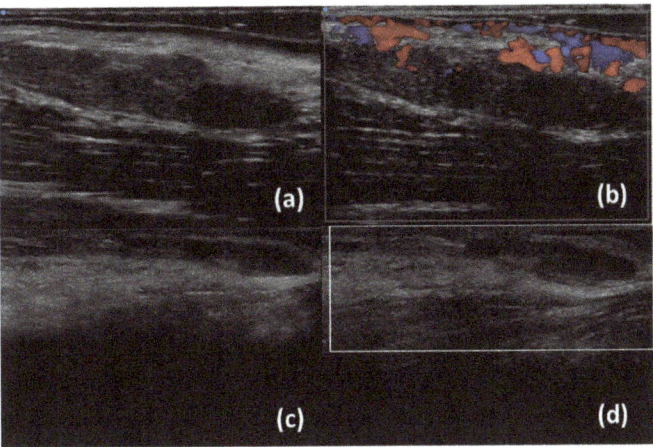

Figure 3. Normal labial salivary glands using UHFUS (**a,b**) and HFUS (**c,d**); B-scale (**a,c**) and Colour Doppler (**b,d**).

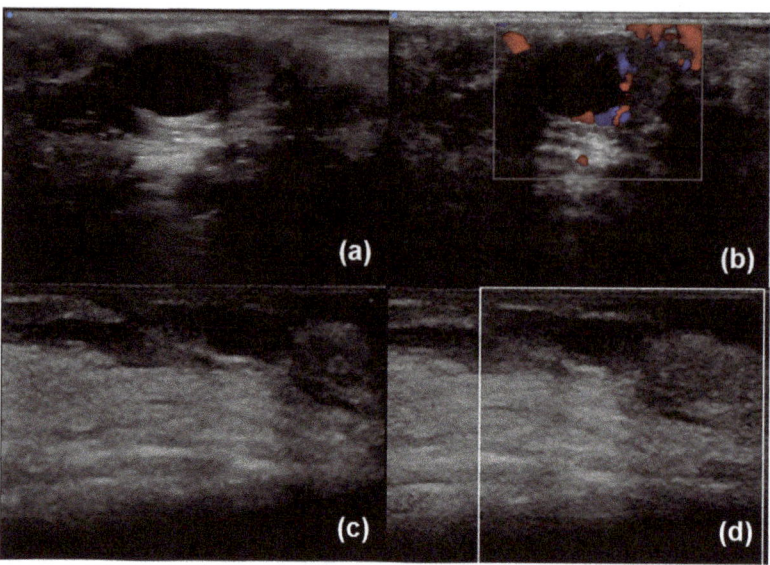

Figure 4. Labial salivary glands with inhomogeneity and a cystic lesion. UHFUS (**a**,**b**) and HFUS (**c**,**d**); B-scale (**a**,**c**) and Colour Doppler (**b**,**d**).

5. Ultrasound of Lacrimal Glands and Labial Salivary Glands

Lacrimal gland ultrasonography (LGUS) is a non-invasive imaging technique used to evaluate the lacrimal glands with several modalities: B-Scale, Doppler, Spectral Doppler, and Shear Wave Elastography (SWE). Table 1 summarizes the most recent and relevant literature studies on LGUS ultrasonography. In greyscale, lacrimal glands of patients with primary Sjögren's Disease may exhibit specific characteristics compared to healthy individuals. These include hypoechoic areas/inhomogeneity with enlargement, suggestive of an inflammatory phase, as well as atrophic changes such as hyperechoic bands, fibrotic changes, or fatty infiltration [19,21,22]. Doppler imaging of lacrimal glands mainly allows for the assessment of high blood flow: in SjD patients, a higher percentage of intraglandular branches of lacrimal artery have been found with a higher Resistivity Index [22,23]. Figures 1 and 2 show normal lacrimal glands and lacrimal glands with inhomogeneity using UHFUS and HFUS. Shear Wave Elastography is an increasingly utilized technique in lacrimal gland ultrasonography to evaluate the elasticity or stiffness of the lacrimal gland. Lacrimal glands often exhibit elevated SWE values, which suggest the presence of fibrotic changes. SWE parameters are associated with several clinical features, including OSDI (Ocular Surface Disease Index), ESSPRI (EULAR Sjögren's Syndrome Patient Reported Index), and the occurrence of dry eye [24–26]. Studies have also demonstrated the utility of ultrasonography in differentiating neoplastic lesions within the lacrimal gland, such as lymphoma or non-epithelial lesions. These lesions typically appear as hypoechoic areas with central and peripheral vascularity [21,27]. Therefore, lacrimal gland ultrasonography can aid in the identification of suspicious lesions for further evaluation. In summary, lacrimal gland ultrasonography can discriminate SjD patients from healthy control, may identify lesions suspicious for lymphoma, and is associated with local disease activity and functional test. It is worth noting that lacrimal glands are located superficially, even if there are currently no studies available on the use of ultra-high frequency ultrasound. Interestingly, ultra-high frequency ultrasound has been employed to assess other eye structures, such as the lacrimal drainage system, highlighting its importance and safety in evaluating ocular pathologies [28–32]. In addition, with conventional ultrasound, lacrimal glands can be frequently undetectable. Conversely, UHFUS, due to a higher resolution and the possibility of performing larger gland scans, may identify small and atrophic glands.

In contrast to lacrimal glands, there is limited research available regarding conventional ultrasonography of labial salivary glands (Table 1). To date, only one study has focused on minor salivary glands, revealing how SWE values in patients with SjD are associated with disease activity measured by the ESSDAI (EULAR Sjögren's Syndrome Disease Activity Index), levels of IgG antibodies, and the presence of hypocomplementemia [33]. Research conducted by our group has yielded insights into the utility of ultra-high frequency ultrasound in assessing labial salivary glands [34]. Figures 3 and 4 show normal LSG and LSG with inhomogeneity and a cystic lesion using UHFUS and HFUS, respectively. UHFUS showed a good reliability to assess glandular inhomogeneity that in turn was associated with histological inflammation and serology. More specifically, in a cross-sectional study including 128 patients with suspected SjD, we found that UHFUS was able to discriminate SjD from no-SjD sicca controls, as LSG inhomogeneity was significantly higher in patients with SjD than in no-SS subjects [35,36]. The study highlighted the optimal feasibility of UHFUS and its high sensitivity in identifying negative patients on subsequent lip biopsy. Interestingly, our preliminary data indicate that UHFUS exhibits a specificity for SjD diagnosis from approximately 65% to 85% depending on the chosen cut-off threshold [35,37]. Furthermore, findings suggestive of lymphoproliferative lesion have been identified; there being very hypoechoic areas and high Doppler signal that were detected in a patient with a more complex inflammatory infiltrate in her biopsy [38]. Eventually, UHFUS may be useful to guide biopsy and to improve sampling of labial salivary glands [20].

Table 1. Major studies on conventional ultrasound of lacrimal gland and labial salivary glands.

Author (Year)	US Modalities	Main Findings
Lacrimal Gland Conventional Ultrasonography		
Giovagnorio et al. (2000) [21]	B-mode Colour Doppler Spectral Doppler	When well visibile, lacrimal glands in SjD patients are enlarged and hypoechoic Presence of Hyperechoic bands in SjD patients Two lymphoma identified with cyst-like lesions RI higher than normal individuals
Bilgili et al. (2004) [23]	Spectral Doppler	Values of RI and PI in normal Lacrimal Artery
De Lucia et al. (2020) [19]	B-mode Colour Doppler	SjD patients have higher proportion of inhomogeneity and fibrous gland appearance
Kim et al. (2022) [22]	B-mode Colour Doppler	SjD patients have higher proportion of intraglandular branch of lacrimal artery, inhomogeneity, hyperechoic bands SjD diagnostic value of intraglandular branch and inhomogeneity
Świecka et al. (2023) [24]	Shear Wave Elastography	SjD diagnostic value of SWE (SjD patients have higher SWE values)
Karadeniz et al. (2023) [25]	Shear Wave Elastography	SjD diagnostic value of SWE (SjD patients have higher SWE values) Correlation of SWE with OSDI and ESSPRI
Yılmaz et al. (2023) [26]	Shear Wave Elastography	SWE values are higher in patients with dry eye
Labial salivary Gland Conventional Ultrasonography		
Wang et al. (2022) [33]	Shear Wave Elastography	SWE values are associated with ESSDAI, IgG values and hypocomplementemia
Labial salivary Gland ultra-high frequency Ultrasonography		
Ferro et al. (2020) [35]	B-mode	SjD diagnostic value (SjD patients have higher inhomogeneity) Associations of inhomogeneity with Ro/SSA+ positivity Correlations of inhomogenity with histological inflammation
Izzetti et al. (2021) [20]	B-mode	Support to the biopsy procedure

SjD = Sjögren's Disease, RI = Resistivity Index, PI = Pulsatility Index, SWE = Shear Wave Elastography, OSDI = Ocular Surface Disease Index, ESSPRI = EULAR Sjogren's Syndrome Patient Reported Index, ESSDAI = EULAR Sjögren's syndrome disease activity index.

6. Conclusions

Ultra-high frequency ultrasound (UHFUS) is a versatile and non-invasive imaging modality that is increasingly employed in patients with Sjögren's Disease for research and clinical purposes. UHFUS, indeed, has the potential to better characterize both normal and pathological findings in the exocrine glands, including lacrimal glands and labial salivary glands. Furthermore, due to its enhanced resolution and associations with microanatomy, UHFUS may contribute to a more comprehensive understanding of glandular abnormalities in SjD. Future biopsy-based prospective clinical studies including a larger patient cohort are warranted to comprehensively define the potential role of ultra-high frequency ultrasound (UHFUS) in both the diagnosis of Sjögren's Disease (SjD) and the phenotyping of affected patients. The comparison between UHFUS findings and histology appears instrumental to better define the correspondence between sonographic and histological biomarkers. Indeed, a comprehensive understanding of glandular involvement in SjD may improve diagnosis, management, and treatment in patients with SjD.

Author Contributions: Conceptualization, G.F. and R.I.; methodology, G.F. and R.I.; software, G.F.; validation, G.F. and R.I.; formal analysis, G.F. and C.B.; investigation, G.F., F.F. and R.I; resources, C.B.; data curation, C.B.; writing—original draft preparation, G.F, R.I. and C.B.; writing—review and editing, G.F., R.I., G.A., V.D., F.F., G.G., M.M. and C.B; visualization, G.F.; supervision, G.F. and R.I.; project administration, C.B. All authors have read and agreed to the published version of the manuscript.

Funding: This research received no external funding.

Institutional Review Board Statement: This study was conducted in accordance with the Declaration of Helsinki and approved by the Institutional Review Board of the University Hospital of Pisa (Comitato Etico Area Vasta Nord-Ovest, CEAVNO) (protocol code 14540 approved on 14 March 2019).

Informed Consent Statement: Informed consent was obtained from all subjects involved in the study.

Data Availability Statement: Data is contained within the article.

Acknowledgments: Images included in this paper were collected from patients participating to an ongoing observational study exploring diagnostic accuracy of UHFUS of labial salivary glands in SjD. We thank all the patients that consented to be involved in the study.

Conflicts of Interest: The authors declare no conflict of interest.

References

1. Cafaro, G.; Bursi, R.; Chatzis, L.G.; Fulvio, G.; Ferro, F.; Bartoloni, E.; Baldini, C. One year in review 2021: Sjögren's syndrome. *Clin. Exp. Rheumatol.* **2021**, *39* (Suppl. S133), 3–13. [CrossRef] [PubMed]
2. Callegher, S.Z.; Giovannini, I.; Zenz, S.; Manfrè, V.; Stradner, M.H.; Hocevar, A.; Gutierrez, M.; Quartuccio, L.; De Vita, S.; Zabotti, A. Sjögren syndrome: Looking forward to the future. *Ther. Adv. Musculoskelet. Dis.* **2022**, *14*, 1–23. [CrossRef]
3. Carotti, M.; Salaffi, F.; Manganelli, P.; Argalia, G. Ultrasonography and Colour Doppler Sonography of Salivary Glands in Primary Sjo¨gren's Syndrome. *Clin. Rheumatol.* **2001**, *20*, 213–219. [CrossRef] [PubMed]
4. Arslan, S.; Durmaz, M.S.; Erdogan, H.; Esmen, S.E.; Turgut, B.; Iyisoy, M.S. Two-Dimensional Shear Wave Elastography in the Assessment of Salivary Gland Involvement in Primary Sjögren's Syndrome. *J. Ultrasound Med.* **2020**, *39*, 949–956. [CrossRef]
5. Hočevar, A.; Rainer, S.; Rozman, B.; Zor, P.; Tomšič, M. Ultrasonographic changes of major salivary glands in primary Sjögren's syndrome: Evaluation of a novel scoring system. *Eur. J. Radiol.* **2007**, *63*, 379–383. [CrossRef]
6. Jousse-Joulin, S.; D'Agostino, M.A.; Nicolas, C.; Naredo, E.; Ohrndorf, S.; Backhaus, M.; Tamborrini, G.; Chary-Valckenaere, I.; Terslev, L.; Iagnocco, A.; et al. Video clip assessment of a salivary gland ultrasound scoring system in Sjögren's syndrome using consensual definitions: An OMERACT ultrasound working group reliability exercise. *Ann. Rheum. Dis.* **2019**, *78*, 967–973. [CrossRef]
7. Hočevar, A.; Bruyn, G.A.; Terslev, L.; De Agustin, J.J.; MacCarter, D.; Chrysidis, S.; Collado, P.; Dejaco, C.; Fana, V.; Filippou, G.; et al. Development of a new ultrasound scoring system to evaluate glandular inflammation in Sjögren's syndrome: An OMERACT reliability exercise. *Rheumatology* **2022**, *61*, 3341–3350. [CrossRef] [PubMed]
8. Deroo, L.; Achten, H.; De Boeck, K.; Genbrugge, E.; Bauters, W.; Roels, D.; Dochy, F.; Creytens, D.; Deprez, J.; Bosch, F.V.D.; et al. The value of separate detection of anti-Ro52, anti-Ro60 and anti-SSB/La reactivities in relation to diagnosis and phenotypes in primary Sjögren's syndrome. *Clin. Exp. Rheumatol.* **2022**, *40*, 2310–2317. [CrossRef] [PubMed]

9. Deroo, L.; Achten, H.; De Boeck, K.; Genbrugge, E.; Bauters, W.; Roels, D.; Dochy, F.; Creytens, D.; De Craemer, A.-S.; Bosch, F.V.D.; et al. Discriminative power of salivary gland ultrasound in relation to symptom-based endotypes in suspected and definite primary Sjögren's Syndrome. *Semin. Arthritis Rheum.* **2022**, *56*, 152075. [CrossRef]
10. Milic, V.; Colic, J.; Cirkovic, A.; Stanojlovic, S.; Damjanov, N. Disease activity and damage in patients with primary Sjögren's syndrome: Prognostic value of salivary gland ultrasonography. *PLoS ONE* **2019**, *14*, e0226498. [CrossRef]
11. Lorenzon, M.; Di Franco, F.T.; Zabotti, A.; Pegolo, E.; Giovannini, I.; Manfrè, V.; Mansutti, E.; De Vita, S.; Zuiani, C.; Girometti, R. Sonographic features of lymphoma of the major salivary glands diagnosed with ultrasound-guided core needle biopsy in Sjögren's syndrome. *Clin. Exp. Rheumatol.* **2021**, *39*, 175–183. [CrossRef] [PubMed]
12. Izzetti, R.; Vitali, S.; Aringhieri, G.; Nisi, M.; Oranges, T.; Dini, V.; Ferro, F.; Baldini, C.; Romanelli, M.; Caramella, D.; et al. Ultra-High Frequency Ultrasound, A Promising Diagnostic Technique: Review of the Literature and Single-Center Experience. *Can. Assoc. Radiol. J.* **2021**, *72*, 418–431. [CrossRef] [PubMed]
13. Fogante, M.; Carboni, N.; Argalia, G. Clinical application of ultra-high frequency ultrasound: Discovering a new imaging frontier. *J. Clin. Ultrasound* **2022**, *50*, 817–825. [CrossRef] [PubMed]
14. Hawez, T.; Graneli, C.; Erlöv, T.; Gottberg, E.; Mitev, R.M.; Hagelsteen, K.; Evertsson, M.; Jansson, T.; Cinthio, M.; Stenström, P. Ultra-High Frequency Ultrasound Imaging of Bowel Wall in Hirschsprung's Disease—Correlation and Agreement Analyses of Histoanatomy. *Diagnostics* **2023**, *13*, 1388. [CrossRef]
15. Obata, H. Anatomy and Histopathology of the Human Lacrimal Gland. *Cornea* **2006**, *25* (Suppl. S1), S82–S89. [CrossRef]
16. Lorber, M. Gross Characteristics of Normal Human Lacrimal Glands. *Ocul. Surf.* **2007**, *5*, 13–22. [CrossRef]
17. Singh, S.; Basu, S. The Human Lacrimal Gland: Historical Perspectives, Current Understanding, and Recent Advances. *Curr. Eye Res.* **2020**, *45*, 1188–1198. [CrossRef]
18. Shen, D.; Ono, K.; Do, Q.; Ohyama, H.; Nakamura, K.; Obata, K.; Ibaragi, S.; Watanabe, K.; Tubbs, R.S.; Iwanaga, J. Clinical anatomy of the inferior labial gland: A narrative review. *Gland. Surg.* **2021**, *10*, 2284–2292. [CrossRef]
19. De Lucia, O.; Zandonella Callegher, S.; De Souza, M.V.; Battafarano, N.; Del Papa, N.; Gerosa, M.; Giovannini, I.; Tullio, A.; Valent, F.; Zabotti, A.; et al. Ultrasound assessment of lacrimal glands: A cross-sectional study in healthy subjects and a preliminary study in primary Sjögren's syndrome patients. *Clin. Exp. Rheumatol.* **2020**, *38* (Suppl. S126), 203–209.
20. Izzetti, R.; Ferro, F.; Vitali, S.; Nisi, M.; Fonzetti, S.; Oranges, T.; Donati, V.; Caramella, D.; Baldini, C.; Gabriele, M. Ultra-high frequency ultrasonography (UHFUS)-guided minor salivary gland biopsy: A promising procedure to optimize labial salivary gland biopsy in Sjögren's syndrome. *J. Oral Pathol. Med.* **2021**, *50*, 485–491. [CrossRef]
21. Giovagnorio, F.; Pace, F.; Giorgi, A. Sonography of lacrimal glands in Sjögren syndrome. *J. Ultrasound Med.* **2000**, *19*, 505–509. [CrossRef]
22. Kim, S.H.; Min, H.K.; Lee, S.-H.; Lee, K.-A.; Kim, H.-R. Ultrasonographic evaluation of lacrimal glands in patients with primary Sjögren's syndrome. *Clin. Exp. Rheumatol.* **2022**, *40*, 2283–2289. [CrossRef] [PubMed]
23. Bilgili, Y.; Taner, P.; Unal, B.; Simsir, I.; Kara, S.A.; Bayram, M.; Alicioglu, B. Doppler sonography of the normal lacrimal gland. *J. Clin. Ultrasound* **2005**, *33*, 123–126. [CrossRef]
24. Świecka, M.; Paluch, Ł.; Pietruski, P.; Maślińska, M.; Zakrzewski, J.; Kwiatkowska, B. Applicability of shear wave elastography for lacrimal gland evaluation in primary Sjögren's syndrome. *Pol. Arch. Intern. Med.* **2023**, *133*, 16397. [CrossRef] [PubMed]
25. Karadeniz, H.; Cerit, M.; Güler, A.A.; Salman, R.B.; Satış, H.; Yıldırım, D.; Göker, B.; Küçük, H.; Öztürk, M.A.; Tufan, A. Lacrimal gland ultrasonography and elastography as a diagnostic and activity tool for primary Sjögren's syndrome. *Int. J. Rheum. Dis.* **2023**, *26*, 1083–1090. [CrossRef]
26. Güneş, I.B.; Yılmaz, H. Evaluation of Main Lacrimal Gland through Shear-wave Ultrasound Elastography in Patients with Low Schirmer Value. *Curr. Med. Imaging* **2023**, *20*, e080623217778. [CrossRef]
27. Lecler, A.; Boucenna, M.; Lafitte, F.; Koskas, P.; Nau, E.; Jacomet, P.V.; Galatoire, O.; Morax, S.; Putterman, M.; Mann, F.; et al. Usefulness of colour Doppler flow imaging in the management of lacrimal gland lesions. *Eur. Radiol.* **2017**, *27*, 779–789. [CrossRef]
28. Bohman, E.; Berggren, J.; Bunke, J.; Albinsson, J.; Engelsberg, K.M.; Dahlstrand, U.M.; Hult, J.; Hasegawa, H.; Cinthio, M.; Sheikh, R.M. Novel Evidence Concerning Lacrimal Sac Movement Using Ultra-High-Frequency Ultrasound Examinations of Lacrimal Drainage Systems. *Ophthalmic Plast. Reconstr. Surg.* **2020**, *37*, 334–340. [CrossRef] [PubMed]
29. Yan, X.; Xiang, N.; Hu, W.; Liu, R.; Luo, B. Characteristics of lacrimal passage diseases by 80-MHz ultrasound biomicroscopy: An observational study. *Graefe's Arch. Clin. Exp. Ophthalmol.* **2020**, *258*, 403–410. [CrossRef] [PubMed]
30. Lim, H.G.; Kim, H.H.; Yoon, C. Synthetic Aperture Imaging Using High-Frequency Convex Array for Ophthalmic Ultrasound Applications. *Sensors* **2021**, *21*, 2275. [CrossRef] [PubMed]
31. Machado, M.A.d.C.; Silva, J.A.F.; Garcia, E.A.; Allemann, N. Ultrasound parameters of normal lacrimal sac and chronic dacryocystitis. *Arq. Bras. Oftalmol.* **2017**, *80*, 172–175. [CrossRef] [PubMed]
32. Luo, B.; Qi, X. Utility of 80-MHz Ultrasound Biomicroscopy and Lacrimal Endoscopy in Chronic Lacrimal Canaliculitis. *J. Ultrasound Med.* **2021**, *40*, 2513–2520. [CrossRef] [PubMed]
33. Wang, X.; Wang, A.; Zhan, X.; Xu, L.; Chang, X.; Dong, F. Value of conventional ultrasound and shear wave elastography in assessing disease activity and prognosis in female patients with Sjögren's syndrome. *Clin. Exp. Rheumatol.* **2022**, *40*, 2350–2356. [CrossRef]
34. Aringhieri, G.; Izzetti, R.; Vitali, S.; Ferro, F.; Gabriele, M.; Baldini, C.; Caramella, D. Ultra-high frequency ultrasound (UHFUS) applications in Sjogren syndrome: Narrative review and current concepts. *Gland. Surg.* **2020**, *9*, 2248–2259. [CrossRef] [PubMed]

35. Ferro, F.; Izzetti, R.; Vitali, S.; Aringhieri, G.; Fonzetti, S.; Donati, V.; Dini, V.; Mosca, M.; Gabriele, M.; Caramella, D.; et al. Ultra-high frequency ultrasonography of labial glands is a highly sensitive tool for the diagnosis of Sjögren's syndrome: A preliminary study. *Clin. Exp. Rheumatol.* **2020**, *38* (Suppl. S126), 210–215.
36. Izzetti, R.; Fulvio, G.; Nisi, M.; Gennai, S.; Graziani, F. Reliability of OMERACT Scoring System in Ultra-High Frequency Ultrasonography of Minor Salivary Glands: Inter-Rater Agreement Study. *J. Imaging* **2022**, *8*, 111. [CrossRef]
37. Fulvio, G.; Ferro, F.; Izzetti, R.; Governato, G.; Fonzetti, S.; La Rocca, G.; García, I.C.N.; Donati, V.; Mosca, M.; Baldini, C. POS1461 advantages of doppler in labial salivary gland ultra-high frequency ultrasound: Correlations with histological inflammation, pSS diagnosis, disease activity, and prognosis. *Ann. Rheum. Dis.* **2023**, *82* (Suppl. S1), 1085. [CrossRef]
38. Fulvio, G.; Donati, V.; Izzetti, R.; Fonzetti, S.; La Rocca, G.; Ferro, F.; Baldini, C. Correspondence between minor salivary glands ultra-high frequency ultrasonography and histology: A case report of severe/atypical lymphoid infiltrate in Sjögren's syndrome. *Ann. Rheum. Dis.* **2022**, *40*, 2474–2475. [CrossRef]

Disclaimer/Publisher's Note: The statements, opinions and data contained in all publications are solely those of the individual author(s) and contributor(s) and not of MDPI and/or the editor(s). MDPI and/or the editor(s) disclaim responsibility for any injury to people or property resulting from any ideas, methods, instructions or products referred to in the content.

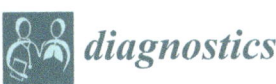

Article

A Computer Program for Assessing Histoanatomical Morphometrics in Ultra-High-Frequency Ultrasound Images of the Bowel Wall in Children: Development and Inter-Observer Variability

Tobias Erlöv [1], Tebin Hawez [2], Christina Granéli [2,3], Maria Evertsson [2,4], Tomas Jansson [4,5], Pernilla Stenström [2,3,*] and Magnus Cinthio [1]

1. Department of Biomedical Engineering, Faculty of Engineering, Lund University, 22363 Lund, Sweden; tobias.erlov@bme.lth.se (T.E.); magnus.cinthio@bme.lth.se (M.C.)
2. Pediatrics, Department of Clinical Sciences, Faculty of Medicine, Lund University, 22185 Lund, Sweden; tebin.hawez@med.lu.se (T.H.); christina.graneli@med.lu.se (C.G.); maria.evertsson@med.lu.se (M.E.)
3. Department of Pediatric Surgery, Skåne University Hospital Lund, 22185 Lund, Sweden
4. Department of Clinical Sciences Lund, Biomedical Engineering, Lund University, 22363 Lund, Sweden; tomas.jansson@med.lu.se
5. Clinical Engineering Skåne, Digitalisering IT/MT, RegionSkåne, 22185 Lund, Sweden
* Correspondence: pernilla.stenstrom@med.lu.se

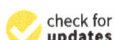

Abstract: Ultra-high-frequency ultrasound (UHFUS) has a reported potential to differentiate between aganglionic and ganglionic bowel wall, referred to as histoanatomical differences. A good correlation between histoanatomy and UHFUS of the bowel wall has been proven. In order to perform more precise and objective histoanatomical morphometrics, the main research objective of this study was to develop a computer program for the assessment and automatic calculation of the histoanatomical morphometrics of the bowel wall in UHFUS images. A computer program for UHFUS diagnostics was developed and presented. A user interface was developed in close collaboration between pediatric surgeons and biomedical engineers, to enable interaction with UHFUS images. Images from ex vivo bowel wall samples of 23 children with recto-sigmoid Hirschsprung's disease were inserted. The program calculated both thickness and amplitudes (image whiteness) within different histoanatomical bowel wall layers. Two observers assessed the images using the program and the inter-observer variability was evaluated. There was an excellent agreement between observers, with an intraclass correlation coefficient range of 0.970–0.998. Bland–Altman plots showed flat and narrow distributions. The mean differences ranged from 0.005 to 0.016 mm in thickness and 0 to 0.7 in amplitude units, corresponding to 1.1–3.6% and 0.0–0.8% from the overall mean. The computer program enables and ensures objective, accurate and time-efficient measurements of histoanatomical thicknesses and amplitudes in UHFUS images of the bowel wall. The program can potentially be used for several bowel wall conditions, accelerating research within UHFUS diagnostics.

Keywords: bowel wall; computer program; histoanatomical morphometrics; ultra-high-frequency ultrasound

Citation: Erlöv, T.; Hawez, T.; Granéli, C.; Evertsson, M.; Jansson, T.; Stenström, P.; Cinthio, M. A Computer Program for Assessing Histoanatomical Morphometrics in Ultra-High-Frequency Ultrasound Images of the Bowel Wall in Children: Development and Inter-Observer Variability. *Diagnostics* **2023**, *13*, 2759. https://doi.org/10.3390/diagnostics13172759

Academic Editors: Rossana Izzetti and Marco Nisi

Received: 1 July 2023
Revised: 4 August 2023
Accepted: 11 August 2023
Published: 25 August 2023

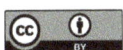

Copyright: © 2023 by the authors. Licensee MDPI, Basel, Switzerland. This article is an open access article distributed under the terms and conditions of the Creative Commons Attribution (CC BY) license (https://creativecommons.org/licenses/by/4.0/).

1. Introduction

Ultrasonography is a diagnostic imaging method based on acoustic echoes and tissue-specific acoustic impedance. The amplitude, i.e., the strength of the reflected ultrasound waves, is described as hyperechoic with higher amplitudes (seen as white areas)—as in fat and collagen—hypoechoic, or anechoic (seen as gray or black areas, respectively) [1,2]. In daily medical use, ultrasound transducers transmitting 2–15 MHz are used, giving a good overview of the organs by imaging tissues to a depth of 2–20 cm. In contrast, UHFUS, with its much higher frequencies (30–50 MHz center frequency), allows for detailed imaging to depths of 0.1–5.0 mm [3,4]. UHFUS has been suggested to be promising for detailed diagnostics in several clinical areas [4–6]. Since the thickness of the bowel wall in small children is reported to be 0.3–2 mm, the use of UHFUS in the diagnosis of bowel diseases has also been suggested [7]. Hirschsprung's disease (HD) is a congenital disease characterized by the absence of ganglia cells within two of the histoanatomical layers of the bowel wall. Currently, diagnosis of HD is by histopathological and immunohistological analyses of tissue biopsies [8], which are time-consuming and costly to perform. In order to replace the use of biopsies both during primary and surgical diagnosis with an instant and secure diagnostic method, the use of UHFUS is being explored [9]. Histoanatomical differences between aganglionic and ganglionic bowel wall have been suggested, and good correlations between histoanatomy and UHFUS of bowel wall specimens from HD patients have been confirmed [10]. Initial clinical observations have shown that UHFUS has the potential to delineate between aganglionic and ganglionic bowel wall [11]. The problem is that the assessment and calculation of histoanatomical measurements within UHFUS images could be both inaccurate and time-consuming, as well as associated with certain observer bias. To obtain reliable measurements of bowel wall layers quickly and easily, avoiding internal variability and limiting observer bias, a computerized assessment of the bowel wall within the UHFUS image is warranted. This would accelerate research by facilitating multiple measurements and enabling collection of amplitude information. Therefore, to be able to more precisely and objectively assess and calculate histoanatomical morphometrics, a computer program for UHFUS diagnostics is required.

The main research objective of the study was to enable the assessment and automatic calculation of the histoanatomical morphometrics of the bowel wall in UHFUS images. The hypothesis was that a computer program would enable the assessment of relevant automatic calculations of the bowel wall's histoanatomical morphometrics and that it would also deliver a high inter-observer correlation.

The main aim of this study was to develop a computer program for the assessment and automatic calculation of the morphometrics of the bowel wall in UHFUS images. The secondary aim was to validate the computer program through inter-observer analyses between users. The main output variable was the ability of the computer program to measure the thicknesses and amplitudes of the bowel wall's histoanatomical layers. The second output variable was the degree of inter-observer variability in the assessment of the thicknesses and amplitudes of the bowel wall.

2. Materials and Methods

2.1. Settings

This was a developmental and validation study performed on UHFUS images of fresh ex vivo bowel wall specimens from children who underwent surgery for HD in a national referral pediatric surgery center for children with HD. The study was part of a larger translational project, involving pediatric surgeons, biomedical engineers and pathologists, and aiming to improve HD diagnostics by the use of UHFUS.

2.2. Tissue Samples and Ultra-High-Frequency Ultrasound Images

All children with recto-sigmoid HD who underwent surgery with resection of the aganglionic bowel segment at a national Swedish referral center for HD, from April 2018 to December 2022, and for whom the guardians' written consent had been obtained, were included in the study. A sample size of 20 was suggested by statisticians at the Department of Swedish Clinical Research Studies Forum South to be required, in accordance with guidelines for sample sizes in agreement analyses [12]. During the study period, a total of 37 children with HD underwent surgery. In accordance with a purposive and systematic sampling method, all these consecutive cases were evaluated for inclusion in the study. Ultimately, 23 of the 37 bowel wall specimens were included because they fulfilled the inclusion criteria by being rectosigmoid HD (<30 cm resected length), and because a successful imaging of both the aganglionic and ganglionic areas of the same specimen had been undertaken without technical obstacles. Of the 37 images, 14 were excluded because of aganglionosis extending more than 30 cm ($n = 8$), or due to an initial lack of standardized settings in the scanning UHFUS program ($n = 6$), leaving 23 images for analysis.

The decision on surgical resection length was based on the pathologist's analysis of intraoperatively taken fresh-frozen biopsies confirming the presence of ganglionic bowel wall. After surgical resection, the retrieved bowel wall segment was pinned to a cork mat and subjected to ex vivo UHFUS imaging from the serosal surface, at sites representing aganglionic and ganglionic bowel wall segments, respectively [11]. The specimen was then fixed in formalin and embedded in paraffin, and the presence of aganglionosis and gangliionosis was confirmed by histopathology (hematoxylin-eosin) and immunohistochemistry (S100 and calretinin) [9,11].

For ultrasound imaging, the Vevo® MD ultrasound scanner, together with the UHF 70 transducer (both FUJIFILM VisualSonics Inc., Toronto, ON, Canada), delivering a center frequency of 50 MHz (bandwidth 29–71 MHz), was used.

Thus, for each patient, UHFUS images of both aganglionic and ganglionic bowel wall were available in the image database. These were exported for one-by-one measurements in the computer program for computerized assessments.

2.3. Computerized Program for Histoanatomical Morphometrics in the Bowel Wall

The computer program, consisting of a user interface in which the user can interact with the ultrasound images, was developed using MATLAB® version 9.13 (R2022b, The MathWorks Inc., Natick, MA, USA) and its tools for user interfaces and functions, respectively, by researchers at the Department of Biomedical Engineering, Lund University. The purpose of the program was: (a) to enable multiple thickness measurements to be taken in a short amount of time; (b) to enable objective measurements of echo amplitudes (image whiteness) within different bowel wall layers in the ultrasound images; (c) to be easy to use by the pediatric surgeons on site; and (d) to be more time-efficient compared to manual measurements using calipers on the ultrasound scanner.

To achieve these aims, the biomedical engineers and the pediatric surgeons worked in close collaboration, improving the user interface and program functionality continuously based on user experience and needs. In order to validate the software and ensure its security, requirements were defined and documented, outlining accomplishments and expected behavior of the program. After each update, the program's new function was verified using simulated images which were assessed according to the specified requirements. In order to ensure that the code did not change during the study, a compiled version of the program was used. The software was developed within a research environment of an international leading research group for UHFUS with considerable experience in computer programming, especially in MATLAB. The engineers' affiliation to one of Sweden's largest research institutions for biomedical engineering secured a solid foundation of technical and experienced resources in computer programming.

2.4. Measurements and Statistical Analysis

The thickness and amplitude of the layers in the bowel wall were measured in all included UHFUS images by two different observers using the computer program. In addition, ratios between measurements in different layers were calculated. The inter-observer variability of the computerized measurements was evaluated using the intraclass correlation coefficient (ICC) for two-way mixed effects, absolute agreement and multiple raters [13]. For testing the hypothesis, ICC values of less than 0.5 indicated poor reliability, values between 0.5 and 0.75 moderate reliability, values between 0.75 and 0.9 good reliability and values greater than 0.90 indicated excellent reliability [13]. In order to visualize agreement strength between observers, Bland–Altman plots were constructed [14]. These show the mean versus difference between observer measurements in each image. A mean level close to 0, and a narrow distribution within $\pm$ 2 SD, was considered to be a strong agreement, while a level with a mean that diverted considerably from 0, and with a wide distribution, was considered to be a poor agreement. Data management and statistical analyses were performed using Microsoft® Excel 365 and MATLAB version 9.13 (R2022b, The MathWorks Inc., Natick, MA, USA). An appointed statistician from the government-supported Clinical Studies Sweden (https://kliniskastudier.se/english (accessed on 30 June 2023)) was consulted, and gave guidance on selecting statistical methods, as well as on the interpretation of results.

2.5. Ethical Considerations

Ethical approval was obtained from the local ethics review board (DNR 2017/769). Oral and written information was given, and the guardians' written consent was obtained.

3. Results

3.1. Computerized Program

The end-product was a semi-automatic program delivering data in the form of mean and standard deviation (SD) on thickness and brightness amplitude (whiteness) of the muscularis externa and muscularis interna, but only amplitude for the submucosa. The thickness of the submucosa was not measured because the inner line of the submucosa could not be determined accurately enough by the use of the UHFUS transducer (70 MHz) (FUJIFILM VisualSonics Inc., Toronto, ON, Canada) with a center frequency of 50 MHz. This was mainly the result of the strong attenuation of high-frequency ultrasound while transducing the bowel wall from the serosa, often rendering the mucosa too deep to image with sufficient quality. For amplitude measurements within the submucosa, the program used a standardized area, calculated from the inner border of the muscularis interna to a delineation at 0.18 mm depth in the underlying submucosa. The program's deliveries after user assessments are shown in Table 1.

Table 1. The program's deliveries after user assessments.

	Thickness	Amplitude
Definition	Number of vertical pixels multiplied with the length of one pixel (in mm)	The unitless value of a pixel representing 'whiteness'
Measurements	Mean, Median, SD (Number of measurements per layer was about 160)	Mean, Median, SD (Number of measurements per layer was about 2000–10,000)
Layers included in analysis	Muscularis externa Muscularis interna	Muscularis externa Muscularis interna Submucosa (first 0.18 mm)

Figure 1 shows the user interface after loading a UHFUS image. A range of interest (ROI) of 5 mm was decided upon for image quality and representation of the bowel wall, including continuity in the bowel wall.

Within the ROI, the inner and outer borders of the muscularis externa and the muscularis interna were marked manually by clicking within the image. The position and spacing between markings were chosen by the user and could be edited easily. At the same time, the software automatically created a full delineation of each layer within the ROI, by interpolating between these markings, and then displaying the layers on screen, see Figure 2.

Once satisfied, the operator stopped adding/editing points and saved the results. The results were displayed on screen, as well as saved in a Microsoft Excel spreadsheet. The thickness of each layer was automatically measured vertically at all lateral positions within the ROI, resulting in a mean, median and SD, based on about 160 measurements per layer. In order to calculate echo amplitudes, all image pixels within the ROI were used, resulting in a mean, median and an SD based on about 2000–10,000 measurements per layer.

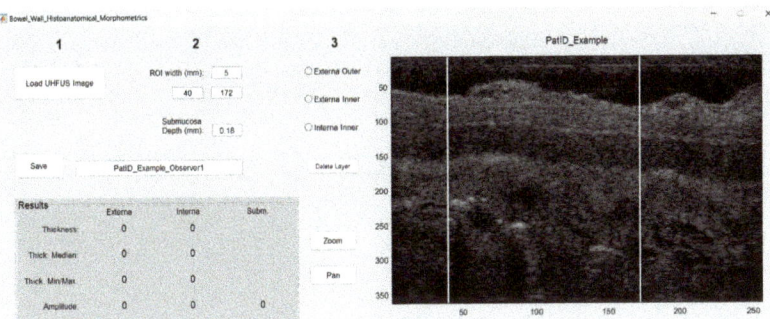

Figure 1. The user interface of the developed program. After loading an image and choosing a suitable range of interest, the user delineates the outer and inner border of the muscularis externa, and the inner border of the muscularis interna, by clicking within the image. The results are shown automatically in parallel to the delineation. Once finished, the user saves the results, and then repeats the process for the next image. Numbers 1–3 in the top refer to the order of how the user is intended to use the program.

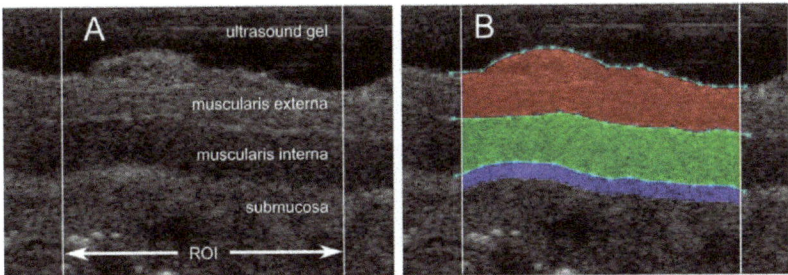

Figure 2. (**A**) Ultrasound image (zoomed) where different layers of the bowel wall are shown, together with the 5 mm wide range of interest. (**B**) The same ultrasound image with user markings (cyan crosses) and the resulting areas of the muscularis externa (red), muscularis interna (green) and submucosa (blue) with a predefined analysis depth of 0.18 mm (blue).

The time required to import images into the program, to map out the histoanatomical layers and to extract all computerized measurements from an image of a bowel segment, took on average 2 min. This is in comparison with manual measurements using the scanner's built-in caliper function, where extraction of three thickness measurements takes approximately 15 min, including selecting, manually measuring the different points, and transferring data from the images to external sheets for manual calculations. In addition, the ultrasound scanner does not permit other manual measurements to be taken, such as echo amplitudes, which the computer program does, which is why more data from images could be extracted by the program.

3.2. Inter-Observer Variability Tests

The results obtained by the computer program for the two observers are summarized in Tables 2 and 3. There was an excellent agreement between observers in all thickness and amplitude measurements with an ICC range of 0.970–0.998. This agreement was also seen in the Bland–Altman plots, with narrow distributions and mean differences ranging from 0.005 to 0.016 mm (1.1–3.6%) from the overall mean for the thicknesses and 0 to 0.7 mm (0.0–0.8%) from the overall mean for amplitudes. Figures 3 and 4 show the Bland–Altman plots for the thicknesses and amplitudes, respectively.

Table 2. The resulting thickness for the two muscle layers and the ratio between them. Presented values are the overall mean and standard deviation (SD); the difference between observers; and the intraclass correlation coefficient (ICC).

	Overall Mean (SD) (mm)	Difference, Mean (SD) (mm)	ICC
Muscularis externa	0.477 (0.185)	0.005 (0.033)	0.992
Muscularis interna	0.439 (0.166)	−0.016 (0.026)	0.992
Ratio (interna/externa)	1.031 (0.479)	−0.014 (0.167)	0.970

Table 3. The resulting amplitudes for the two muscle layers and the ratio between them. Presented values are the overall mean and standard deviation (SD); the difference between observers; and the intraclass correlation coefficient (ICC). Muscularis interna (int), Muscularis externa (ext), submucosa (sub). a.u.—arbitrary units.

	Overall Mean (SD) (a.u.)	Difference Mean (SD) (a.u.)	ICC
Muscularis externa	118.2 (12.5)	−0.1 (1.1)	0.998
Muscularis interna	87.2 (13.4)	−0.7 (1.2)	0.997
Submucosa	107.7 (14.0)	−0.2 (1.5)	0.997
Ratio int./ext.	0.738 (0.090)	−0.005 (0.011)	0.995
Ratio sub./ext.	0.917 (0.124)	0.000 (0.015)	0.996
Ratio int./sub.	0.810 (0.082)	−0.006 (0.017)	0.988

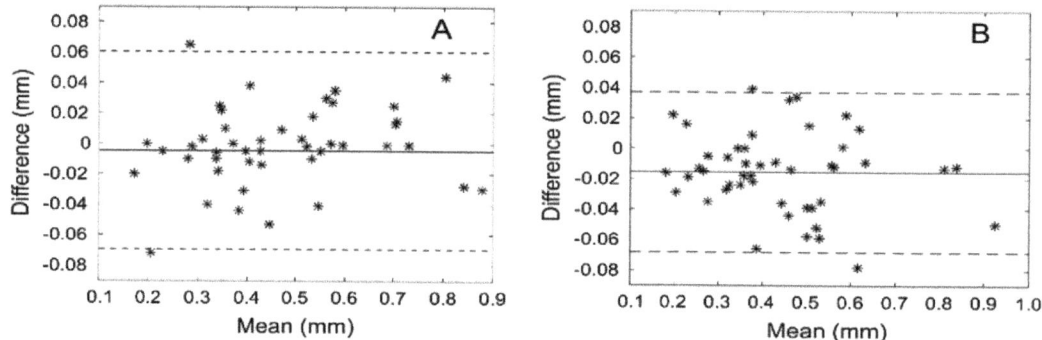

Figure 3. Bland-Altman plots that show the differences between users' measured thicknesses against their mean for muscularis externa (**A**) and muscularis interna (**B**) mm—millimeters.

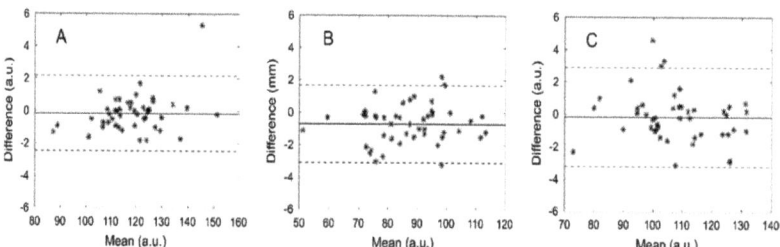

Figure 4. Bland-Altman plots that show the differences between users' measured amplitudes against their mean for muscularis externa (**A**), muscularis interna (**B**) and submucosa (**C**) a.u.—albitrary units.

4. Discussion

The aim of this developmental study was to describe the construction and evaluation of a computer program for measuring the thickness and ultrasound echo amplitudes in layers of the bowel wall. The purpose of this semiautomatic program was to enable and ensure more objective, accurate and time-efficient on-site measurements. This was achieved by automatically obtaining a maximum number of thickness and amplitude measurements (from all available image columns/pixels) within the chosen ROI, while keeping the user interaction to a minimum. The results show excellent agreement between observers, suggesting that the results provided by the computer program are observer-invariant. The program was deemed to be easy to use, as well as time-efficient.

Furthermore, the computer program enables automatic measurement of ultrasound-derived, tissue-specific parameters based on amplitude information, which is not currently possible with manual measurements. In this study, the average amplitude of each layer was measured. Besides being tissue-specific, this parameter is dependent upon several other factors, including the choice of scanner, transducer and settings. Therefore, a ratio between amplitudes in different layers could be a more relevant parameter, compensating for many of these undesired dependencies. However, there are several other amplitude-based parameters that have been shown to be robust and valuable for tissue characterization, including kurtosis, skewness and Nakagami-m distribution [2,3], that could be incorporated into the program. Hence, the use of computerized measurements is considered to be an asset for future work within this project, both from a scientific and a practical point of view.

The time efficiency of the computer program was found to be an advantage. Although times may vary depending on patient/image and on user experience, the developed program shows clear advantages in terms of user-operation time and the number of measurements per unit of time, compared to multiple manual measurements using an ultrasound scanner. Furthermore, the ultrasound scanner does not allow other manual measurements to be taken, such as echo amplitudes, but the computer program does.

The use of UHFUS to investigate the structure of the bowel wall has previously shown promise with regards to the delineation between aganglionosis and ganglionosis in patients with HD [11]. Research into the use of UHFUS in primary diagnostics of the bowel wall is ongoing [10]. Insertion of images into computer programs, as in this study, will enable more data to be assessed in a safe setting compared to data collected manually. Certainly, within the software of the Vevo® MD, manual measurements of histoanatomical layers are possible. However, such manual assessment is time consuming, and the number of measurements needed to correspond accurately to the computerized calculation has not been evaluated. To be able to include both assessments in one program—thickness and amplitude measurements—is considered to be a tremendous advantage compared to manual calculations. In addition, the programmed calculations save observer time. Each assessment, collecting all data required, took on average just 2 min.

Despite several advantages of computer calculations, it should be noted that the quality of images is of the utmost concern and that the examiner's competence constitutes the main determining factor for all measurements. This study only addressed the inter-observer variability, not any inter-examiner's variability that might be associated with the ultrasound scanning itself. Although computerized measurements might reduce potential variations in measurements between ultrasound images acquired by two different examiners, examiner-dependent variations are difficult to correct by such means and would be better addressed by the use of other methods. A potential variation between examiners could be interesting to investigate in future studies. Saving images for computerized assessment also makes fully blinded testing feasible. Comparisons of agreement in assessments of aganglionic and ganglionic tissues, respectively, were not undertaken since all single measurements indicated high agreements. However, this could be of interest in future studies comparing UHFUS features of aganglionic and ganglionic bowel wall.

One strength of this study is the novelty of the technique, since no automatic assessment by a computer program for bowel wall assessment using UHFUS has been proposed previously. The program was developed in close collaboration between end users who are well-experienced clinicians operating daily on bowel walls, and biomedical engineers with substantial experience in constructing and implementing similar programs in other imaging applications. Several adjustments of the computerized program were made during the development process, following repeated discussions about combined clinical relevance and future research topics, with respect to detailed amplitude analyses and testing. Another strength of our study is the fact that the developed program could potentially be used not only for assessment of the bowel wall in children, but also for adults, and in several additional conditions, e.g., delineations of inflammatory bowel disease, and in endo-luminal UHFUS imaging.

A limitation of our study is that the computer program does not enable calculations of the whole bowel wall thickness to be made. This was because the UHF 70 transducer generally provided poor image quality at the depth of the mucosa. A program is under development which includes possibilities to also explore the full thickness of the bowel wall using a 30 MHz center frequency transducer (UHF 48, bandwidth 20–46 MHz, FUJIFILM VisualSonics Inc., Toronto, ON, Canada). For interested UHFUS users, the plan is to make the program for automatic assessment of UHFUS images available in future (after validation of different center frequencies) within a complete user package, including instructions.

5. Conclusions

This computer program enables and ensures more objective, accurate and time-efficient on-site measurements of the histoanatomical layers of the bowel wall. It also provides unique possibilities to quantify amplitudes in different bowel wall layers assessed by UHFUS imaging. The inter-variability analyses show excellent agreement between observers, suggesting that the results provided by the program are observer-invariant. The computer program was deemed to be easy to use, as well as time-efficient.

Author Contributions: Conceptualization, C.G., T.J., M.C. and P.S.; Data curation, T.E., M.E., T.H., C.G., M.C. and P.S.; Formal analysis, T.E., T.H., M.C. and P.S.; Funding acquisition, M.C. and P.S.; Investigation, T.E., T.H., C.G. and P.S.; Methodology, T.E., T.J., M.C. and P.S.; Project administration, P.S.; Resources, M.C. and P.S.; Software, T.E. and T.H.; Supervision, M.C. and P.S.; Validation, T.E., T.H. and P.S.; Visualization, T.E.; Writing—original draft, T.E. and P.S.; Writing—review and editing, T.H., C.G., M.E., T.J. and M.C. All authors have read and agreed to the published version of the manuscript.

Funding: This research was funded by the Swedish Regional Research Funding (ALF) 43901, Region Skåne, Skåne University Hospital's Funding 95908 (SUS Fonder och Stiftelser), Swedish Research Council Starting grants 2021-01569 and Swedish Research Council Project grants 2017-3993. Open access funding was provided by Lund University, Sweden.

Institutional Review Board Statement: The study was conducted in accordance with the Declaration of Helsinki and approved by the Local Ethics Committee at Lund University (approval 17 November 2017/769) and the National Ethics Authority (approval 2023-01833-01) for studies involving humans.

Informed Consent Statement: Informed consent was obtained by proxy from parents to all children involved in the study.

Data Availability Statement: The data that support the findings of this study are available from the corresponding author (P.S.) upon request.

Conflicts of Interest: The authors declare no conflict of interest.

References

1. Malagi, A.V.; Kandasamy, D.; Pushpam, D.; Khare, K.; Sharma, R.; Kumar, R.; Bakhshi, S.; Mehndiratta, A. IVIM-DKI with parametric reconstruction method for lymph node evaluation and characterization in lymphoma: A preliminary study comparison with FDG-PET/CT. *Results Eng.* **2023**, *17*, 100928. [CrossRef]
2. Mamou, J.; Coron, A.; Oelze, M.L.; Saegusa-Beecroft, E.; Hata, M.; Lee, P.; Machi, J.; Yanagihara, E.; Laugier, P.; Feleppa, E.J. Three-dimensional high-frequency backscatter and envelope quantification of can-cerous human lymph nodes. *Ultrasound. Med. Biol.* **2011**, *37*, 345–357. [CrossRef]

3. Izzetti, R.; Vitali, S.; Aringhieri, G.; Nisi, M.; Oranges, T.; Dini, V.; Ferro, F.; Baldini, C.; Romanelli, M.; Caramella, D.; et al. Ultra-High Frequency Ultrasound, A Promising Diagnostic Technique: Review of the Literature and Single-Center Experience. *Can. Assoc. Radiol. J.* **2020**, *72*, 418–431. [CrossRef] [PubMed]
4. Izzetti, R.; Vitali, S.; Aringhieri, G.; Oranges, T.; Dini, V.; Nisi, M.; Graziani, F.; Gabriele, M.; Caramella, D. Discovering a new anatomy: Exploration of oral mucosa with ultra-high frequency ultrasound. *Dentomaxillofac. Radiol.* **2020**, *49*, 20190318. [CrossRef] [PubMed]
5. Russo, A.; Reginelli, A.; Lacasella, G.V.; Grassi, E.; Karaboue, M.A.A.; Quarto, T.; Busetto, G.M.; Aliprandi, A.; Grassi, R.; Berritto, D. Clinical Application of Ultra-High-Frequency Ultrasound. *J. Pers. Med.* **2022**, *12*, 1733. [CrossRef] [PubMed]
6. Boczar, D.; Forte, A.J.; Serrano, L.P.; Trigg, S.D.; Clendenen, S.R. Use of Ultra-high-frequency Ultrasound on Diagnosis and Management of Lipofibromatous Hamartoma: A Technical Report. *Cureus* **2019**, *11*, e5808. [CrossRef] [PubMed]
7. Granéli, C.; Erlöv, T.; Mitev, R.M.; Kasselaki, I.; Hagelsteen, K.; Gisselsson, D.; Jansson, T.; Cinthio, M.; Stenström, P. Ultra high frequency ultrasonography to distinguish ganglionic from aganglionic bowel wall in Hirschsprung disease: A first report. *J. Pediatr. Surg.* **2021**, *56*, 2281–2285. [CrossRef] [PubMed]
8. Kyrklund, K.; Sloots, C.E.J.; de Blaauw, I.; Bjørnland, K.; Rolle, U.; Cavalieri, D.; Francalanci, P.; Fusaro, F.; Lemli, A.; Schwarzer, N.; et al. ERNICA guidelines for the management of rectosigmoid Hirschsprung's disease. *Orphanet J. Rare Dis.* **2020**, *15*, 164. [CrossRef] [PubMed]
9. Hawez, T.; Graneli, C.; Erlöv, T.; Gottberg, E.; Mitev, R.M.; Hagelsteen, K.; Evertsson, M.; Jansson, T.; Cinthio, M.; Stenström, P. Ultra-High Frequency Ultrasound Imaging of Bowel Wall in Hirschsprung's Disease—Correlation and Agreement Analyses of Histoanatomy. *Diagnostics* **2023**, *13*, 1388. [CrossRef] [PubMed]
10. Evertsson, M.; Graneli, C.; Vernersson, A.; Wiaczek, O.; Hagelsteen, K.; Erlöv, T.; Cinthio, M.; Stenström, P. Design of a Pediatric Rectal Ultrasound Probe Intended for Ultra-High Frequency Ultrasound Diagnostics. *Diagnostics* **2023**, *13*, 1667. [CrossRef] [PubMed]
11. Beltman, L.; Windster, J.D.; Roelofs, J.J.T.H.; van der Voorn, J.P.; Derikx, J.P.M.; Bakx, R. Diagnostic accuracy of calretinin and acetylcholinesterase staining of rectal suction biopsies in Hirschsprung disease examined by unexperienced pathologists. *Virchows Arch.* **2022**, *481*, 245–252. [CrossRef] [PubMed]
12. Gerke, O.; Pedersen, A.K.; Debrabant, B.; Halekoh, U.; Möller, S. Sample size determination in method comparison and observer variability studies. *J. Clin. Monit. Comput.* **2022**, *36*, 1241–1243. [CrossRef] [PubMed]
13. Koo, T.K.; Li, M.Y. A Guideline of Selecting and Reporting Intraclass Correlation Coefficients for Reliability Research. *J. Chiropr. Med.* **2016**, *15*, 155–163. [CrossRef]
14. Bland, J.M.; Altman, D.G. Statistical methods for assessing agreement between two methods of clinical measurement. *Lancet* **1986**, *1*, 307–310. [CrossRef]

Disclaimer/Publisher's Note: The statements, opinions and data contained in all publications are solely those of the individual author(s) and contributor(s) and not of MDPI and/or the editor(s). MDPI and/or the editor(s) disclaim responsibility for any injury to people or property resulting from any ideas, methods, instructions or products referred to in the content.

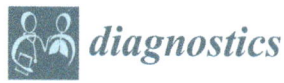

Article

Ultra-High-Frequency Ultrasound as an Innovative Imaging Evaluation of Hyaluronic Acid Filler in Nasolabial Folds

Giorgia Salvia [1,*,†], Nicola Zerbinati [2,†], Flavia Manzo Margiotta [1], Alessandra Michelucci [1], Giammarco Granieri [1], Cristian Fidanzi [1], Riccardo Morganti [3], Marco Romanelli [1] and Valentina Dini [1]

[1] Department of Dermatology, University of Pisa, 56126 Pisa, Italy; manzomargiottaflavia@gmail.com (F.M.M.); alessandra.michelucci@gmail.com (A.M.); giammarcogranieri@gmail.com (G.G.); cri.fidanzi@outlook.it (C.F.); romanellimarco60@gmail.com (M.R.); valentinadini74@gmail.com (V.D.)
[2] Dermatologic Unit, Department of Medicine and Surgery, University of Insubria, 21100 Varese, Italy; nicola.zerbinati@uninsubria.it
[3] Section of Statistics, Department of Clinical and Experimental Medicine, University of Pisa, 56126 Pisa, Italy; r.morganti@ao-pisa.toscana.it
* Correspondence: giorgia.salvia2@gmail.com
† These authors contributed equally to this work.

Abstract: Dermal hyaluronic acid (HA) fillers are used for nasolabial fold correction, but no study is still available on the use of ultra-high-frequency ultrasound (UHFUS) with 70 MHz probes for the evaluation of HA distribution and wrinkle amelioration. We selected 13 patients who received HA filler, evaluated before (Time (T) 0) and after injection (T1), and after 24 weeks (T2). The dermal thickness and distribution of HA were registered, as well as the Wrinkle Severity Rating Scale (WSRS), Global Aesthetic Improvement Scale (GAIS), and wrinkle 3D fullness. The UHFUS dermal thickness was increased by 11% for both sides at T1 and by 7.4% and 6.8% for the right and left side, respectively, at T2 ($p < 0.01$). The 3D wrinkle fullness showed a T1 increase (+0.59 cc and +0.79 cc for the right and left side, respectively) with a T2 maintenance of 45% of the T1 fullness (p-value < 0.001). The only clinical score significantly modified was WSRS, with a reduction of 56% at T1 and of 47.1% at T2 (p-value < 0.001). Our study then demonstrated the efficacy of UHFUS in the assessment of nasolabial fold correction, representing also the first multi-modal evaluation of HA persistence and its visual subsequent aesthetic results.

Keywords: filler; ultra-high-frequency ultrasound; hyaluronic acid; aesthetic medicine

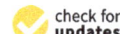

1. Introduction

The process of aging influences the appearance of the skin by producing both microscopic and macroscopic transformations that lead to a decrease in volume [1]. Various factors, including environmental conditions and personal habits such as smoking, play a role in skin aging and drive the subsequent alterations in the extracellular matrix of the dermis, resorption of bony structures, gravity, and a decrease in and redistribution of adipose tissue [2]. Additionally, a reduction in hyaluronic acid levels accompanies skin aging, which can expedite dehydration, loss of elasticity, and the formation of wrinkles. In recent decades, there has been a growing emphasis on appearance and the notion of beauty, leading to the expansion of the field of aesthetic medicine. This field is dedicated to modifying aesthetic appearance by addressing various conditions through both invasive and minimally invasive procedures, with some of the most recent ones also involving bioartificial injectable products [3]. With the emergence of advanced technologies, today's physicians have the opportunity to address these changes with a variety of techniques.

Regarding non-permanent injectable products, hyaluronic acid (HA)-based dermal fillers are among the most widely used, due to their effectiveness and safety compared to permanent surgical cosmetic procedures [4]. HA is a non-sulfated glycosaminoglycan,

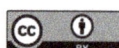

widely distributed in connective, epithelial, and neural tissues; in the skin, it confers flexibility and hydration through its ability to bind and retain water molecules [5]. HA-based dermal fillers are used to restore volume loss, fill in fine lines and wrinkles, increase lip volume or define lip contour, and perform various procedures such as chin augmentation, nose reshaping, mid-facial volumization, lip enhancement, and wrinkle correction [6]. HA-based dermal fillers then represent an ideal aesthetic tool since they are safe and effective, biocompatible, easy to inject and distribute, and easy to remove if necessary [7]. This type of filler can be easily removed in the event of complications or dissatisfaction with the aesthetic result by injecting commercially available hyaluronidase into the concerned area [1]. The aesthetic result of HA dermal filler injections is closely related to the permanence of the product and its redistribution in the tissues. The literature provides evidence on the detected tissue integration in ultrasound (US) images as early as 1 month after injection [8]. Although there are several theories regarding the interaction between HA filler and tissue components, there is still little scientific evidence on the matter, and few data are available on the instrumental detection of long-term permanence of fillers [9]. High-frequency ultrasound (HFUS) is a non-invasive method for the analysis of skin and subcutaneous tissue composition that can detect tissue composition and potential changes [6]. HFUS provides clear imaging of the dermis and hypodermis layers, but it is limited in accurately visualizing the epidermis, except for the palmar and plantar surfaces. This restriction makes HFUS inadequate for detecting the smallest structures and capturing the finest details. In contrast, ultra-high-frequency ultrasound (UHFUS) operates at frequencies above 20 megahertz (MHz), significantly higher than the frequencies used in conventional US systems that typically range from 2 to 18 MHz; therefore, it is particularly valuable in the field of dermatology. One of the key advantages of UHFUS in dermatology is its ability to identify microscopic structures. It can effectively visualize sebaceous glands, hair erector muscles, and hair follicles, providing valuable insights into various dermatological conditions and facilitating accurate diagnoses [10]. By revealing these intricate structures, UHFUS enhances the understanding of skin pathologies and aids in determining appropriate treatment approaches. For instance, UHFUS has demonstrated its efficacy in the field of dermato-oncology, particularly in relation to melanoma, a type of skin cancer known for its poor prognosis and persistently underestimated incidence [11]. The literature data point out that US evaluation with a 70 MHz probe allowed the non-invasive measurement of melanoma thickness, which showed an excellent correlation with Breslow thickness [12]. Moreover, the use of UHFUS has shown a promising role in the evaluation of chronic ulcers [13] and in the pre-operative characterization of basal cell carcinoma [14].

To date, numerous clinical studies have also been published on the vascular, musculoskeletal, and intraoral applications of UHFUS [13]. However, there is a lack of studies regarding the use of UHFUS in the field of aesthetic medicine. The aim of our study was then to use, for the first time in the literature, a UHFUS probe of 70 MHz to evaluate the distribution pattern and permanence of an HA filler for nasolabial fold correction, correlating the results with a panel of validated aesthetic scores and clinical images obtained from the selected population.

2. Material and Methods

We performed a single-center prospective cohort study, involving a population of patients followed by the Unit of Dermatology, University of Pisa, Pisa (Italy), from May 2022 to December 2022. A total of 13 subjects were enrolled in this study, all with written informed consent. The eligibility criteria for enrollment in the study were as follows: participants had to be over 18 years of age and exhibit visible and moderate–severe nasolabial wrinkles. Throughout the duration of the study, patients were required to refrain from any cosmetic procedures involving the face, minimize exposure to UV radiation without using sunscreen, and use contraception if they were women of childbearing age. Individuals who had undergone cosmetic correction procedures within the past six months or permanent procedures were not included in the study. The exclusion criteria included significant skin diseases, trauma and genetic defects of the face, allergies or hypersensitivity to the product being tested, presence of neoplasms or severe clinical conditions such as neurological disorders, recent treatment with antithrombotic or antiplatelet drugs within the week preceding the study, pregnancy or breastfeeding, and a tendency to develop hypertrophic, atrophic, or keloid scars. All the selected patients presented with moderate to severe nasolabial folds and received an injective treatment with HA filler into each side of the nasolabial folds, ranging from 0.6 to 1 mL at a concentration of 25 mg/mL. In particular, the HA filler used in this study was a cross-linked sodium hyaluronate, of non-animal origin, stabilized in a phosphate buffer with pH 7. No anesthetic products were applied on the treated areas before filler injection. All the anamnestic information of our population was obtained from our electronic database. Clinical and UHFUS evaluations were performed at Week (W) 0, as well as before (T0) and after injection (T1). A third evaluation was then carried out at W24 (T24). Moreover, at W24, patients filled out a questionnaire on the side effects occurring in the 2 weeks following the injection. Aesthetic evaluation was based on the Wrinkle Severity Rating Scale (WSRS) and Global Aesthetic Improvement Scale (GAIS), calculated by a well-trained investigator who also obtained clinical images using a 3D image system, VECTRA® H2 (Canfield Scientific, Inc., Parsippany, NJ, USA) and its vector analysis program, Markerless Tracking. Through 3D photographs, a differential volumetric assessment in cubic centimeters (cc) was obtained. US images were taken using a linear 70 MHz probe (B-MODE), which was positioned transversally at the midpoint of both nasolabial folds, perpendicular to the skin. Each image was analyzed by two experienced operators to assess quantitative dermal thickness, obtained by measuring in millimeters (mm) the distance between the dermo-epidermal junction and the subcutaneous tissue.

Categorical data were described with absolute and relative (%) frequency, while continuous data were summarized with mean and standard deviation. To compare repeated measures of the dermal thickness and WSRS variables, ANOVA for repeated measures was applied, while, to compare paired data of the GAIS and delta fullness variables, a t-test for paired data was performed. Significance was set at 0.05, and all analyses were carried out using SPSS v.28 software.

3. Results

Population Features

Our population consisted of 12/13 females (92%) and 1/13 male (8%), with a mean age of 51.6 years (59.6–43.8). Overall, 3/13 patients (23%) had phototype 1 on the Fitzpatrick scale, 3/13 patients (23%) showed phototype 2, and 7/13 patients (54%) had phototype 3. A history of sunburn and clinical signs of photodamage were registered in 11/13 patients (84.6%). Furthermore, 8/13 patients (61.5%) were smokers or former smokers. The mean BMI was 22.9 (19.2–26.6). No comorbidities were reported by our population.

At baseline (Time (T) 0), the severity of pre-filler wrinkles measured by WSRS was 3.4 (±0.8) for both right and left wrinkles. The mean dermal thickness measured by UHFUS was 2.04 mm (±0.09 mm) and 2.05 mm (±0.1 mm) for the right and left nasolabial folds, respectively. The mean volume of filler injected in the right nasolabial fold was 0.51 mL (±0.20 mL), and that in the left was 0.52 mL (±0.18 mL). Following the injection (T1), the severity of wrinkles measured by the WSRS was 1.5 (±0.7) on the right and 1.5 (±0.5) on the left, thus recording a significant reduction of 56% (p-value < 0.001). The overall judgment of improvement in cosmetic appearance using the GAIS score, even if not statistically significant, registered an amelioration to 1.6 (±0.8) on the right and 1.7 (±0.8) on the left. On UHFUS, there was an increase in mean dermal thickness to 2.28 mm (±0.15 mm) on the right and 2.27 mm (±0.15 mm) on the left, registering an increase of 11% in both thicknesses that resulted statistically significant (p-value < 0.001). The average degree of diffusion of HA-based materials was 2.6 (±0.4) for the right side and 2.2 (±0.1) for the left side. Furthermore, the volume assessment performed through the 3D photographs showed a significant average increase of +0.59 cc (±0.33 cc) and +0.79 cc (±0.39 cc) for the right and left side, respectively (p-value < 0.01). At W24 (T2), the severity of wrinkles measured using the WSRS was 1.8 (±0.6) for the right wrinkles and 1.7 (±0.6) for the left wrinkles. Therefore, the severity of wrinkles at 6 months showed a reduction of 47.1% (p-value < 0.001). The overall judgment of the improvement of the aesthetic aspect using the GAIS score, even if not statistically significant, registered an amelioration to 1.7 (±0.8) on the right and 1.8 (±0.7) on the left, thus maintaining 94% of the result obtained at baseline, immediately after the injection of the filler. Moreover, UHFUS detected a mean dermal thickness of 2.19 mm (±0.14 mm) on both sides, with subsequent statistically significant thickness increases of 7.4% and 6.8% from the baseline for the right and left sides, respectively (p-value < 0.01). Furthermore, the volume assessment performed through the 3D photographs showed mean increases of +0.26 cc (±0.13 cc) and +0.36 cc (±0.21 cc) for the right and left sides, respectively, thus maintaining 45% of the result obtained at baseline, immediately after the injection of the filler (p < 0.001).

4. Discussion

Dermal fillers are widely used in aesthetic medicine with the main purpose of filling wrinkles, creating volume, and correcting age-related tissue loss [4]. A vast range of dermal fillers are available on the market, which differ in composition, duration of effect, ease of administration, complications, and limitations [15]. US is a non-invasive imaging method that allows a real-time evaluation of both pathological lesions and healthy skin, and it is also able to detect exogenous materials. Their echogenicity depends on their composition; tissue augmentation products with a predominantly hydrophilic component usually appear as anechoic areas, while synthetic materials, such as silicon oil or polymethylmethacrylate, tend to be hyperechoic [16]. HA is a polysaccharide composed of repeating units of disaccharides D-glucuronic acid and N-acetyl-D-glucosamine linked by a 28 glucuronidic β (1→3) bond, representing a fundamental component of the extracellular matrix, synovial fluid, and vitreous humor [17]. HA dermal fillers are widely used due to their physicochemical characteristics and biological properties, as well as their efficacy and easy management of adverse effects [18]. After the injection into the skin, HA initiates a mild inflammatory response at the interface with the host tissue. This initial reaction is subsequently succeeded by a progressive formation of fibrous tissue, which firmly secures the gel to the host tissue, effectively obstructing any displacement of the product [15]. However, the main limitation of this procedure is the limited permanence of the product (from 3 up to 12 months) [19], which affects the final aesthetic outcome. The longevity of HA fillers is determined by particle size, manufacturing processes, and consequent characteristics of the product, volume, location of injection, and host metabolism [15]. A previous study evaluated how dermal HA fillers could be observed and followed over time using a 25 MHz US probe and magnetic resonance imaging, pointing out the usefulness of the two combined techniques; however, the probe used had too low of a frequency to ensure optimal visualization of the dermis, thus necessitating another adjuvant imaging technique [20]. In another study, nasolabial wrinkles were evaluated with a 20 MHz probe after HA injection, which identified the injected HA as hypoechogenic or anechogenic areas that were well demarcated and homogeneous in the skin [6]. The study by Quiao et al. represented the first long-term evaluation of nasolabial HA filler and an important validation of the use of ultrasound for follow-up assessment [9]. Using a traditional 20 MHz probe, it is possible to identify the dermis and hypodermis, while the epidermis is poorly characterized. Traditional HFUS has limitations in accurately measuring skin thickness and identifying the dermal–epidermal junction [21]. On the contrary, the UHFUS 70 MHz probe precisely identifies the epidermis and obtains a more precise characterization of the dermis, attaining images with sub-millimeter precision of all the skin structures. UHFUS has demonstrated its ability to establish correlations between ultrasound images and histology with a high degree of specificity. This advanced technology enables the differentiation between healthy and pathological tissues, providing comparable accuracy to traditional biopsy methods. In particular, the epidermis of healthy patients displays a superficial hyperechogenic layer, an inferior hypoechogenic layer, and a hyperechogenic line delimiting it from the dermis [10].

The dermis appears as a hyperechogenic band, due to its collagen content, while the hypodermis presents hypoechoic fatty lobules and hyperechoic fibrous septae in between the lobules [22]. Thanks to the sub-millimeter precision and high resolution of the UHFUS images, we were able to determine the presence and distribution of the HA dermal filler and to determine the dermal thickness after injection and 6 months later (Figures 1 and 2). Immediately after the injection of HA filler, a thorough examination of the ultrasound images revealed the presence of an inhomogeneous region within the treated area. This region displayed multiple anechoic oval areas, indicating the presence of fluid-filled cavities or voids. The overall appearance was characterized by an uneven distribution of the filler material. However, as the post-treatment period progressed, significant changes were observed over the course of 24 weeks. The previously identified inhomogeneous region began to exhibit a more uniform and homogeneous pattern. The anechoic oval areas, which had initially appeared scattered and unevenly distributed, gradually merged and became less pronounced (Figures 1 and 2). Multiple descriptions of ultrasound images following the injection of HA can be found in the existing literature. However, it is important to note that these studies were conducted using lower-frequency probes, which can account for the observed discrepancies between our study and the previously reported data. Urdiales-Gálvez F et al. reported a globular distribution of HA filler at the ultrasound evaluation (12–18 MHz) performed after the injection and a heterogeneous pattern composed of alternating anechoic/hyperechoic after one month [23]. The ultrasound analysis conducted by Jiang involved the examination of 94 patients who received nasolabial fold filling [24], and ultrasound imaging was performed using 15 MHz frequency. In the study, HA dermal filler was predominantly observed as an anechoic structure with a distinct boundary, efficient sound transmission, consistent internal echo, and the absence of noticeable blood flow signals. The authors noted that, when HA dispersed into the surrounding tissue, it typically manifested as a hypoechoic structure. These anechoic or hypoechoic regions displayed an irregular distribution within the layered tissue, often forming a grid-like or honeycomb-like pattern. The different uses of US technology within the realm of aesthetic medicine have been explored in the literature, with one notable area of focus being the examination of US characteristics associated with volume-enhancing products [16]. In particular, it has been confirmed that fillers containing a hydrophilic component typically exhibit hypo- or anechoic patterns, appearing as subcutaneous pseudocystic deposits. This literature review also showed that the manifestations of face-filling materials under US are inconsistent due to different anatomical injection sites, different product characteristics, and, above all, different ultrasound probe frequencies. We can conclude that our data are comparable to those already found in the literature, and that the differences we observed depend mainly on the possibility of obtaining more detailed images thanks to the higher resolution of the 70 MHz probe.

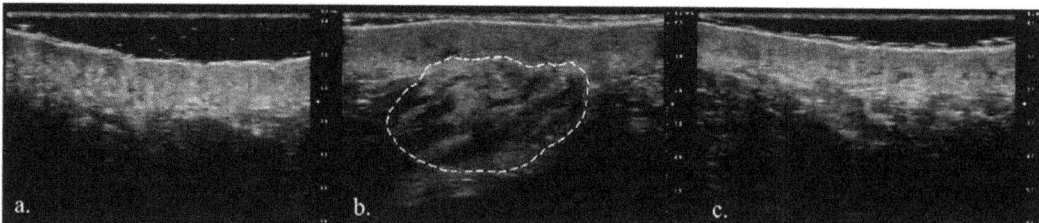

Figure 1. (a) Ultra-high-frequency ultrasound (UHFUS) of a 45-year-old patient's nasolabial area before hyaluronic acid (HA) filler injection; (b) UHFUS of nasolabial area after HA filler injection (dashed yellow line), with the HA filler visible as anechogenic areas in the dermis; (c) UHFUS 6 months after the injection.

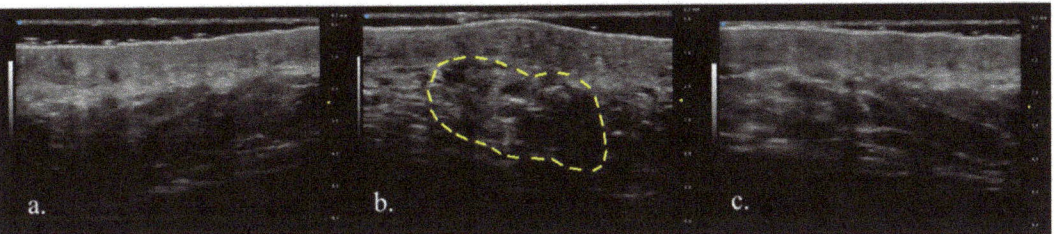

Figure 2. (a) Ultra-high-frequency ultrasound (UHFUS) of nasolabial area before hyaluronic acid (HA) filler injection, (b) after HA filler injection with the yellow dashed lines indicating the injected HA filler, and (c) 6 months after injection of a 58-year-old patient.

Our study then represents further proof of the role of UHFUS as a non-invasive method in the field of aesthetic medicine, due to its ability to obtain precise dimensional evaluations and high-resolution images [25]. The potential applications of UHFUS in the field of cosmetic medicine remain largely unexplored. For example, one potential area of implementation involves the prospect of conducting echo-guided procedures using UHFUS. There are cases in the literature of complications from HA fillers treated with UHFUS-guided hyaluronidase injection, which ensured the safety of the procedure and the possibility of real-time monitoring [26]. Larger studies are needed to prove the superiority of the UHFUS-guided procedure. Moreover, UHFUS is considered as a valuable diagnostic tool in many fields other than dermatology, such as oral medicine and musculoskeletal anatomy [27].

To date, there is a lack of published research specifically focusing on the use of UHFUS for assessing the long-term durability of HA fillers in the skin. However, our study aimed to address this gap and provide insights into the persistence of HA fillers over an extended period. In our investigation, we were able to identify the presence of HA filler six months after injection using UHFUS. This finding is consistent with another study which used a 20 MHz probe to examine the longevity of HA filler six months post injection [9]. Their results align with ours, indicating that HA fillers can maintain their presence in the skin for at least half a year.

Furthermore, Fino et al. conducted a comparative analysis of two types of HA fillers for the treatment of nasolabial wrinkles. Their research determined that the average duration of both products was approximately 9.5 months [28]. This evidence suggests that HA fillers can provide noticeable effects for a considerable period. In contrast, Kalmanson et al. reported a particular case of a patient who exhibited persistent HA filler in the zygomatic area 2.5 years after the initial injection. The persistence was confirmed through magnetic resonance imaging (MRI) [18]. This exceptional case underscores the possibility of HA fillers demonstrating a prolonged presence in specific circumstances. Nevertheless, its important to note that these findings are based on a limited number of studies with relatively small sample sizes and varying follow-up durations. Consequently, further research involving larger and more diverse populations, as well as longer follow-up periods, is necessary to establish a precise understanding of the permanence and durability of these dermal fillers. UHFUS was not only used to assess the presence and distribution pattern of the HA filler, but also led to the quantification of dermal thickness at each follow-up visit. We registered a slight reduction in dermal thickness at 6 months compared to the measurement after the injection; however, dermal thickness remained higher than baseline values. We can consequently deduce that, 6 months later, the HA is integrated but still present. These results confirm the bio-integration of injected HA and its subsequent heterogeneous distribution, thus indicating degradation and reabsorption in the tissue [9,23]. Limited research exists in the literature that has specifically investigated dermal thickness through ultrasound following the administration of HA dermal filler. In a recently conducted study led by Bravo BSF, researchers examined the effects of a single session of a combined hybrid filler, consisting of HA and calcium hydroxyapatite, on dermal thickness. The study focused on 15 participants with mild to moderate sagging in the jawline, ranging in age from 32 to 63 years. US analysis was performed immediately before the procedure and at 30, 90, and 120 days post treatment. The assessment of dermal thickness in the preauricular regions was carried out using an HF-US device equipped with a linear 18 MHz probe. The ultrasound evaluation encompassed two areas: the treated area (right preauricular region) and a small untreated area on the left preauricular region, serving as the control in this study. After the results analysis, it emerged that the intra-patient comparison showed a significant increase in dermal thickness on the treated side. Furthermore, in the US evaluation conducted by Qiao et al. [9], dermal thickness was measured, and the results indicated an increase in dermal thickness and a lower echogenicity at 2 weeks and 24 weeks after the administration of HA filler. The decrease in dermal thickness at 48 weeks compared to 24 weeks post injection indicates the possibility of diffusion, reabsorption, degradation, or fragmentation of the fillers within the skin tissues. To obtain a clinical assessment of the severity of nasolabial wrinkles and the cosmetic improvement achieved, we used WSRS and GAIS. The WSRS is a validated clinical outcome instrument, widely used for the assessment of facial wrinkles and effectiveness of soft-tissue augmentation [29], while GAIS is a five-point scale ranging from much improved (1) to much worse (5). A previous meta-analysis by Stefura T et al. [30] regarding tissue filler for the nasolabial area reported a mean improvement of 1.21 in the WSRS score at 6 months and an increase from a GAIS score of 2.2 one month after filler injection to a score of 2.32 after six months. In our group, we registered a significant difference of 1.6 between baseline and 6 months follow-up in the WSRS score, reporting a substantial stability of the aesthetic outcome at 6 months, measured using GAIS. To visually evaluate both scores, we referred to 3D photographs of the patient's face using a 3D image system, VECTRA® H2 (Canfield Scientific, Inc. Parsippany, NJ, USA). By using the 3D images, we were able to achieve a level of precision and detail that traditional 2D imaging methods would not have provided, Moreover, the use of 3D images enabled us to conduct a volumetric assessment of the nasolabial folds and provided valuable insight into the maintenance of results over time. The data indicated that, after a 6-month period following the initial injection, 45% of the initially achieved results were notably still maintained (Table 1). This speaks to the effectiveness and durability of the injection, underlining its positive impact on the patient's facial aesthetics. This additional method of evaluation proves very useful in aesthetic medicine, especially in procedures involving volume modification, which can, thus, be measured precisely and objectively. The relationship between UHFUS images and 3D imaging will require additional investigation in forthcoming research.

Table 1. Delta fullness comparison. Statistics: mean, standard deviation (sd).

Delta Fullness	Mean	Sd	p-Value
Between T1 and T0 dx	0.59	0.34	<0.001
Between T24w and T1 dx	−0.47	0.41	
Between T1 and T0 sx	0.79	0.39	<0.001
Between T24w and T1 sx	−0.38	0.30	

The overall view of the dermal thickness measured with UHFUS and the reduction in WSRS score can be appreciated in Figure 3.

This study had some limitations, including the inherent challenge of achieving complete standardization both in the injection process and in the imaging evaluation. Regarding the later aspect, to advance the application of ultrasound in aesthetic medicine, it is necessary to establish new, objective, and replicable evaluation scales. Over time, the study of larger patient cohorts will allow the development of ultrasound evaluation metrics to assess the efficacy of hyaluronic acid fillers. In fact, the sample size employed in this study was relatively small, which should be taken into consideration when interpreting the results. In future research, exploring the relationship between the dermal response to hyaluronic acid injection and individual factors, such as smoking habits and the skin's history of sunburn, could provide valuable insights. This avenue of investigation holds potential for uncovering correlations and understanding how these factors might influence the dermis's reaction to hyaluronic acid.

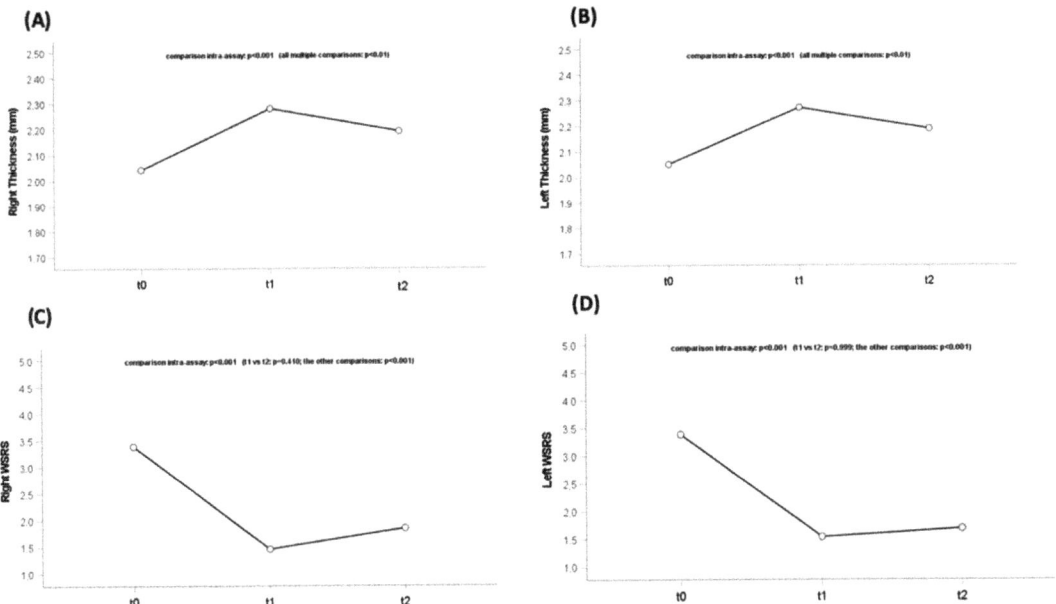

Figure 3. Dermal thickness modifications and statistical differences in the (A) right and (B) left nasolabial folds. WSRS modifications and statistical differences in the (C) right and (D) left nasolabial folds. WSRS: Wrinkle Severity Rating Scale.

5. Conclusions

Our study represents the first experience in the assessment of nasolabial fold correction through an UHFUS with 70 MHz probe. The possibility of acquiring exceptionally high-resolution images presents the opportunity, for the first time in the literature, to identify anatomical landmarks and HA dermal filler with unparalleled precision, allowing for meticulous descriptions with an accuracy down to the millimeter scale. Moreover, it represents the first multi-modal aesthetic assessment of nasolabial folds amelioration using US evaluation of HA persistence, validated clinical scores, and 3D images of the subsequent visual aesthetic results. An additional novelty of this approach is the possibility of accurately visualizing the anatomical sites where fillers are injected, which opens up interesting prospects for future progress. These include the implementation of echo-guided filler injections, which can significantly minimize the risks of severe adverse events. Additionally, the ability to perform echo-guided dissolution with hyaluronidase becomes a viable option, further enhancing safety and accuracy in aesthetic procedures. It is crucial to emphasize the considerable potential for the deepening and expansion of the role of UHFUS in aesthetic medicine. To conclude, we propose the use of UHFUS for the follow-up of patients undergoing HA filler injections, due to the low invasiveness of the diagnostic technique and the high precision in detecting the deposition of the selected product.

Author Contributions: Conceptualization, V.D., M.R. and N.Z.; methodology, V.D., M.R. and N.Z.; validation, V.D., M.R. and N.Z.; formal analysis, R.M.; investigation, G.S., A.M., G.G. and C.F.; data curation, G.S. and F.M.M.; writing—original draft preparation, G.S., A.M. and F.M.M.; writing—review and editing: G.S., A.M. and F.M.M.; visualization, R.M. and G.G.; supervision, V.D., M.R. and N.Z.; project administration, V.D. All authors have read and agreed to the published version of the manuscript.

Funding: This research received no external funding.

Institutional Review Board Statement: The study was conducted in accordance with the Declaration of Helsinki, and approved by the Institutional Review Board (or Ethics Committee) of UO Dermatology, AOUP, Pisa (SUS1-AD ASTRA, 8 July 2019).

Informed Consent Statement: All patients in this manuscript gave written informed consent for participation in the study and for the use of their de-identified, anonymized, aggregated data and case details (including photographs) for publication.

Data Availability Statement: The data presented in this study are available on request from the corresponding author. The data are not publicly available due to privacy reasons.

Conflicts of Interest: The authors declare no conflict of interest.

Abbreviations

GAIS	Global Aesthetic Improvement Scale
HA	Hyaluronic acid
MHz	Megahertz
UHFUS	Ultra-high-frequency ultrasound
WSRS	Wrinkle Severity Rating Scale

References

1. Brandt, F.S.; Cazzaniga, A. Hyaluronic acid gel fillers in the management of facial aging. *Clin. Interv. Aging* **2008**, *3*, 153–159.
2. Wongprasert, P.; Dreiss, C.A.; Murray, G. Evaluating hyaluronic acid dermal fillers: A critique of current characterization methods. *Dermatol. Ther.* **2022**, *35*, e15453. [CrossRef]
3. Laurano, R.; Boffito, M.; Cassino, C.; Liberti, F.; Ciardelli, G.; Chiono, V. Design of Injectable Bioartificial Hydrogels by Green Chemistry for Mini-Invasive Applications in the Biomedical or Aesthetic Medicine Fields. *Gels* **2023**, *9*, 59. [CrossRef] [PubMed]
4. Vasvani, S.; Kulkarni, P.; Rawtani, D. Hyaluronic acid: A review on its biology, aspects of drug delivery, route of administrations and a special emphasis on its approved marketed products and recent clinical studies. *Int. J. Biol. Macromol.* **2020**, *151*, 1012–1029. [CrossRef] [PubMed]
5. Maytin, E.V. Hyaluronan: More than just a wrinkle filler. *Glycobiology* **2016**, *26*, 553–559. [CrossRef] [PubMed]
6. Bukhari, S.N.A.; Roswandi, N.L.; Waqas, M.; Habib, H.; Hussain, F.; Khan, S.; Sohail, M.; Ramli, N.A.; Thu, H.E.; Hussain, Z. Hyaluronic acid, a promising skin rejuvenating biomedicine: A review of recent updates and pre-clinical and clinical investigations on cosmetic and nutricosmetic effects. *Int. J. Biol. Macromol.* **2018**, *120 Pt B*, 1682–1695. [CrossRef]
7. Safran, T.; Swift, A.; Cotofana, S.; Nikolis, A. Evaluating safety in hyaluronic acid lip injections. *Expert Opin. Drug Saf.* **2021**, *20*, 1473–1486. [CrossRef]
8. Urdiales-Gálvez, F.; Barres-Caballer, J.; Carrasco-Sánchez, S. Ultrasound assessment of tissue integration of the crosslinked hyaluronic acid filler VYC-25L in facial lower-third aesthetic treat-ment: A prospective multicenter study. *J. Cosmet. Dermatol.* **2020**, *20*, 1439–1449. [CrossRef]
9. Qiao, J.; Jia, Q.N.; Jin, H.Z.; Li, F.; He, C.-X.; Yang, J.; Zuo, Y.-G.; Fu, L.-Q. Long-Term Follow-Up of Longevity and Diffusion Pattern of Hyaluronic Acid in Nasolabial Fold Correction through High-Frequency Ultrasound. *Plast. Reconstr. Surg.* **2019**, *144*, 189e–196e. [CrossRef]
10. Granieri, G.; Oranges, T.; Morganti, R.; Janowska, A.; Romanelli, M.; Manni, E.; Dini, V. Ultra-high frequency ultrasound detection of the dermo-epidermal junction: Its potential role in dermatology. *Exp. Dermatol.* **2022**, *31*, 1863–1871. [CrossRef]
11. Fidanzi, C.; D'Erme, A.M.; Janowska, A.; Dini, V.; Romanelli, M.; Margiotta, F.M.; Viacava, P.; Bagnoni, G. Epidemiology of melanoma: The importance of correctly reporting to the cancer registries. *Eur. J. Cancer Prev.* **2022**, *31*, 385–387. [CrossRef]
12. Oranges, T.; Janowska, A.; Scatena, C.; Faita, F.; Di Lascio, N.; Izzetti, R.; Fidanzi, C.; Romanelli, M.; Dini, V. Ultra-High Frequency Ultrasound in Melanoma Management: A New Combined Ultrasonographic-Histopathological Approach. *J. Ultrasound Med.* **2023**, *42*, 99–108. [CrossRef] [PubMed]
13. Izzetti, R.; Oranges, T.; Janowska, A.; Gabriele, M.; Graziani, F.; Romanelli, M. The Application of Ultra-High-Frequency Ultrasound in Dermatology and Wound Management. *Int. J. Low Extrem. Wounds* **2020**, *19*, 334–340. [CrossRef] [PubMed]

14. Janowska, A.; Oranges, T.; Granieri, G.; Romanelli, M.; Fidanzi, C.; Iannone, M.; Dini, V. Non-invasive imaging techniques in presurgical margin assessment of basal cell carcinoma: Current evidence. *Skin Res. Technol.* **2023**, *29*, e13271. [CrossRef] [PubMed]
15. Herrmann, J.L.; Hoffmann, R.K.; Ward, C.E.; Schulman, J.M.; Grekin, R.C. Biochemistry, Physiology, and Tissue Interactions of Contemporary Biodegradable Injectable Dermal Fillers. *Dermatol. Surg.* **2018**, *44* (Suppl. S1), S19–S31. [CrossRef]
16. Wortsman, X. Common Applications of Ultrasound in Cosmetic and Plastic Surgery. In *Atlas of Dermatologic Ultrasound*, 1st ed.; Springer International Publishing: Berlin/Heidelberg, Germany, 2018; pp. 181–189.
17. Liang, J.; Jiang, D.; Noble, P.W. Hyaluronan as a therapeutic target in human diseases. *Adv. Drug Deliv. Rev.* **2016**, *97*, 186–203. [CrossRef]
18. King, M.; Convery, C.; Davies, E. This month's guideline: The Use of Hyaluronidase in Aesthetic Practice (v2.4). *J. Clin. Aesthetic Dermatol.* **2018**, *11*, E61–E68.
19. Kalmanson, O.A.; Misch, E.S.; Terella, A. Hyaluronic acid fillers may be longer-lasting than previously described: A case report of delayed filler-associated facial cellulitis. *JPRAS Open* **2022**, *33*, 37–41. [CrossRef]
20. Josse, G.; Haftek, M.; Gensanne, D.; Turlier, V.; Mas, A.; Lagarde, J.; Schmitt, A. Follow up study of dermal hyaluronic acid injection by high frequency ultrasound and magnetic resonance imaging. *J. Dermatol. Sci.* **2010**, *57*, 214–216. [CrossRef]
21. Schneider, S.L.; Kohli, I.; Hamzavi, I.H.; Council, M.L.; Rossi, A.M.; Ozog, D.M. Emerging imaging technologies in dermatology: Part II: Applications and limitations. *J. Am. Acad. Dermatol.* **2019**, *80*, 1121–1131. [CrossRef]
22. Wortsman, X. Practical applications of ultrasound in dermatology. *Clin. Dermatol.* **2021**, *39*, 605–623. [CrossRef] [PubMed]
23. Urdiales-Gálvez, F.; De Cabo-Francés, F.M.; Bové, I. Ultrasound patterns of different dermal filler materials used in aesthetics. *J. Cosmet. Dermatol.* **2021**, *20*, 1541–1548. [CrossRef] [PubMed]
24. Jiang, L.; Yuan, L.; Li, Z.; Su, X.; Hu, J.; Chai, H. High-Frequency Ultrasound of Facial Filler Materials in the Nasolabial Groove. *Aesthetic Plast. Surg.* **2022**, *46*, 2972–2978. [CrossRef] [PubMed]
25. Gan, L.M.; Grönros, J.; Hägg, U.; Wikström, J.; Theodoropoulos, C.; Friberg, P.; Fritsche-Danielson, R. Non-invasive real-time imaging of atherosclerosis in mice using ultrasound biomicroscopy. *Atherosclerosis* **2007**, *190*, 313–320. [CrossRef]
26. Quezada-Gaón, N.; Wortsman, X. Ultrasound-guided hyaluronidase injection in cosmetic complications. *J. Eur. Acad. Dermatol. Venereol.* **2016**, *30*, e39–e40. [CrossRef] [PubMed]
27. Izzetti, R.; Vitali, S.; Aringhieri, G.; Nisi, M.; Oranges, T.; Dini, V.; Ferro, F.; Baldini, C.; Romanelli, M.; Caramella, D.; et al. Ultra-High Frequency Ultrasound, A Promising Diagnostic Technique: Review of the Literature and Single-Center Experience. *Can. Assoc. Radiol. J.* **2021**, *72*, 418–431. [CrossRef]
28. Fino, P.; Toscani, M.; Grippaudo, F.R.; Giordan, N.; Scuderi, N. Randomized Double-Blind Controlled Study on the Safety and Efficacy of a Novel Injectable Cross-linked Hyaluronic Gel for the Correction of Moderate-to-Severe Nasolabial Wrinkles. *Aesthetic Plast. Surg.* **2019**, *43*, 470–479. [CrossRef]
29. Day, D.J.; Littler, C.M.; Swift, R.W.; Gottlieb, S. The wrinkle severity rating scale: A validation study. *Am. J. Clin. Dermatol.* **2004**, *5*, 49–52. [CrossRef]
30. Stefura, T.; Kacprzyk, A.; Droś, J.; Krzysztofik, M.; Skomarovska, O.; Fijałkowska, M.; Koziej, M. Tissue Fillers for the Nasolabial Fold Area: A Systematic Review and Meta-Analysis of Randomized Clinical Trials. *Aesthetic Plast. Surg.* **2021**, *45*, 2300–2316. [CrossRef]

Disclaimer/Publisher's Note: The statements, opinions and data contained in all publications are solely those of the individual author(s) and contributor(s) and not of MDPI and/or the editor(s). MDPI and/or the editor(s) disclaim responsibility for any injury to people or property resulting from any ideas, methods, instructions or products referred to in the content.

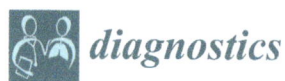

Article

Ultra-High Frequency UltraSound (UHFUS) Assessment of Barrier Function in Moderate-to-Severe Atopic Dermatitis during Dupilumab Treatment

Valentina Dini [1], Michela Iannone [1], Alessandra Michelucci [1,*], Flavia Manzo Margiotta [1], Giammarco Granieri [1], Giorgia Salvia [1], Teresa Oranges [2], Agata Janowska [1], Riccardo Morganti [3] and Marco Romanelli [1]

1. Department of Dermatology, University of Pisa, 56126 Pisa, Italy; valentina.dini@unipi.it (V.D.); drmichelaiannone@gmail.com (M.I.); manzomargiottaflavia@gmail.com (F.M.M.); giammarcogranieri@gmail.com (G.G.); giorgia.salvia2@gmail.com (G.S.); dottoressajanowska@gmail.com (A.J.); marco.romanelli@unipi.it (M.R.)
2. Unit of Dermatology, Department of Pediatrics, IRCCS Meyer Children's Hospital, 50139 Florence, Italy; teresa.oranges@gmail.com
3. Statistical Support to Clinical Trials Department, University of Pisa, 56126 Pisa, Italy; r.morganti@ao-pisa.toscana.it
* Correspondence: alessandra.michelucci@gmail.com

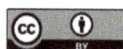

Citation: Dini, V.; Iannone, M.; Michelucci, A.; Manzo Margiotta, F.; Granieri, G.; Salvia, G.; Oranges, T.; Janowska, A.; Morganti, R.; Romanelli, M. Ultra-High Frequency UltraSound (UHFUS) Assessment of Barrier Function in Moderate-to-Severe Atopic Dermatitis during Dupilumab Treatment. *Diagnostics* 2023, *13*, 2721. https://doi.org/10.3390/diagnostics13172721

Academic Editor: Francesco Inchingolo

Received: 18 July 2023
Revised: 11 August 2023
Accepted: 13 August 2023
Published: 22 August 2023

Copyright: © 2023 by the authors. Licensee MDPI, Basel, Switzerland. This article is an open access article distributed under the terms and conditions of the Creative Commons Attribution (CC BY) license (https://creativecommons.org/licenses/by/4.0/).

Abstract: Atopic dermatitis (AD) is a chronic multifactorial inflammatory disease characterized by intense itching and inflammatory eczematous lesions. Biological disease-modifying drugs, such as dupilumab are recommended for patients with moderate-to-severe AD, refractory to systemic immunosuppressive therapies. Disease monitoring is performed by clinical scores. Since 1970, however, the use of ultrasound and particularly high-frequency ultrasound (HFUS), has identified alterations in dermal echogenicity, called the subepidermal low-echogenic band (SLEB), that correlates with disease severity and response to treatment. We enrolled 18 patients with moderate-to-severe AD, divided into two groups: twelve patients in the dupilumab treatment (Group A) and six patients in standard treatment, from February 2019 to November 2019. We performed ultra-high frequency ultrasound (UHFUS) evaluation of lesional and non-lesional skin, focusing on SLEB average thicknesses measurement, epidermal thickness, and vascular signal in correlation with objective disease scores (EASI, IGA), patient's reported scores (Sleep Quality NRS and Itch NRS), and TEWL and corneometry at baseline (T0), after 1 month (T1) and 2 months (T2). The SLEB average thickness measurement, vascular signal, and epidermal thickness showed a statistically significant reduction in lesional skin of the biological treatment group and no significant reduction in non-lesional skin in both groups. In the lesional skin of the standard treatment group, only epidermal thickness showed a statistically significant reduction. Our study demonstrates that SLEB measurement, vascular signals, and epidermal thickness could be used as objective parameters in monitoring the AD treatment response, while the presence of SLEB in non-lesional skin could be used as a marker of subclinical inflammation and could predict development of clinical lesions, suggesting a pro-active therapy. Further follow-up and research are needed to clarify the association of SLEB decrease/disappearance with a reduction of flares/prolongment of the disease remission time.

Keywords: atopic dermatitis; ultra-high frequency ultrasound; SLEB; dupilumab; corneometry

1. Introduction

Atopic dermatitis (AD) is a chronic, relapsing cutaneous inflammatory disease characterized by the interaction of genetic factors, environmental factors, immune abnormalities, and comorbidities [1]. In developed countries, AD affects one-fifth of the population and has been identified as the most common inflammatory skin disease. In particular, it has been demonstrated that AD affects approximately 5 to over 20 percent of children worldwide, with higher rates in Africa, Oceania, and the Asia–Pacific region rather than in Northern/Eastern Europe [2,3]. The onset of the disease frequently occurs before the age of five years, with early onset in the first six months of life that seems to be associated with severe disease and with a slight preponderance of prevalence in female children [4]. Clinical features include intense itching and inflammatory eczematous lesions [5]. Diagnosis of AD is based on a typical clinical picture without diagnostic markers; practical aspects of management, such as duration of treatment, criteria for switching, and determination of severity, are insufficient. Disease severity is determined using scales such as the Atopic Dermatitis Score Index (SCORAD), the Eczema Area and Severity Index (EASI), or the Investigator Global Assessment (IGA), which measures the degree of erythema, induration/papule/edema, abrasions, and lichenification according to the physician and the degree of itching and sleep disturbance according to the patient [6].

The chronic nature of the disease means that long-term treatment strategies are necessary, which entails high global healthcare costs and significant psychosocial implications for patients and their relatives [7]. In particular, AD imposes a significant economic burden on healthcare systems, including direct medical costs of diagnosis and treatment, along with indirect costs related to productivity loss and intangible costs, such as reduced quality of life and psychological distress [8]. Efforts to address the economic burden of AD should focus on early diagnosis, effective treatments, patient education, and supportive care. Investing in the management of AD can lead to better patient outcomes, improved quality of life, and potentially reduced long-term healthcare costs.

The optimal management of AD is based on a multimodal approach that involves, first, correct patient education on the importance of skin hydration, avoidance of trigger factors, and implementation of the skin barrier function, highlighting that pharmacologic treatment of skin inflammation represents a second step that cannot ignore the first one. Although there is no definitive cure, the disease can be controlled with appropriate treatment. Current therapy recommendations include topical moisturizers to restore epidermal barrier function, topical corticosteroids (TCS) to control the acute outbreak, topical calcineurin inhibitors (TCI) for sensitive skin areas and long-term use, and phototherapy (preferably UVB 311 nm or UVA1) as adjuvant therapy [9]. In severe refractory cases, systemic immunosuppressive treatments such as cyclosporine, methotrexate, azathioprine, and mycophenolic acid are recommended. Biologic disease modifiers such as dupilumab are recommended "for patients with moderate to severe AD for whom local treatment is inadequate and other systemic treatments are undesirable" [10]. In particular, dupilumab is a human monoclonal antibody able to inhibit IL-4 and IL-13 signaling through a link to the IL-4R-alpha and IL-13R-alpha-1 subunits of the receptor [11]. The blocking of IL-4 is responsible for under-stimulating B-cell differentiation and IgE production [12], leading to the regulation of receptor signaling downstream of the JAKSTAT pathway, with the subsequent activation of tyrosine kinases 2 and Januskinase (JAK) 1/2, resulting in gene expression regulation [13]. In particular, JAK-STAT activation is able to down-regulate skin-barrier proteins and interfere with keratinocyte differentiation, defeating the decrease of skin barrier function caused by the down-regulation of the filaggrin protein [14].

Moreover, AD shows a chronic and relapsing course, with several flares of the disease, which usually undergo spontaneous remission in cases of mild disease, while moderate to severe dermatitis rarely clears without treatment. The monitoring of the flares is mainly clinical, but several non-invasive methods have been proposed for objective evaluation of the disease, independently from the chosen therapy. The first studies on non-invasive assessment of skin biophysical parameters were published as early as the late 1990s. Transepidermal water loss (TEWL) and corneometry were the most evaluated parameters [15]. TEWL is a critical parameter that measures the amount of water lost through the epidermis to the external environment. A healthy skin barrier effectively retains moisture, preventing excessive water loss and maintaining skin hydration. However, in AD, the disrupted barrier function results in elevated TEWL levels, contributing to the hallmark symptoms of dry and itchy skin [16]. Excessive TEWL exacerbates the inflammatory response in AD by triggering a cascade of immune reactions. It also weakens the skin's ability to heal, perpetuating skin lesions and further compromising the barrier function. Therefore, understanding and managing TEWL play a crucial role in the treatment and management of AD. On the other side, corneometry is a non-invasive technique used to assess the skin's hydration levels, primarily by measuring the electrical capacitance of the skin surface. The principle behind corneometry is based on the fact that water is a potent electrical conductor, and changes in skin hydration affect its electrical properties; therefore, by measuring the skin's electrical capacitance, corneometry provides a quantitative evaluation of its hydration status [17]. Corneometry has become an important tool in the evaluation and management of AD, since it allows dermatologists to objectively measure and monitor the hydration status of the skin, providing valuable insights into disease severity and treatment response [18]. In patients with active AD flares, corneometry often reveals significantly lower hydration values, indicating decreased skin moisture content. Monitoring hydration levels during treatment can help clinicians assess the efficacy of topical moisturizers and systemic therapies, such as immunomodulators and corticosteroids [19]. For all these reasons, corneometry has been established as a valid tool also for the identification of individuals at risk of developing AD, as early changes in skin hydration may precede the appearance of clinical symptoms.

Another non-invasive diagnostic method was explored in 1979, when Alexander and Miller Skin introduced ultrasound into dermatology to measure skin thickness. Since the development of high-frequency ultrasonography (HF-US) and its application in the non-invasive monitoring of inflammatory skin diseases, significant advancements have been made in understanding and diagnosing conditions such as psoriasis, eczema, and atopic dermatitis (AD). One prominent feature observed in these inflammatory skin diseases is the presence of a subepidermal low-echogenic band (SLEB), which indicates skin edema and infiltration by inflammatory cells, resulting in increased distance between collagen fibers [20]. Research has demonstrated a correlation between the thickness of the SLEB and the severity of AD, making it a valuable objective parameter for monitoring the disease's course [21]. Moreover, studies using HF-US have revealed that non-lesional AD skin exhibits a thinner SLEB compared to healthy controls, suggesting the presence of subclinical eczematous lesions [22,23]. These findings underscore the potential of HF-US as a non-invasive diagnostic tool and its utility in monitoring AD patients over time. Despite the promising developments in using HF-US for disease monitoring, there is a notable gap in the literature regarding a multimodal assessment of changes in the skin barrier function following various systemic and/or biological therapies used for managing AD. This area of research remains relatively unexplored, and there is a need for more comprehensive studies to investigate the impact of different treatment modalities on the skin barrier function in AD patients. A multimodal assessment would entail integrating data from HF-US with other diagnostic techniques, such as dermatological assessments, biopsies, and measurements of biomarkers related to skin barrier function. By combining these approaches, researchers and clinicians could gain a more comprehensive understanding of how specific therapies affect the skin barrier in AD patients and whether these changes correlate with treatment response and disease outcome. Such studies would not only advance our knowledge of the underlying mechanisms of AD but also provide valuable insights for tailoring personalized treatment plans for patients. Additionally, understanding the impact of different therapies on the skin barrier could lead to the development of novel treatment strategies targeting the restoration of barrier integrity, ultimately improving the management and quality of life for AD patients.

Since then, new applications of high-frequency ultrasonography (HF-US) have been developed, including non-invasive monitoring of inflammatory skin diseases. In inflammatory skin diseases (psoriasis, eczema, AD), a subepidermal echogenic or hypoechogenic band (SLEB) is observed, and the average skin echogenicity is reduced; SLEB shows skin edema and infiltration by inflammatory cells with increased distance between collagen fibers [20]. It has been demonstrated that SLEB thickness correlates with the severity of

AD and can be used as an objective parameter to monitor the course of the disease [21]. Moreover, HF-US studies reported a thinner SLEB in non-lesional AD skin compared to higher cutaneous US in controls, with a thinner SLEB that may generally indicate a subclinical eczematous lesion [22,23]. Even if non-invasive diagnostic has then been shown to represent an opportunity for the follow-up of AD patients, curiously, there are still no studies in the literature that perform a multimodal assessment of the changes in the barrier function following the various systemic and/or biological therapies available for the management of AD.

2. Materials and Methods

A prospective study was conducted from February 2019 to November 2019 at the Department of Dermatology of the University of Pisa, Pisa, Italy, on AD patients who were followed with non-invasive measurements of affected and unaffected skin. The study was conducted under the 1964 Declaration of Helsinki and all subsequent amendments, and all patients provided informed consent. Eligible subjects were patients aged ≥ 18 years affected by the classic phenotype of moderate to severe AD; subjects with erythrodermic or prurigo nodularis forms were excluded, as well as patients who were lost to follow-up, or who had any biologic treatment interruption, or the switching from biologic therapy to another biologic therapy. The patients were divided into two groups: Group A included those patients in the biological treatment, while Group B consisted of patients treated with standard treatment. For Group A, we included all patients who received Dupilumab 300 mg administered subcutaneous according to the dosing schedule at week 0, 4, and then every 2 weeks. Clinical and instrumental evaluations were performed at baseline (T0), after 1 month (T1), and 2 months (T2). At each visit, an objective examination based on classic disease scores (EASI, IGA) and patient-reported scores (NRS sleep quality, NRS itching) was performed. For each patient, instrumental examinations were performed on the lesional skin of the antecubital cavity and on the non-lesional skin of the contralateral antecubital cavity not affected by eczematous lesions. TEWL and corneometry were measured by Dermalab® COMBO (Cortex Technology, Hadsund, Danmark) according to EEMCO Group guidelines (European Expert Group on Efficacy Measurement of Cosmetics and Other Topical Products). Each assessment was always conducted under identical environmental conditions after 15–30 min of acclimation; TEWL was expressed in international units ($g/m^2/h$) and ranged from 0 to 250 $g/m^2/h$ (normal values were 0–25 $g/m^2/h$). Corneometry was expressed in microsimens (μS) and ranged from 0 to 9999 μS. Depending on the instrument settings, eight measurements were taken and the average value automatically generated by the software was taken into account. To further investigate skin barrier function and inflammation, an ultra-high frequency ultrasound (UHFUS) was performed on a VEVO MD® (FUJIFILM VisualSonics, Toronto, Ontario, Canada) using a 70 MHz ultrasound probe with a frequency range of 29–71 MHz, axial resolution of 30 µm, lateral resolution of 65 µm, depth of 10 mm and maximum width of 9.7 mm (B MODE 31, C-MODE speed 1.9 cm/s). Longitudinal ultrasound probe video clips, transverse ultrasound probe video clips, and color Doppler studies (both longitudinal and transverse) at a standard di 1.9 cm/s were performed for each skin area under examination. Ultrasonography was performed using a sufficient amount of ultrasound gel between the probe and the skin. The probe was held perpendicular to the skin with minimal pressure and moved manually. Two dermatologists trained in skin ultrasonography practiced ultrasonography and imaging. For each ultrasound video clip, SLEB, epidermis and dermis thickness were measured using RadiAnt DICOM Viewer® software (Medixant, v.5.0.1.21910) and displayed in millimeters. Three trained operators chose the three most significative frames in each image, both longitudinal and transverse, and they practiced three measurements of each parameter. The final value was calculated as the average of the three measurements for both images.

The level of vascularization, evaluated both in longitudinal and transverse axes, was assessed using color Doppler imaging at a standard rate of 1.9 cm/s. For each image, the vascularization level was determined in a 2.0 mm depth window. The same settings were used for images of healthy skin. Color Doppler signal was assessed in quantitative scores from 0 to 3: 0—none; 1—weak (physiological); 2—moderate; 3—strong. The final numerical score was calculated by average longitudinal and transverse image scores. All categorical data were described by absolute and relative (%) frequency, and continuous data by mean and standard deviation. To evaluate the differences between groups in terms of clinical scores and non-invasive measurements, ANOVA for repeated measures was performed. Significance was fixed at 0.05, and all analyses were carried out with SPSS v.28 technology.

3. Results

A total of 18 subjects, 11/18 (61%) males and 7/18 (39%) females, with a mean BMI of 24.6 kg/m^2 affected by eczematous lesions of the classic clinical form of AD were included in the study. Age ranged from 20 to 77 years, the mean age was 46 years and the standard deviation was 18. 10/18 patients (55%) presented phototype II and 8/18 (45%) phototype III. Group A included 12/18 (66.7%) patients who were treated with dupilumab, while Group B included 6/18 (33.3%) patients who were treated as follows: 1/12 (8.3%) with cyclosporine, 1/12 (8.3%) with ultraviolet phototherapy, 3/12 (25%) with TCI, and 1/12 (8.3%) with TCS. The mean values and standard deviations of clinical parameters, ultrasound parameters, TEWL, and corneometry at T0, T1, and T2 are reported in Table 1 for patients who received biological treatment (Group A) and in Table 2 for patients who received standard treatment (Group B). The two groups displayed some clinical differences at baseline, since Group A moved from a mean EASI of 28.425 (sd: 12.339) and IGA of 3.250 (sd: 0.452), while Group B from a mean EASI of 12.050 (sd: 7.584) and IGA of 2.167 (sd: 0.753). Also the quality of life of patients of Group A was more compromised, with a mean DLQI of 12.750 (sd: 6.426), itch-NRS of 8.5 (sd: 1.382), and sleep-NRS of 5.750 (sd: 3.019); on the other side, Group B showed a mean DLQI of 9.833 (sd: 6.494), an itch-NRS of 6.667 (sd: 1.033), and sleep-NRS of 3.333 (sd: 2.944). Focusing on UHFUS measurements, Group A presented an initial lesional skin SLEB of 0.291 mm(sd: 0.126), non-lesional skin SLEB of 0.053 mm (sd: 0.040), a lesional skin epidermic thickness of 0.177 mm (sd: 0.030), a non-lesional skin epidermic thickness of 0.146 mm (sd: 0.027), a lesional skin dermis thickness of 1.749 mm (sd: 0.480), a non-lesional skin dermis thickness of 1.559 mm (sd: 0.451), a lesional skin vascularization of 2.292 (sd: 0.480), and a non-lesional skin vascularization of 0.750 (sd: 0.584). Results from Group B were similar, with some lower values as well as the clinical ones. Indeed, we registered an initial lesional skin SLEB of 0.195 mm (sd: 0.085), non-lesional skin SLEB of 0.038 mm (sd: 0.049), a lesional skin epidermic thickness of 0.171 mm (sd: 0.055), a non-lesional skin epidermic thickness of 0.138 mm (sd: 0.044), a lesional skin dermis thickness of 1.544 mm (sd: 0.273), a non-lesional skin dermis thickness of 1.311 mm (sd: 0.345), a lesional skin vascularization of 2.167 (sd: 0.516), and a non-lesional skin vascularization of 0.583 (sd: 0.492). TEWL measurements pointed out a mean value of lesional skin TEWL of 40.833 (sd: 22.904) in Group A and of 40.983 (sd: 21.505) in Group B, while non-lesional skin TEWL showed a mean value of 16.067 (sd: 11.271) in Group A and of 28,417 (sd: 22.668) in Group B. To conclude baseline measurements, mean lesional skin corneometry of Group A was 131.00 (sd: 68,621) vs. 248.33 (sd: 257.498) in Group B; furthermore, the mean non-lesional skin corneometry of Group A was 107,333 (sd: 39,919) vs. 194.50 (sd: 1496.020) in Group B.

Table 1. Mean values (sd) for patients in biological treatment (Group A), evaluated at baseline (t0), after 1 month (t1) and 2 months (t2).

Time Line	t0		t1		t2		
PARAMETERS	Mean	SD	Mean	SD	Mean	SD	p-Value
EASI	28.425	12.339	9.875	9.360	8.033	8.815	<0.001
IGA	3.250	0.452	1.833	0.718	1.750	0.866	<0.001
DLQI	12.750	6.426	3.667	3.284	3.417	3.942	0.001
Sleep-NRS	5.750	3.019	1.167	1.946	2.417	2.778	0.002
Itch-NRS	8.500	1.382	3.250	2.340	3.333	2.309	<0.001
Lesional skin SLEB (mm)	0.291	0.126	0.103	0.072	0.085	0.100	<0.001
Non-lesional skin SLEB (mm)	0.053	0.040	0.057	0.080	0.030	0.035	ns
Lesional skin epidermic thickness (mm)	0.177	0.030	0.156	0.037	0.148	0.028	0.002
Non-lesional skin epidermic thickness (mm)	0.146	0.027	0.142	0.023	0.138	0.020	ns
Lesional skin dermis thickness (mm)	1.749	0.480	1.656	0.690	1.607	0.678	ns
Non-lesional skin dermis thickness (mm)	1.559	0.451	1.650	0.567	1.589	0.527	ns
Lesional skin vascularization	2.292	0.450	1.292	0.450	1.042	0.396	<0.001
Non-lesional skin vascularization	0.750	0.584	0.625	0.483	0.625	0.483	ns
Lesion skin TEWL	40.833	22.904	29.250	12.624	28.150	12.697	ns
Non-lesional skin TEWL	16.067	11.271	21.583	15.967	14.392	9.104	ns
Lesion skin corneometry	131.000	68.621	132.667	81.615	103.833	37.365	ns
Non-lesional skin corneometry	107.333	39.919	119.667	83.049	101.167	33.526	ns

Eczema Area and Severity Index (EASI), Investigator's Global Assessment (IGA), Dermatology Life Quality Index (DLQI), Numerical Rating Scale (NRS), Subepidermal Low-Echogenic Band (SLEB), Transepidermal water loss (TEWL).

Table 2. Mean values (sd) for patients in standard treatment (Group B) evaluated at baseline (t0), after 1 month (t1) and 2 months (t2).

Time Line	t0		t1		t2		
PARAMETERS	Mean	SD	Mean	SD	Mean	SD	p-Value
EASI	12.050	7.584	6.183	3.945	5.667	5.297	0.020
IGA	2167	0.753	1.667	0.816	1.500	1.049	0.063
DLQI	9833	6.494	4.667	3.011	1.667	1.506	0.083
Sleep-NRS	3333	2.944	1.833	2.483	1.667	2.338	ns
Itch-NRS	6667	1.033	2.833	2.927	3.333	2.338	0.033
Lesional skin SLEB (mm)	0.195	0.085	0.146	0.084	0.139	0.159	ns
Non-lesional skin SLEB (mm)	0.038	0.049	0.050	0.045	0.044	0.040	ns
Lesional skin epidermic thickness (mm)	0.171	0.055	0.168	0.023	0.149	0.034	0.043
Non-lesional skin epidermic thickness (mm)	0.138	0.044	0.127	0.024	0.146	0.019	ns
Lesional skin dermis thickness (mm)	1.544	0.273	1.387	0.200	1.360	0.329	ns
Non-lesional skin dermis thickness (mm)	1.311	0.345	1.341	0.282	1.306	0.374	ns
Lesional skin vascularization	2.167	0.516	1.583	0.585	1.500	0.837	ns
Non-lesional skin vascularization	0.583	0.492	0.667	0.753	0.750	0.274	ns

Table 2. Cont.

Time Line	t0		t1		t2		
PARAMETERS	Mean	SD	Mean	SD	Mean	SD	p-Value
Lesion skin TEWL	40.983	21,505	28,367	8.641	46,350	25,401	ns
Not-lesional skin TEWL	28,417	22,668	26,000	17,535	41,100	14,846	ns
Lesion skin corneometry	248,333	257,498	117,667	95,406	151,000	62,846	ns
Not-lesional skin corneometry	194,500	146,020	158,000	101,052	166,167	76,583	ns

Eczema Area and Severity Index (EASI), Investigator's Global Assessment (IGA), Dermatology Life Quality Index (DLQI), Numerical Rating Scale (NRS), subepidermal low-echogenic band (SLEB), transepidermal water loss (TEWL).

For Group A, a significant reduction in the objective clinical parameters of EASI, IGA (p-value < 0.001) was found, as well as an improvement in the quality of life measured through DLQI (p-value 0.001) and both Itch NRS (p-value < 0.001) and Sleep-NRS (p-value = 0.002). Similar results were obtained in Group B, with a slighter reduction of EASI (p-value = 0.02), IGA (p-value = 0.063), DLQI (p-value = 0.083), and Itch NRS (p-value = 0.033), while Sleep-NRS did not reach a statistically significant improvement. Focusing on non-invasive measurements, none of the two groups presented a significant reduction in TEWL and corneometry. Conversely, UHFUS evaluations pointed out differences in Group A in terms of mean lesional skin SLEB (p-value = 0.001), lesional skin epidermic thickness (p-value = 0.002), and lesional skin vascularization measured through Doppler (p-value < 0.001). In the standard treatment Group B, only the epidermal thickness of lesional skin showed a statistically significant decrease (p-value = 0.043). Non-lesional skin parameters did not display any significant modifications in either Group A or in Group B.

4. Discussion

Patients affected by moderate to severe forms of AD often require systemic treatment to achieve adequate disease control independently from a correct and optimal topical therapy [24,25]. On the contrary, a recent meta-analysis demonstrated that mild to moderate forms of AD can benefit from intermittent therapy with moderate- to high-potency TCS or TCI, which was able to reduce the risk of flares after the disease control achieved with continuous use of the agents [26]. In any case, a re-evaluation of patients to exclude concurrent diseases or conditions that may influence the response (e.g., infection, contact dermatitis) is considered a good clinical practice before the start of any systemic therapy, as well continuous monitoring of the clinical response after the choice of the first-line therapy. Dupilumab is a fully human monoclonal antibody approved for the treatment of adults and children with moderate to severe AD not correctly controlled with topical and/or systemic therapies, displaying a favorable safety profile that does not typically require a serum monitoring as non-targeted immunosuppressive agents [27]. Efficacy of dupilumab has been shown in multiple work and real life-experiences, such as a recent network meta-analysis of 74 randomized trials (more than 8000 patients), which declared dupilumab as the most effective treatment in achieving a 75 percent reduction in the EASI (EASI-75) score (risk ratio 3.04, 95% CI 2.51–3.69) and improving the Patient-Oriented Eczema Measure (POEM) score (mean difference 7.3, 95% CI 6.61–8.00) during short-term follow-up when compared with placebo [28]. Moreover, the long-term safety of dupilumab was evaluated in a randomized, double-blind, multicenter trial (LIBERTY AD CHRONOS) on 740 patients [27], who experienced similarly rated adverse events both when treated with dupilumab or receiving placebo plus topical corticosteroids (83 to 88 percent). Beyond its therapeutic efficacy, recent research has shed light on the impact of dupilumab on skin modification, particularly in relation to the skin barrier function and overall cutaneous health. Indeed, research investigating the effects of dupilumab on skin modification at the histological and molecular levels has revealed promising findings. Biopsy studies have shown that dupilumab treatment reduces epidermal thickness, parakeratosis, and spongiosis, all of which are associated with AD severity [29]. Additionally, gene expression analysis has demonstrated that dupilumab shifts the transcriptome of lesional skin toward a more non-pathological phenotype. This means that dupilumab reduces the expression of genes involved in type 2 inflammation and epidermal hyperplasia while increasing the expression of genes associated with epidermal differentiation, barrier function, and lipid metabolism [30]. Even if monitoring of therapeutic response can be frequently performed through a clinical evaluation and correct dialogue with the patient, the study of residual inflammation and skin modification, which can lead to new flares, is not easily performed during the clinical practice. From a molecular point of view, non-lesional skin of AD patients does not have the structure of normal skin from healthy controls [31], with deep differences in terms of the general skin barrier function, qualitative and quantitative changes in dendritic cell populations, and lymphocytic infiltration. In particular, clinical severity seems to be related to the mean number of infiltrating dendritic cells as well as disease recurrence was demonstrated to be driven by the repopulation of cutaneous inflammatory dendritic cells [32]. All this molecular evidence suggests that there is still limited knowledge on managing subclinical inflammation, and few studies have been performed on managing clinical responses through non-invasive dermatological instruments. UHFUS allows the clinician to obtain real-time images with the possibility of performing measurements of physiological and pathological aspects of the skin. According to data presented in the literature, dermal echogenicity is influenced by collagen fiber location and water content [33–35]. Damage to collagen fibers leads to a reduction in the echogenicity of the dermis, which is visible in different inflammatory diseases due to swelling of the skin and inflammatory cell infiltration. Although SLEB is not a specific parameter for any skin disease, its changes over time have important prognostic value, especially for patients with chronic skin diseases such as psoriasis and AD. SLEB thickness in AD correlates with histopathological aspects such as epidermal hyperplasia and hyperkeratosis, levels of parakeratosis and spongiosis, and inflammatory cell infiltration [36,37]. Moving from these assumptions, it is not surprising that even in our work, UHFUS measurements have revealed a parallel reduction in skin thickness and inflammation in response to dupilumab therapy. The most valuable result of our study is that SLEB scores, vascular signals, and epidermal thickness were much more significantly reduced in patients receiving biological treatment compared to patients with standard treatment. The results obtained from this study support the possibility of considering SLEB as an objective parameter for monitoring treatment efficacy in AD [20]. In particular, as can be seen from Figure 1, there is a parallel reduction in SLEB, vascular signs, and epidermal thickness in the lesional skin of both treated groups. These results can be explained by the ability of biological drugs to gradually shift lesion transcriptomes toward a non-pathological phenotype, reducing the expression of genes involved in type 2 inflammation and epidermal hyperplasia and increasing the expression of epidermal differentiation, barrier, and lipid metabolism genes [29]. According to the literature, SLEB at baseline was measurable on the affected skin in 100% of patients with AD [21–23]. In 72.2% of patients with AD, SLEB could also be detected on non-lesional skin. These data are significantly higher than those reported in the literature and can be explained by considering that ultrasound was performed using a 70 MHz probe (UHFUS), with an axial resolution of 30 µm and transverse resolution of 65 µm, which enable better skin resolution [22,23]. A statistically significant decrease in SLEB correlates with AD severity and may be an indicator of treatment effectiveness. The presence of a hypoechogenic band also in the perilesional skin of AD subjects would support the idea that there are subclinical eczematous reactions predictive of disease reactivation [23]. Particularly, the persistence of subclinical inflammation could identify patients who need to change or intensify therapy, as previously indicated in the literature [38,39]. In the lesional skin of patients with AD, a moderately-intensive vascular signal was detected in 100% of cases at baseline and not detected at T1 and T2. Physiological patterns of vascularization at baseline and follow-up visits were detected in non-lesional skin. A statistically significant decrease in vascular signal from baseline to T1 and T2 represents a useful marker of clinical inflammation. Data on vascular signals in AD affected and non-affected skin has been poorly evaluated in the literature. Conversely, vascular signals have been used to assess angiogenesis and malignant and metastatic potential in pigmented skin lesions and as a marker of clinical inflammation in psoriasis and hidradenitis suppurativa [40]. In AD, the vascular signal can be a useful marker of clinical inflammation, but unlike SLEB, it cannot be considered a marker of subclinical inflammation. Studies have shown that angiogenesis is increased in the lesional skin of individuals with AD, and the increased blood vessel density and vascular permeability contribute to skin redness and edema observed in AD flare-ups [41]. Additionally, the newly formed blood vessels facilitate the recruitment of immune cells to the affected skin, amplifying the inflammatory response even through vascular endothelial growth factor (VEGF), one of the key angiogenic factors implicated in AD and whose levels are Increased in AD skin lesions [42]. In Figure 2, there is a representation of the clinical and UHFUS evolution of a patient treated with dupilumab during the different time sets of our study, with a clear reduction of the vascular signal measured through the Doppler function.

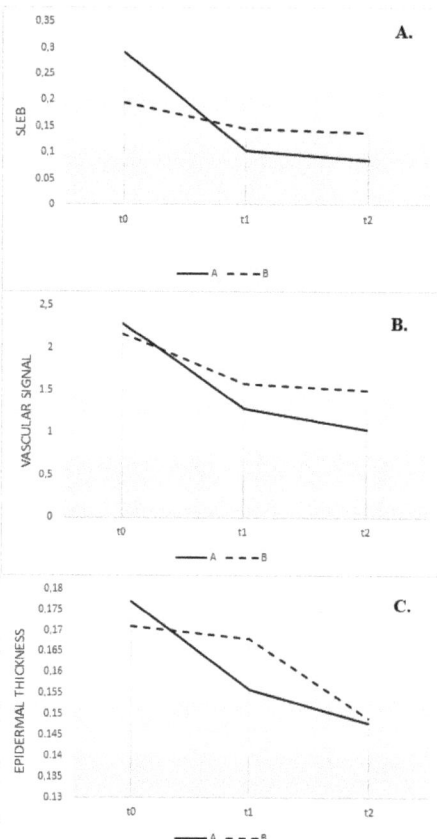

Figure 1. Subepidermal low-echogenic band (SLEB) reduction in lesional skin of the two groups, evaluated at baseline (t0), after 1 month (t1) and 2 months (t2) (**A**); the vascular signal in lesional skin of the two groups, evaluated at baseline (t0), after 1 month (t1) and 2 months (t2) (**B**); epidermal thickness in lesional skin of the two groups, evaluated at baseline (t0), after 1 month (t1) and 2 months (t2) (**C**).

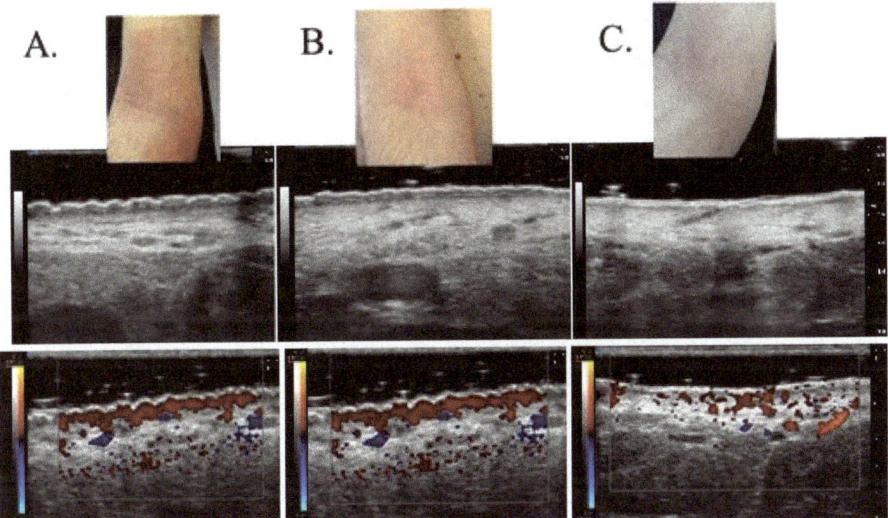

Figure 2. Clinical and UHFUS examination of a patient treated with dupilumab evaluated at baseline (t0) (**A**), after 1 month (t1) (**B**) and 2 months (t2) (**C**).

5. Conclusions

Our study displays a few limitations. The first one is represented by the differences in some clinical parameters at T0 between the two selected groups. However, the differences in the two groups can be easily explained by taking into account that Group A included patient candidates for the biologic therapy, which in Italy can be prescribed in adults patients only in the presence of a high burden of the disease measured through the classical clinical score of EASI that, consequently, leads to differences even in terms of IGA and quality of life indexes [43,44]. Another limitation is represented by the sample size. We expect that this pilot study can be expanded to achieve a higher level of statistical significance. It would also be interesting to include patients with different AD severity to objectify the correlation between clinical severity assessment and ultrasound parameters. Our study shows that SLEB measurements, vascular signals, and epidermal thickness can be used as objective parameters to monitor treatment efficacy in AD. To date, treatment monitoring has always been based on clinical remission of active lesions, but the presence of SLEB in non-lesional skin can be used as a marker of subclinical inflammation and can predict the development of clinical lesions, requiring active treatment. In conclusion, SLEB is a non-invasive, safe, and reproducible parameter, and it seems appropriate to combine ultrasound features of lesional and non-lesional skin with clinical scores to assess disease severity. Further investigations are needed to clarify the relationship between a decrease or disappearance of SLEB and a reduction in flares and prolongment of disease remission time. Combining UHFUS with clinical scores allows for a comprehensive evaluation of disease activity, guiding treatment decisions for better patient outcomes. Although this pilot study shows promising results, further research and larger-scale studies are necessary to validate the utility of UHFUS in routine clinical practice. The integration of advanced imaging techniques like UHFUS holds great potential to revolutionize AD management, leading to more effective and personalized treatment approaches for patients affected by this challenging skin condition.

Author Contributions: Conceptualization: V.D. and M.R.; Methodology: V.D. and M.R.; Validation: V.D., A.J., M.R. and T.O.; Formal Analysis: R.M. and M.I.; Investigation: M.I., A.M. and F.M.M.; Data Curation: M.I. and G.G.; Writing—Original Draft Preparation: M.I., V.D. and T.O.; Writing—Review

& Editing: M.I., A.M., G.S. and F.M.M.; Visualization: A.J., R.M. and G.G.; Supervision: V.D. and M.R.; Project Administration: V.D. All authors have read and agreed to the published version of the manuscript.

Funding: This research received no external funding.

Institutional Review Board Statement: The study was conducted in accordance with the Declaration of Helsinki, and approved by the Institutional Review Board (or Ethics Committee) of UO Dermatology, AOUP, Pisa (SUS1-AD ASTRA, 8 July 2019).

Informed Consent Statement: All patients in this manuscript have given written informed consent for participation in the study and the use of their de-identified, anonymized, aggregated data and their case details (including photographs) for publication.

Data Availability Statement: The data presented in this study are available on request from the corresponding author. The data are not publicly available due to privacy reasons.

Conflicts of Interest: The authors declare no conflict of interest.

References

1. Iannone, M.; Tonini, G.; Janowska, A.; Dini, V.; Romanelli, M. Definition of treatment goals in terms of clinician-reported disease severity and patient-reported outcomes in moderate-to-severe adult atopic dermatitis: A systematic review. *Curr. Med. Res. Opin.* **2021**, *37*, 1295–1301. [CrossRef] [PubMed]
2. Williams, H.; Robertson, C.; Stewart, A.; Aït-Khaled, N.; Anabwani, G.; Anderson, R.; Asher, I.; Beasley, R.; Björkstén, B.; Burr, M.; et al. Worldwide variations in the prevalence of symptoms of atopic eczema in the International Study of Asthma and Allergies in Childhood. *J. Allergy Clin. Immunol.* **1999**, *103*, 125. [CrossRef] [PubMed]
3. Odhiambo, J.A.; Williams, H.C.; Clayton, T.O.; Robertson, C.F.; Asher, M.I.; ISAAC Phase Three Study Group. Global variations in prevalence of eczema symptoms in children from ISAAC Phase Three. *J. Allergy Clin. Immunol.* **2009**, *124*, 1251. [CrossRef] [PubMed]
4. Sacotte, R.; Silverberg, J.I. Epidemiology of adult atopic dermatitis. *Clin. Dermatol.* **2018**, *36*, 595–605. [CrossRef] [PubMed]
5. Weidinger, S.; Novak, N. Atopic dermatitis. *Lancet* **2016**, *387*, 1109–1122. [CrossRef]
6. Calzavara Pinton, P.; Cristaudo, A.; Foti, C.; Canonica, G.W.; Balato, N.; Costanzo, A.; DEPità, O.; DESimone, C.; Patruno, C.; Pellacani, G.; et al. Diagnosis and management of moderate to severe adult atopic dermatitis: A Consensus by the Italian Society of Dermatology and Venereology (SIDeMaST), the Italian Association of Hospital Dermatologists (ADOI), the Italian Society of Allergy, Asthma and Clinical Immunology (SIAAIC), and the Italian Society of Allergological, Environmental and Occupational Dermatology (SIDAPA). *G. Ital. Dermatol. Venereol.* **2018**, *153*, 133–145.
7. Weidinger, S.; Beck, L.A.; Bieber, T.; Kabashima, K.; Irvine, A.D. Atopic dermatitis. *Nat. Rev. Dis. Primers.* **2018**, *4*, 1. [CrossRef]
8. Drucker, A.M.; Wang, A.R.; Li, W.Q.; Sevetson, E.; Block, J.K.; Qureshi, A.A. The Burden of Atopic Dermatitis: Summary of a Report for the National Eczema Association. *J. Investig. Dermatol.* **2017**, *137*, 26–30. [CrossRef]
9. Wollenberg, A.; Barbarot, S.; Bieber, T.; Christen-Zaech, S.; Deleuran, M.; Fink-Wagner, A.; Gieler, U.; Girolomoni, G.; Lau, S.; Muraro, A.; et al. Consensus-based European guidelines for treatment of atopic eczema (atopic dermatitis) in adults and children: Part I. *J. Eur. Acad. Dermatol. Venereol.* **2018**, *32*, 657–682, Erratum in *J. Eur. Acad. Dermatol. Venereol.* **2019**, *33*, 1436. [CrossRef]
10. Wollenberg, A.; Barbarot, S.; Bieber, T.; Christen-Zaech, S.; Deleuran, M.; Fink-Wagner, A.; Gieler, U.; Girolomoni, G.; Lau, S.; Muraro, A.; et al. Consensus-based European guidelines for treatment of atopic eczema (atopic dermatitis) in adults and children: Part II. *J. Eur. Acad. Dermatol. Venereol.* **2018**, *32*, 850–878. [CrossRef]
11. Harb, H.; Chatila, T.A. Mechanisms of Dupilumab. *Clin. Exp. Allergy* **2020**, *50*, 5–14. [CrossRef]
12. McKenzie, A.N.; Culpepper, J.A.; De Waal Malefyt, R.; Briere, F.; Punnonen, J.; Aversa, G.; Sato, A.; Dang, W.; Cocks, B.G.; Menon, S. Interleukin 13, a T-cell-derived cytokine that regulates human monocyte and B-cell function. *Proc. Natl. Acad. Sci. USA* **1993**, *90*, 3735–3739. [CrossRef] [PubMed]
13. Bao, L.; Zhang, H.; Chan, L.S. The involvement of the JAK-STAT signaling pathway in chronic inflammatory skin disease atopic dermatitis. *Jak-Stat* **2013**, *2*, e24137. [CrossRef]
14. Esche, C.; De Benedetto, A.; Beck, L.A. Keratinocytes in atopic dermatitis: Inflammatory signals. *Curr. Allergy Asthma Rep.* **2004**, *4*, 276–284. [CrossRef] [PubMed]
15. Vanbever, R.; Fouchard, D.; Jadoul, A.; De Morre, N.; Préat, V.; Marty, J.P. In vivo noninvasive evaluation of hairless rat skin after high-voltage pulse exposure. *Skin Pharmacol. Appl. Skin Physiol.* **1998**, *11*, 23–34. [CrossRef]
16. Kelleher, M.; Dunn-Galvin, A.; Hourihane, J.O.; Murray, D.; Campbell, L.E.; McLean, W.H.I.; Irvine, A.D. Skin barrier dysfunction measured by transepidermal water loss at 2 days and 2 months predates and predicts atopic dermatitis at 1 year. *J. Allergy Clin. Immunol.* **2015**, *135*, 930–935.e1. [CrossRef] [PubMed]
17. Osseiran, S.; Cruz, J.D.; Jeong, S.; Wang, H.; Fthenakis, C.; Evans, C.L. Characterizing stratum corneum structure, barrier function, and chemical content of human skin with coherent Raman scattering imaging. *Biomed. Opt. Express* **2018**, *9*, 6425–6443. [CrossRef]

18. Werner, Y. The water content of the stratum corneum in patients with atopic dermatitis. Measurement with the Corneometer CM 420. *Acta Derm.-Venereol.* **1986**, *66*, 281–284.
19. Kircik, L.H. Transepidermal water loss (TEWL) and corneometry with hydrogel vehicle in the treatment of atopic dermatitis: A randomized, investigator-blind pilot study. *J. Drugs Dermatol.* **2012**, *11*, 180–184.
20. Polańska, A.; Dańczak-Pazdrowska, A.; Jałowska, M.; Żaba, R.; Adamski, Z. Current applications of high-frequency ultrasonography in dermatology. *Postepy Dermatol. Alergol.* **2017**, *34*, 535–542. [CrossRef]
21. Polańska, A.; Dańczak-Pazdrowska, A.; Silny, W.; Woźniak, A.; Maksin, K.; Jenerowicz, D.; Janicka-Jedyńska, M. Comparison between high-frequency ultrasonography (Dermascan C, version 3) and histopathology in atopic dermatitis. *Skin Res. Technol.* **2013**, *19*, 432–437. [CrossRef] [PubMed]
22. Izzetti, R.; Vitali, S.; Aringhieri, G.; Nisi, M.; Oranges, T.; Dini, V.; Ferro, F.; Baldini, C.; Romanelli, M.; Caramella, D.; et al. Ultra-High Frequency Ultrasound, A Promising Diagnostic Technique: Review of the Literature and Single-Center Experience. *Can. Assoc. Radiol. J.* **2021**, *72*, 418–431. [CrossRef]
23. Sabău, M.; Boca, A.N.; Ilies, R.F.; Tătaru, A. Potential of high-frequency ultrasonography in the management of atopic dermatitis. *Exp. Ther. Med.* **2019**, *17*, 1073–1077. [CrossRef] [PubMed]
24. Simpson, E.L.; Bruin-Weller, M.; Flohr, C.; Ardern-Jones, M.R.; Barbarot, S.; Deleuran, M.; Bieber, T.; Vestergaard, C.; Brown, S.J.; Cork, M.J.; et al. When does atopic dermatitis warrant systemic therapy? Recommendations from an expert panel of the International Eczema Council. *J. Am. Acad. Dermatol.* **2017**, *77*, 623. [CrossRef]
25. Roekevisch, E.; Spuls, P.I.; Kuester, D.; Limpens, J.; Schmitt, J. Efficacy and safety of systemic treatments for moderate-to-severe atopic dermatitis: A systematic review. *J. Allergy Clin Immunol.* **2014**, *133*, 429. [CrossRef] [PubMed]
26. Schmitt, J.; von Kobyletzki, L.; Svensson, A.; Apfelbacher, C. Efficacy and tolerability of proactive treatment with topical corticosteroids and calcineurin inhibitors for atopic eczema: Systematic review and meta-analysis of randomized controlled trials. *Br. J. Dermatol.* **2011**, *164*, 415. [CrossRef]
27. Blauvelt, A.; de Bruin-Weller, M.; Gooderham, M.; Cather, J.C.; Weisman, J.; Pariser, D.; Simpson, E.L.; Papp, K.A.; Hong, H.C.H.; Rubel, D.; et al. Long-term management of moderate-to-severe atopic dermatitis with dupilumab and concomitant topical corticosteroids (LIBERTY AD CHRONOS): A 1-year, randomised, double-blinded, placebo-controlled, phase 3 trial. *Lancet* **2017**, *389*, 2287. [CrossRef]
28. Sawangjit, R.; Dilokthornsakul, P.; Lloyd-Lavery, A.; Lai, N.M.; Dellavalle, R.; Chaiyakunapruk, N. Systemic treatments for eczema: A network meta-analysis. *Cochrane Database Syst. Rev.* **2020**, *9*, CD013206. [CrossRef]
29. Guttman-Yassky, E.; Bissonnette, R.; Ungar, B.; Suárez-Fariñas, M.; Ardeleanu, M.; Esaki, H.; Suprun, M.; Estrada, Y.; Xu, H.; Peng, X.; et al. Dupilumab progressively improves systemic and cutaneous abnormalities in patients with atopic dermatitis. *J. Allergy Clin. Immunol.* **2019**, *143*, 155–172. [CrossRef]
30. Hamilton, J.D.; Suárez-Fariñas, M.; Dhingra, N.; Cardinale, I.; Li, X.; Kostic, A.; Ming, J.E.; Radin, A.R.; Krueger, J.G.; Graham, N.; et al. Dupilumab improves the molecular signature in skin of patients with moderate-to-severe atopic dermatitis. *J. Allergy Clin. Immunol.* **2014**, *134*, 1293–1300. [CrossRef]
31. Mihm, M.C., Jr.; Soter, N.A.; Dvorak, H.F.; Austen, K.F. The structure of normal skin and the morphology of atopic eczema. *J. Investig. Dermatol.* **1976**, *67*, 305–312. [CrossRef] [PubMed]
32. Suárez-Fariñas, M.; Tintle, S.J.; Shemer, A.; Chiricozzi, A.; Nograles, K.; Cardinale, I.; Duan, S.; Bowcock, A.M.; Krueger, J.G.; Guttman-Yassky, E. Nonlesional atopic dermatitis skin is characterized by broad terminal differentiation defects and variable immune abnormalities. *J. Allergy Clin. Immunol.* **2011**, *127*, 954–964. [CrossRef] [PubMed]
33. Fornage, B.D.; McGavran, M.H.; Duvic, M.; Waldron, C.A. Imaging of the skin with 20-MHz US. *Radiology* **1993**, *189*, 69–76. [CrossRef]
34. Gutierrez, M.; Wortsman, X.; Filippucci, E.; De Angelis, R.; Filosa, G.; Grassi, W. High-frequency sonography in the evaluation of psoriasis: Nail and skin involvement. *J. Ultrasound Med.* **2009**, *28*, 1569–1574. [CrossRef]
35. Marina, M.E.; Botar Jid, C.; Roman, I.I.; Mihu, C.M.; Tătaru, A.D. Ultrasonography in psoriatic disease. *Med. Ultrason.* **2015**, *17*, 377–382. [CrossRef] [PubMed]
36. Yazdanparast, T.; Yazdani, K.; Humbert, P.; Khatami, A.; Nasrollahi, S.A.; Firouzabadi, L.I.; Firooz, A. Biophysical Measurements and Ultrasonographic Findings in Chronic Dermatitis in Comparison with Uninvolved Skin. *Indian J. Dermatol.* **2019**, *64*, 90–96.
37. Polańska, A.; Jenerowicz, D.; Paszyńska, E.; Żaba, R.; Adamski, Z.; Dańczak-Pazdrowska, A. High-Frequency Ultrasonography-Possibilities and Perspectives of the Use of 20 MHz in Teledermatology. *Front. Med.* **2021**, *8*, 619965. [CrossRef] [PubMed]
38. Dańczak-Pazdrowska, A.; Polańska, A.; Silny, W.; Sadowska, A.; Osmola-Mańkowska, A.; Czarnecka-Operacz, M.; Zaba, R.; Jenerowicz, D. Seemingly healthy skin in atopic dermatitis: Observations with the use of high-frequency ultrasonography, preliminary study. *Skin Res. Technol.* **2012**, *18*, 162–167. [CrossRef]
39. Osmola-Mańkowska, A.; Polańska, A.; Silny, W.; Żaba, R.; Adamski, Z.; Dańczak-Pazdrowska, A. Topical tacrolimus vs medium-dose ultraviolet A1 phototherapy in the treatment of atopic dermatitis-A preliminary study in relation to parameters of the epidermal barrier function and high-frequency ultrasonography. *Eur. Rev. Med. Pharmacol. Sci.* **2014**, *18*, 3927–3934.
40. Jasaitiene, D.; Valiukeviciene, S.; Linkeviciute, G.; Raisutis, R.; Jasiuniene, E.; Kazys, R. Principles of high-frequency ultrasonography for investigation of skin pathology. *J. Eur. Acad. Dermatol. Venereol.* **2011**, *25*, 375–382. [CrossRef]
41. Lee, H.J.; Hong, Y.J.; Kim, M. Angiogenesis in Chronic Inflammatory Skin Disorders. *Int. J. Mol. Sci.* **2021**, *22*, 12035. [CrossRef] [PubMed]

42. Genovese, A.; Detoraki, A.; Granata, F.; Galdiero, M.R.; Spadaro, G.; Marone, G. Angiogenesis, lymphangiogenesis and atopic dermatitis. *Chem. Immunol. Allergy* **2012**, *96*, 50–60. [CrossRef] [PubMed]
43. Agenzia Italiana del Farmaco. DETERMINA 24 Novembre 2020. Regime di Rimborsabilita' e Prezzo a Seguito di Nuove Indicazioni Terapeutiche e Riclassificazione del Medicinale per uso Umano «Dupixent», ai sensi dell;art. 8, Comma 10, della Legge 24 Dicembre 1993, n. 537. (Determina n. DG/1204/2020). (20A06599). Available online: https://www.gazzettaufficiale.it/atto/serie_generale/caricaDettaglioAtto/originario?atto.dataPubblicazioneGazzetta=2020-12-09&atto.codiceRedazionale=20A06601&elenco30giorni=true (accessed on 24 November 2020).
44. Fargnoli, M.C.; Esposito, M.; Ferrucci, S.; Girolomoni, G.; Offidani, A.; Patrizi, A.; Peris, K.; Costanzo, A.; Malara, G.; Pellacani, G.; et al. Real-life experience on effectiveness and safety of dupilumab in adult patients with moderate-to-severe atopic dermatitis. *J. Dermatol. Treat.* **2021**, *32*, 507–513. [CrossRef] [PubMed]

Disclaimer/Publisher's Note: The statements, opinions and data contained in all publications are solely those of the individual author(s) and contributor(s) and not of MDPI and/or the editor(s). MDPI and/or the editor(s) disclaim responsibility for any injury to people or property resulting from any ideas, methods, instructions or products referred to in the content.

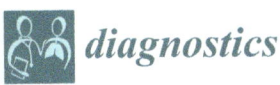

Article

Assessment and Monitoring of Nail Psoriasis with Ultra-High Frequency Ultrasound: Preliminary Results

Alessandra Michelucci [1,†], Valentina Dini [1,*,†], Giorgia Salvia [1], Giammarco Granieri [1], Flavia Manzo Margiotta [1], Salvatore Panduri [1], Riccardo Morganti [2] and Marco Romanelli [1]

1 Department of Dermatology, University of Pisa, 56126 Pisa, Italy; alessandra.michelucci@gmail.com (A.M.); giorgia.salvia2@gmail.com (G.S.); giammarcogranieri@gmail.com (G.G.); manzomargiottaflavia@gmail.com (F.M.M.); salvatore.panduri@ao.pisa.toscana.it (S.P.); marco.romanelli@unipi.it (M.R.)
2 Statistical Support to Clinical Trials Department, University of Pisa, 56126 Pisa, Italy; r.morganti@ao-pisa.toscana.it
* Correspondence: valentinadini74@gmail.com or valentina.dini@unipi.it; Tel.: +39-347-893-9729
† These authors contributed equally to this work.

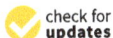

Citation: Michelucci, A.; Dini, V.; Salvia, G.; Granieri, G.; Manzo Margiotta, F.; Panduri, S.; Morganti, R.; Romanelli, M. Assessment and Monitoring of Nail Psoriasis with Ultra-High Frequency Ultrasound: Preliminary Results. *Diagnostics* **2023**, *13*, 2716. https://doi.org/10.3390/diagnostics13162716

Academic Editors: Francesco Inchingolo and Mariano Scaglione

Received: 26 June 2023
Revised: 25 July 2023
Accepted: 12 August 2023
Published: 21 August 2023

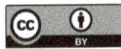

Copyright: © 2023 by the authors. Licensee MDPI, Basel, Switzerland. This article is an open access article distributed under the terms and conditions of the Creative Commons Attribution (CC BY) license (https://creativecommons.org/licenses/by/4.0/).

Abstract: Psoriatic onychopathy is one of the clinical presentations of psoriasis and a well-known risk factor for the development of psoriatic arthritis. High-frequency ultrasounds (HFUS > 20 MHz) have recently been used to evaluate the nail apparatus of healthy and psoriatic subjects. The aim of our study was to detect by means of ultra-high-frequency ultrasound (UHFUS 70–100 MHz) alterations of the nail bed and matrix in patients with psoriatic onychopathy and to monitor these parameters during the treatment with monoclonal antibody (mAb). We enrolled 10 patients with psoriatic onychopathy and naive to previous biologic therapies. Patients were evaluated at baseline, after 1 month and after 3 months from the beginning of mAb therapy by a complete clinical assessment and US evaluation. A UHFUS examination with a 70 MHz probe was performed on the thumbnail (I), the index fingernail (II) and the nail with greater clinical impairment (W). The following measurements were analyzed: nail plate thickness (A), nail bed thickness (B), nail insertion length (C), nail matrix length (D) and nail matrix thickness (E). Among the various parameters analyzed, some measures showed a statistically significant decrease with p-value < 0.05 (t0 WA = 0.52 mm vs. t2 WA = 0.42 mm; t0 WB = 2.8 mm vs. t2 WB = 2.4 mm; t0 WE = 0.76 mm vs. t2 WE = 0.64 mm; t0 IIA = 0.49 mm vs. t2 IIA = 0.39 mm). In conclusion, UHFUS could represent a viable imaging technique for the real-time evaluation and monitoring of psoriatic onychopathy, thus supporting the clinical parameters and revealing any subclinical signs of early drug response.

Keywords: psoriasis; ultra-high-frequency ultrasound; onycopathy; monoclonal antibodies

1. Introduction

Psoriasis is a chronic multisystemic and polymorphous inflammatory disease. In addition to the classic cutaneous presentation, represented by erythematous–desquamative lesions, the nail and musculoskeletal system could also be involved. The nail impairment can represent the exclusive clinical manifestation of the disease or, more frequently, it can be associated with cutaneous involvement [1,2]. Moreover, psoriatic onycopathy is a recognized risk factor for the development of psoriatic arthritis in patients with psoriasis. The nail apparatus is considered a link between the joint and the skin [3]. Since psoriasis often precedes psoriatic arthritis symptoms, dermatologists play a unique position in identifying psoriatic arthritis before the development of permanent joint damage [4]. Nail psoriasis severity index (NAPSI) is a clinical, standardized index used for quantifying the severity of nail psoriasis, analyzing nail matrix and bed alterations. Lesions involving the matrix are pitting, leuconichia, friability of the nail plate and red spots on the nail lunula. Lesions of the nail bed, on the other hand, are the oil-drop stain, onycholysis, subungual hyperkeratosis, splinter hemorrhages, Beau's lines and trachyonychia [5]. Although it is not a validated index, it remains the reference system in clinical trials regarding psoriatic onychopathy [6].

To date, the use of ultrasound (US) in the research field of psoriasis has focused on the role of US in the study of joints, tendons and entheses of patients with psoriatic arthritis. The development of devices provided with high-resolution probes and highly sensitive power Doppler (PD) allow detailed study of tissue morphostructural features and accurate assessment of minute changes in blood flow [7–9].

However, more recently, US imaging has been widely used for the evaluation of nail unit features [10]. Therefore, the use of a high-frequency ultrasound (HFUS), with >20 MHz probe, has also been employed in the descriptive analysis of various nail diseases, including psoriatic onychopathy [11,12]. In the early stages of psoriatic onychopathy, a loss of the typical hyperechogenicity of the ventral portion of the nail plate can be observed. As the disease progresses, more pronounced and distinctive changes become evident in the US images. In the more advanced stages of psoriatic onychopathy, the trilaminar aspect of the nail plate, which is characteristic of healthy nails, becomes completely lost. This profound transformation is a clear indicator of the severity of the disease and reflects the extent of nail involvement: in more advanced stages of disease, the nail plate appears as a thickened, wavy, hyperechoic and inhomogeneous layer [13,14].

The use of a ultra-high-frequency ultrasonography (UHFUS) with a 70 MHz probe allows to examine the more superficial cutaneous and adnexal features with a spatial resolution in the order of 30 µm, thus offering new capabilities for the exploration of different cutaneous and non-cutaneous districts, including nails and oral mucosa [15–18]. There are no data in the literature regarding an evaluation of the nail system of patients with psoriatic onychopathy by UHFUS. Nail psoriasis represents a difficult-to-treat site for the clinician; the various options available in addition to topical therapy include the use of conventional systemic therapy (systemic retinoids, methotrexate and cyclosporine) or biologics and synthetic targeted disease-modifying drugs. Biologics, such as tumor necrosis factor (TNF)-alpha inhibitors, Interleukin (IL)-17 inhibitors and IL-23 inhibitors, have demonstrated remarkable efficacy in treating psoriatic nail disease by specifically targeting key inflammatory pathways involved in the condition. These targeted therapies offer a more favorable safety profile compared to conventional systemic agents, as they are designed to selectively interfere with the underlying disease process while minimizing the impact on the immune system [19,20]. To date, monitoring of treatment response is based exclusively on clinical assessment; however, US could represent a repeatable, noninvasive imaging technique that can be used for objective assessment of treatment efficacy.

The aim of the study was to evaluate the role of UHFUS in the assessment of psoriatic onychopathy and in the therapeutic response of naive patients treated with biological therapy compared to clinical score and patient's quality of life. Finding a correlation between nail dystrophies, evaluated by NAPSI and US findings means developing a new and more objective way to identify and quantify the presence of nail involvement before its clinical appearance.

Moreover, UHFUS imaging could monitor US nail features improvement during the treatment and reveal any subclinical signs of drug effectiveness and nail psoriasis relapse.

2. Materials and Method

We conducted a prospective single-center study enrolling 10 patients with psoriasis and psoriatic onychopathy, in the absence of psoriatic arthritis, who started therapy with monoclonal antibodies (mAb) directed against TNF-alpha, (IL)-17 and IL-23. The patients were naive to previous conventional and biologic systemic therapies and were evaluated at baseline and after 1 month and after 3 months from the beginning of biologic therapy. At each visit, the clinical investigation was performed by a dermatologist expert in psoriasis who collected a photographic record of the patient and assessed clinical disease parameters such as the psoriasis area severity index (PASI), NAPSI, modified (m)-NAPSI calculated on the nail with major clinical alterations and dermatology life quality index (DLQI) [21–23]. For the US examination of the nail apparatus, a UHFUS with a 70 MHz probe was used (Vevo MD®® FUJIFILM VisualSonics, Toronto, ON, Canada). UHFUS investigation was performed by a dermatologist expert in UHFUS blinded from the clinical diagnosis. The fingernail examination was performed in a seated position with hands placed on a table. The proper distance of the probe from the skin, to permit imaging of superficial structures, was maintained with an appropriate amount of gel [23]. The fingernail apparatus was assessed in B-MODE with a longitudinal section on the middle point of the lamina. For each patient, the first (I) and second fingers (II) of the right hand and the nail with the worst clinical aspect (W) were examined. The following parameters were measured three times by the same operator who performed the UHFUS examination and the average value of the three measurements was recorded (Figure 1)

- Nail plate thickness: measured as the maximum distance between the dorsal and ventral hyperechoic plates of the nail (measure A).
- Nail bed thickness: measured as the maximum distance between the ventral plate of the nail and the edge of the phalangeal bone (measure B).
- Nail plate insertion: the non-visible part of the nail plate measured from its proximal point to its distal point (measure C).
- Nail matrix length: measured from the insertion of the nail plate to the proximal point of the matrix (measure D).
- Nail matrix thickness: measured at the point of maximum matrix thickness (measure E).

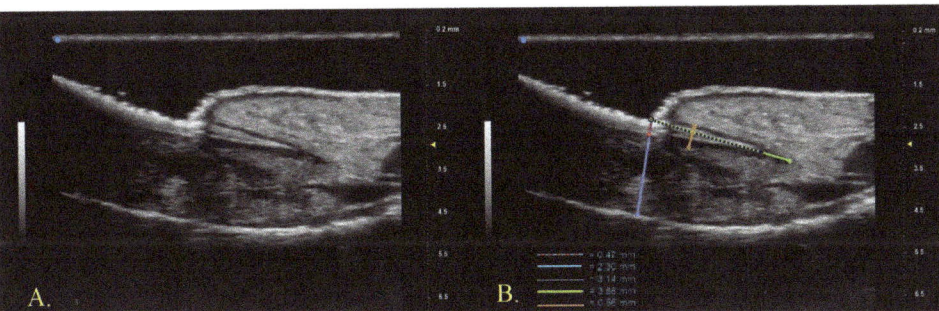

Figure 1. (**A**). UHFUS nail morphology; (**B**). UHFUS structural features measured: nail plate thickness, red-blue dotted line (measure A); nail bed thickness, blue line (measure B); nail plate insertion, purple-green dotted line (measure C); nail matrix length, green line (measure D); nail matrix thickness, orange line (measure E).

The target sample size was 10 patients, which provides 80% power at the 5% level of significance and an effect size equal to 0.1 between mean IIA at baseline and mean IIA at 3 months, with a standard deviation equal to 0.1.

Categorical data were described with absolute and relative (%) frequency and continuous data were summarized with mean and standard deviation. To compare repeated measures (t0, t1, t2) of the factors ANOVA for repeated measures was applied followed by multiple comparisons with the Bonferroni method. The significance was set at 0.05 and all analyses were carried out by SPSS v.28 technology.

3. Results

Our population consisted of 8/10 males (80%) and 2/10 females (20%), with a mean age of 51 years (39–63). In total, 7/10 patients (70%) were smokers or former smokers. The mean BMI was 26.7 (20.1–33.3). The mean time of disease was 18 years (5–31). All patients were naive to previous biologic therapies: three patients were treated with Adalimumab (anti TNF-alpha mAb); two patients started therapy with Ixekizumab (anti IL-17 mAb); four patients started therapy with Bimekizumab (anti IL-17A/F mAb); and one patient was treated with Tildrakizumab (anti IL-23 mAb). The clinical and US features evaluated at baseline (t0), after 1 month (t1) and after 3 months (t2) are shown in Table 1. At baseline, patients had a mean PASI of 17.5, a mean NAPSI of 40.6, an m-NAPSI calculated on the nail with major clinical changes of 9.6 and a DLQI of 12.6. A statistically significant (p-value < 0.05) improvement in the analyzed clinical parameters (mean PASI = 0.4; mean NAPSI = 22.9; mean m-NAPSI = 4.9; mean DLQI = 0) was detected after 3 months from the start of therapy. Among the various US parameters analyzed, some measures showed a statistically significant decrease with p-value < 0.05 (t0 WA = 0.52 mm vs. t2 WA = 0.42 mm; t0 WB = 2.8 mm vs. t2 WB = 2.4 mm; t0 WE = 0.76 mm vs. t2 WE = 0.64 mm; t0 IIA = 0.49 mm vs. t2 IIA = 0.39 mm). The other parameters showed a decreasing trend (measures IA, IB; IE, IIB, IIE) or an increasing trend (measures IC, ID, IIC, IIE, WC, WD) during the treatment. The results obtained from the comparison between repeated measures (t0, t1, t2) using multiple comparisons by the Bonferroni method are reported in Table 2.

Table 1. Comparison between repeated measures ANOVA. Statistics: mean (sd). Psoriasis area severity index (PASI), NAPSI, modified (m)-NAPSI, dermatology life quality index (DLQI), thumbnail (I), index fingernail (II) nail with worst clinical impairment (W), nail plate thickness (A), nail bed thickness (B), nail insertion length (C), nail matrix length (D) and nail matrix thickness (E).

Factor	t0	t1	t2	p-Value
PASI	17.5 (14.2)	5 (3.6)	0.4 (0.6)	0.017
NAPSI	40.6 (25.2)	40.6 (25.2)	22.9 (7.8)	0.032
mNAPSI	9.6 (4.1)	9.6 (4.1)	4.9 (1.8)	0.003
DLQI	12.6 (7.2)	3.4 (2.3)	0 (0)	<0.001
I A	0.47 (0.19)	0.46 (0.15)	0.38 (0.11)	0.109
I B	3.1 (0.7)	2.9 (1)	2.6 (0.3)	0.147
I C	3.9 (1.4)	4.3 (0.7)	4.1 (1.1)	0.506
I D	4.4 (1.3)	4.7 (0.7)	4.6 (1)	0.459
I E	0.66 (0.22)	0.61 (0.13)	0.58 (0.11)	0.236
II A	0.49 (0.14)	0.47 (0.16)	0.39 (0.07)	0.032
II B	2.8 (0.3)	2.8 (0.4)	2.6 (0.3)	0.057
II C	4.1 (1.3)	4.4 (1.1)	4.5 (1.1)	0.087
II D	4.9 (1.3)	5.3 (1.2)	5 (1.1)	0.448
II E	0.74 (0.25)	0.68 (0.19)	0.64 (0.13)	0.295
W A	0.52 (0.15)	0.48 (0.1)	0.42 (0.1)	0.039
W B	2.8 (0.3)	2.7 (0.5)	2.4 (0.3)	0.003
W C	4 (1.2)	4.2 (1.1)	4.1 (1.1)	0.275
W D	4.8 (1.1)	4.9 (1)	5.3 (1.1)	0.293
W E	0.76 (0.2)	0.71 (0.17)	0.64 (0.13)	0.025

Table 2. Multiple comparisons by Bonferroni method. Statistics: *p*-value. Psoriasis area severity index (PASI), NAPSI, modified (m)-NAPSI, dermatology life quality index (DLQI), thumbnail (I), index fingernail (II) nail with worst clinical impairment (W), nail plate thickness (A), nail bed thickness (B), nail insertion length (C), nail matrix length (D) and nail matrix thickness (E). Not evaluable (ne).

Factor	t0 vs. t1	t0 vs. t2	t1 vs. t2
PASI	0.022	0.014	0.010
NAPSI	ne	0.097	0.097
mNAPSI	ne	0.010	0.010
DLQI	0.010	0.001	0.003
II A	0.662	0.038	0.138
W A	0.478	0.054	0.061
W B	0.682	0.002	0.208
W E	0.868	0.040	0.144

4. Discussion

The diagnosis of nail psoriasis is usually clinical and the only severity index of psoriatic onychopathy is a strictly clinical and unvalidated score, called NAPSI. Our interest in researching US changes in the nail bed, lamina and matrix would allow us to identify an objective imaging score in addition to using NAPSI to assess the level of disease severity. To date, the application of US in psoriasis research has primarily concentrated on its role in investigating joints, tendons and entheses in patients with psoriatic arthritis. The advances in technology have led to the development of devices equipped with high-resolution probes and highly sensitive PD capabilities, enabling a more in-depth examination of tissue morphostructural characteristics and precise evaluation of minute changes in blood flow. Despite these significant advancements, the application of US in other aspects of psoriasis research still remains poorly investigated. With the introduction of UHFUS, attention has shifted towards exploring its usefulness in assessing nail psoriasis, with initial studies suggesting its potential to provide valuable insights into the severity and response to the treatment of psoriatic nail disease.

The healthy nail plate was described by HFUS examination (20 MHz) as two parallel hyperechogenic bands (railways sign), defined as the ventral and dorsal lamina of the nail plate. Between them, a hypoechogenic linear layer was detectable. The cuticle appeared as a proximally localized structure with echogenicity comparable to that of the ventral and dorsal lamina [24]. US changes of the nail plate in a patient with psoriatic onychopathy were detectable by a loss of echogenicity of the ventral plate in the early stage, and the involvement of the dorsal lamina with a complete loss of the trilaminar aspect in the advanced stages [25]. The qualitative severity of psoriatic nail alteration could be assessed ultrasonographically according to the classification presented by Wortsman et al.: type I was defined as focal, point-like hyperechoic involvement of the ventral plate; type II as continuous loss of the borders of the ventral plate; type III as the identification of wavy plates; and type IV as the complete loss of definition of both plates [26]. Also, in our study conducted with a UHFUS probe (70 MHz), we detected a trilaminar structure of the nail plate. However, the middle band presented a predominantly hypoechogenic and not totally anechogenic appearance, unlike studies in the literature.

The thickness of a normal plate varied between 0.3 and 0.65 mm [27]. Szymoniak-Lipska et al., in 2021, reported an average value in a population of healthy subjects of index fingernail plate thickness of 0.42 evaluated with a 20 MHz probe [24]. Gisondi et al. in 2012 identified with an 18 MHz probe that the average nail plate thickness of patients with psoriatic onychopathy and an average NAPSI of 18 was 0.9 mm and 0.82 mm for the thumbnail and the fingernail, respectively [28]. In another study, Idolazzi et al. identified, with an 18 MHz probe, an average value of 0.64 in a population of patients with psoriatic onychopathy with a mean NAPSI of 12.2 [11]. They also found a linear correlation between NAPSI and nail plate and bed thickness. Ally Essayed et al. identified the cut off for the diagnosis of nail psoriasis in a nail plate thickness above 0.63 mm and 0.61 mm for the thumb and the index finger, respectively (sensitivity 72% and 60% and specificity 70% and 88%, respectively) [29]. Our study collected data from a group of patients with a mean NAPSI of 40.6 and mNAPSI of 9.6 and reported mean values of nail plate thickness of 0.47 and 0.49 for the thumbnail and the index fingernail, respectively. Also, in our study, we found a correlation between higher mNAPSI and increased nail plate thickness: the plate thickness of the nail with major clinical changes was 0.52 mm.

The healthy nail bed appeared as a hypoechogenic structure localized between the ventral nail plate and the periosteum of the distal phalanx, with a thickness that ranged from 0.7 to 6.5 mm [27]. The study conducted by Ally Essayed et al. in 2015 identified a thickness of the nail bed above 1.85 mm and 1.89 mm, for the thumbnail bed and the index fingernail, respectively, to define nail psoriasis [29]. However, there was no agreement about the thickness of the nail bed to define a pathological condition. Another study identified nail bed thickness above 2.0 mm as a cut-off point for the diagnosis of psoriatic changes [30]. In more advanced stages, an increase in the distance between the ventral plate and the bony margin of the distal phalanx (>2.5 mm) was detectable [25]. Gisondi et al. in 2012 identified a mean thumbnail bed thickness of 2.95 mm in a population of patients with psoriatic onychopathy and a mean NAPSI of 18 [28]. Idolazzi et al. identified, with an 18 MHz probe, an average value of 2.5 in a population of patients with psoriatic onychopathy with a mean NAPSI of 12.2 [11]. Finally, it has been shown that nail bed thickness and plate thickness were higher in patients with psoriasis and psoriatic arthritis, with or without nail clinical involvement, compared to healthy nails [31,32].

Our study reported mean values of nail bed thickness of 3.1 mm and 2.8 mm for the thumbnail and the index fingernail, respectively. Compared to the previous study our results in terms of mean plate and bed thickness reported some differences that could be associated with the higher mean NAPSI and mNAPSI values of our population, as well as the use of UHFUS with greater axial resolution and the landmarks used for measurement. Establishing a correlation between nail dystrophies, as assessed by NAPSI, and US findings represent a significant advancement in the field of psoriasis research. Such a correlation could give new insight into the development of a novel and more objective scoring system for measuring disease severity related to nail involvement. Unlike traditional subjective assessments, UHFUS would provide a standardized and quantifiable measure of the extent and severity of nail psoriasis, leading to more accurate disease monitoring and treatment evaluation.

Few studies were reported in the literature regarding US monitoring of the nail system in subjects with psoriatic onychopathy undergoing systemic therapy. One study showed that 6 months of methotrexate therapy was able to reduce nail plate, bed and matrix thickness in patients with psoriatic onychopathy [33]. A second study revealed a reduction in matrix and nail bed thickness of patients with psoriatic onychopathy treated with acitretin [34]. There were no data in the literature regarding US monitoring of nail features with a 70 MHz probe in patients treated with mAb. Our study demonstrated that treatment with mAb anti-TNF-alpha and anti-IL determined a decrease in the nail plate and bed thickness. The statistically significant reduction in clinical parameters over time was associated with a statistically significant reduction in the nail plate thickness value of the index finger (t0 IIA = 0.49 mm vs. t2 IIA = 0.39 mm) and the finger with major clinical impairment (t0 WA = 0.52 mm vs. t2 WA = 0.42 mm) as well as a reduction in the nail bed measurement of the finger with major clinical alterations (t0 WB = 2.8 mm vs. t2 WB = 2.4 mm). The measures of lamina thickness and nail bed thickness of the other nail fingers also showed a tendency to decrease over time. UHFUS imaging's role in monitoring the improvement of US nail features during systemic treatment is particularly promising. As an innovative biologic therapy, mAb anti-TNF-alpha and anti-IL have shown considerable efficacy in treating psoriasis, including nail psoriasis. UHFUS imaging could act as a valuable tool in assessing treatment response, allowing clinicians to visualize and objectively measure the changes in nail structures over time. This monitoring capability could help in personalizing therapeutic approaches to optimize patient outcomes. Additionally, the early detection of subclinical signs of drug effectiveness and potential nail psoriasis relapse with UHFUS imaging is a significant advancement. Identifying signs of treatment response or relapse earlier than traditional clinical assessments may enable prompt adjustments to therapy, ensuring patients receive the most effective and timely interventions.

The proximal nail fold was described by studies in the literature as a structure with lower echogenicity than the ventral and dorsal plates of the nail plate [24]. In contrast, examination with a 70 MHz probe allowed precise identification of the appearance of the nail plate insertion in the distal phalanx. The dorsal and ventral plates continued beyond the cuticle as two hyperechogenic bands that converged proximally with a hypoechogenic layer in the middle. The sharpness and linearity of the US bands were higher in subjects with fewer detectable clinical changes (lower NAPSI and m-NAPSI). No data regarding the measurement of nail plate insertion length in the distal phalanx were available in the literature. The data found from our study showed that the clinical improvement detectable by a reduction in NAPSI and m-NAPSI due to treatment was associated with elongation and increased linearity of the nail plate insertion (Figure 2).

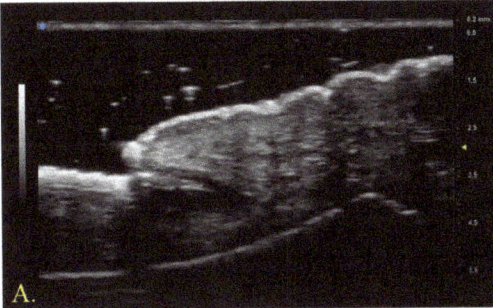 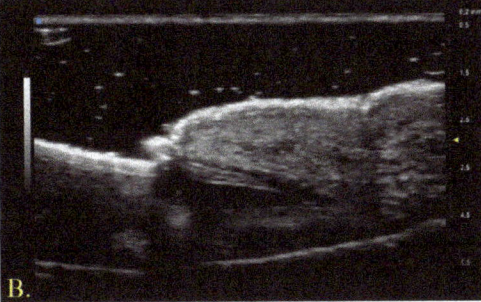

Figure 2. UHFUS (70 MHz) examination of nail apparatus, evaluated at baseline (**A**) and after 3 months of Ixekizumab (**B**).

It could be hypothesized that the inflammatory state of the matrix and the periungual tissues of patients with psoriatic onychopathy caused an increase in the level of mechanical compression in the nail insertion determining qualitative and quantitative US alterations. The improvement of these parameters during the treatment with anti-IL mAbs, able to reduce the inflammatory burden, would support our hypothesis, although further studies are needed to confirm these preliminary data.

The matrix was defined as a hypoechoic structure with blurred borders, near the nail fold, 1–5.3 mm long, detectable in a minority of subjects and variable in different types of fingers. The matrix was identified with more precision in the fourth and fifth fingers and more often in female patients [24]. Our study defined the nail matrix as a hypoechogenic structure that surrounded the nail insertion in the distal phalanx, whose linearity and US sharpness were higher in patients with lower nail changes at baseline and after treatment with mAb. In our study, we also measured nail matrix length reporting higher values for patients with fewer clinical alterations at baseline and after treatment with mAb. US studies in patients with nail PsO also revealed significantly increased thickness of nail matrix compared to healthy nails. In particular, Krajewska-Włodarczyk reported mean nail matrix thickness values of 1.96 mm in patients with psoriatic onychopathy obtained with a linear probe with a frequency ranging from 12 to 48 MHz. [35] The importance of an objective assessment of nail matrix impairment was related to the association between the involvement of the distal interphalangeal joint and the nail root inflammation. Psoriatic arthritis is a complex condition that involves not only the skin but also the musculoskeletal system. Recent advancements in US measurements gave new insight into the evaluation of nail alterations in subjects with psoriatic arthritis, offering valuable insights into the disease's underlying pathophysiology. In the pathophysiology of psoriatic arthritis, the central role of TNF-α and IL-17 had been highlighted. MAbs directed against these molecules had shown potential efficacy in reducing early signs of psoriatic arthritis activity, representing a significant clinical–therapeutic challenge. Optimizing the early management of psoriasis patients through targeted biologic therapies could potentially prevent or slow down the progression of arthritis, leading to better long-term outcomes and improving the quality of life for affected individuals. Nail involvement in psoriasis patients has been recognized as a significant risk factor for developing psoriatic arthritis, emphasizing the importance of nail assessments in dermatological practice. Dermatologists play a pivotal role in the early detection of psoriatic arthritis, as psoriasis often precedes joint manifestations. Recognizing patients before permanent joint damage occurs is crucial for initiating timely and appropriate interventions to improve patient outcomes. However, the possibility that psoriatic nail disease may be related to enthesis microdamage or mechanically stressed tissues still awaits confirmation by high-resolution imaging [36]. Our study reported a mean nail matrix thickness value of 0.66 mm for the thumbnail, 0.74 mm for the index fingernail and 0.76 mm for the fingernail with major clinical impairment. A statistically significant reduction was found for matrix thickness of the nail with greater clinical changes after 3 months of therapy (t0WE 0.76 mm vs. t2WE 0.64 mm). The differences observed between our values and those presented in the literature are likely related to the differences in the population analyzed (higher NAPSI and mNAPSI), the different US frequencies used, and the landmarks chosen to perform the measurement. As in the case of nail insertion, it is possible to hypothesize that the inflammatory burden of the periungual tissues is able to cause alterations such as quantitative changes at the level of the nail matrix. The decrease in inflammatory load following treatment would reduce mechanical and inflammatory compression at the level of the matrix, leading to its elongation and decrease in thickness, as well as an improvement in its sharpness, evaluated by US examination. Finally, our study demonstrated that treatment with mAb determines an improvement in US nail features even before a reduction in the corresponding clinical index: after one month of therapy, a decreasing trend in measures A, B, E and an increasing trend in measures C and D in the absence of a change in clinical values were detected for all the fingernails analyzed.

5. Conclusions

Several studies in the literature reported the use of HFUS in assessing the severity of psoriatic nail disease and its correlation with clinical parameters (mNAPSI or NAPSI) following the introduction of pharmacological therapy. We presented, for the first time, the preliminary results obtained using UHFUS as an objective parameter for psoriatic onychopathy assessment and monitoring, able to support clinical evaluation in future clinical trials and studies. Moreover, UHFUS would allow early assessment of nail changes even before clinical changes are detectable. From our study, the measurements of the nail apparatus obtained through UHFUS showed a correlation with the clinical improvement of psoriatic nail disease, sometimes even anticipating it. For example, during the first month of therapy, a significant reduction in nail plate thickness was observed in the absence of an obvious clinical improvement in NAPSI and mNAPSI. Therefore, we believe that this tool can be used to identify subclinical modifications that are not directly detectable during a dermatological clinical examination. The clinical improvement becomes evident months after the start of therapy, raising the suspicion of a lack of therapeutic response. However, changes in UHFUS parameters appearing earlier could be suggestive of an initial response to pharmacological therapy and could guide the decision to maintain a particular pharmacological treatment. Furthermore, evaluating a larger number of patients on different pharmacological therapies could reveal, through intergroup analysis, which drug can provide a faster and more effective improvement in psoriatic nail disease. This would also guide the initial choice of pharmacological treatment. Finally, because of the close anatomical relationship between the enthesis and the nail root, the evidence of early US changes in patients with early psoriatic arthritis could play a role in the early management and prevention of irreversible joint damage. Nails are integral components of the musculoskeletal system, acting as a link between the joints and the integument. Therefore, understanding nail alterations could offer valuable clues about the underlying joint disease and support early diagnosis and disease management. Collaborative efforts between dermatologists, rheumatologists, and other healthcare professionals are crucial in ensuring comprehensive care for patients affected by psoriasis and psoriatic arthritis. The main limitation of this study is related to the small sample and the absence of a comparison between the different treatment outcomes. In conclusion, the incorporation of UHFUS imaging in the evaluation of nail psoriasis represents a promising step towards more precise and objective disease assessment. It has the potential to revolutionize the way we understand, diagnose, and treat nail psoriasis, ultimately leading to better patient care and improved long-term outcomes. As research in this area continues to evolve, we can expect UHFUS imaging to play a pivotal role in shaping the future of psoriasis management. Further investigations with prolonged observation time and a greater number of patients will be necessary to confirm the suggested hypotheses.

Author Contributions: Conceptualization: V.D. and M.R.; Methodology: V.D. and M.R.; Validation: V.D., M.R. and S.P.; Formal Analysis: R.M. and S.P.; Investigation: A.M., G.S. and G.G.; Data Curation: G.S. and F.M.M.; Writing—Original Draft Preparation: A.M., G.S. and F.M.M.; Writing—Review and Editing: A.M., G.S. and F.M.M.; Visualization: S.P., R.M. and G.G.; Supervision: V.D. and M.R.; Project Administration: V.D. All authors have read and agreed to the published version of the manuscript.

Funding: This research received no external funding.

Institutional Review Board Statement: The study was conducted in accordance with the Declaration of Helsinki, and approved by the Institutional Review Board (or Ethics Committee) of UO Dermatology, AOUP, Pisa (SUS1-AD ASTRA, 08/07/2019).

Informed Consent Statement: All patients in this manuscript have given written informed consent for participation in the study and the use of their de-identified, anonymized, aggregated data and their case details (including photographs) for publication.

Data Availability Statement: Data Availability Statement: The data presented in this study are available on request from the corresponding author. The data are not publicly available due to privacy reasons.

Conflicts of Interest: The authors declare no conflict of interest.

References

1. Griffiths, C.E.M.; Armstrong, A.W.; Gudjonsson, J.E.; Barker, J.N.W.N. Psoriasis. *Lancet* **2021**, *397*, 1301–1315. [CrossRef] [PubMed]
2. Canal-García, E.; Bosch-Amate, X.; Belinchón, I.; Puig, L. Nail Psoriasis. *Actas Dermosifiliogr.* **2022**, *113*, 481–490. [CrossRef] [PubMed]
3. Scher, J.U.; Ogdie, A.; Merola, J.F.; Ritchlin, C. Preventing psoriatic arthritis: Focusing on patients with psoriasis at increased risk of transition. *Nat. Rev. Rheumatol.* **2019**, *15*, 153–166. [CrossRef]
4. Messina, F.; Valenti, M.; Malagoli, P.; Dattola, A.; Gisondi, P.; Burlando, M.; Dapavo, P.; Dini, V.; Franchi, C.; Loconsole, F.; et al. Early predictors of psoriatic arthritis: A Delphi-based consensus from Italian dermatology centers. *Ital. J. Dermatol. Venerol.* **2022**, *157*, 231–234. [CrossRef] [PubMed]
5. Battista, T.; Scalvenzi, M.; Martora, F.; Potestio, L.; Megna, M. Nail Psoriasis: An Updated Review of Currently Available Systemic Treatments. *Clin Cosmet Investig Dermatol.* **2023**, *16*, 1899–1932. [CrossRef]
6. Rich, P.; Scher, R.K. Nail Psoriasis Severity Index: A useful tool for evaluation of nail psoriasis. *J. Am. Acad. Dermatol.* **2003**, *49*, 206–212. [CrossRef]
7. Gutierrez, M.; Filippucci, E.; De Angelis, R.; Filosa, G.; Kane, D.; Grassi, W. A sonographic spectrum of psoriatic arthritis: "The five targets". *Clin. Rheumatol.* **2010**, *29*, 133–142. [CrossRef]
8. Tan, A.L.; McGonagle, D. Imaging of seronegative spondyloarthritis. *Best. Pract. Res. Clin. Rheumatol.* **2008**, *22*, 1045–1059. [CrossRef]
9. Mease, P.J.; Armstrong, A.W. Managing patients with psoriatic disease: The diagnosis and pharmacologic treatment of psoriatic arthritis in patients with psoriasis. *Drugs* **2014**, *74*, 423–441. [CrossRef]

10. Aluja Jaramillo, F.; Quiasúa Mejía, D.C.; Martínez Ordúz, H.M.; González Ardila, C. Nail unit ultrasound: A complete guide of the nail diseases. *J. Ultrasound.* **2017**, *20*, 181–192. [CrossRef]
11. Idolazzi, L.; Zabotti, A.; Fassio, A.; Errichetti, E.; Benini, C.; Vantaggiato, E.; Rossini, M.; De Vita, S.; Viapiana, O. The ultrasonographic study of the nail reveals differences in patients affected by inflammatory and degenerative conditions. *Clin. Rheumatol.* **2019**, *38*, 913–920. [CrossRef] [PubMed]
12. Moreno, M.; Lisbona, M.P.; Gallardo, F.; Deza, G.; Ferran, M.; Pontes, C.; Luelmo, J.; Maymó, J.; Gratacós, J. Ultrasound Assessment of Psoriatic Onychopathy: A Cross-sectional Study Comparing Psoriatic Onychopathy with Onychomycosis. *Acta Derm. Venereol.* **2019**, *99*, 164–169. [CrossRef] [PubMed]
13. Krajewska-Włodarczyk, M.; Owczarczyk-Saczonek, A. Usefulness of Ultrasound Examination in the Assessment of the Nail Apparatus in Psoriasis. *Int. J. Env. Res. Public. Health* **2022**, *19*, 5611. [CrossRef]
14. Cunha, J.S.; Qureshi, A.A.; Reginato, A.M. Nail Enthesis Ultrasound in Psoriasis and Psoriatic Arthritis: A Report from the 2016 GRAPPA Annual Meeting. *J. Rheumatol.* **2017**, *44*, 688–690. [CrossRef]
15. Berritto, D.; Iacobellis, F.; Rossi, C.; Reginelli, A.; Cappabianca, S.; Grassi, R. Ultra high-frequency ultrasound: New capabilities for nail anatomy exploration. *J. Dermatol.* **2017**, *44*, 43–46. [CrossRef] [PubMed]
16. Dini, V.; Janowska, A.; Faita, F.; Panduri, S.; Benincasa, B.B.; Izzetti, R.; Romanelli, M.; Oranges, T. Ultra-high-frequency ultrasound monitoring of plaque psoriasis during Ixekizumab treatment. *Ski. Res. Technol.* **2021**, *27*, 277–282. [CrossRef] [PubMed]
17. Izzetti, R.; Vitali, S.; Aringhieri, G.; Nisi, M.; Oranges, T.; Dini, V.; Ferro, F.; Baldini, C.; Romanelli, M.; Caramella, D.; et al. Ultra-High Frequency Ultrasound, A Promising Diagnostic Technique: Review of the Literature and Single-Center Experience. *Can. Assoc. Radiol. J.* **2021**, *72*, 418–431. [CrossRef]
18. Faita, F.; Oranges, T.; Di Lascio, N.; Ciompi, F.; Vitali, S.; Aringhieri, G.; Janowska, A.; Romanelli, M.; Dini, V. Ultra-high-frequency ultrasound and machine learning approaches for the differential diagnosis of melanocytic lesions. *Exp. Dermatol.* **2022**, *31*, 94–98. [CrossRef]
19. Sarma, N. Evidence and Suggested Therapeutic Approach in Psoriasis of Difficult-to-treat Areas: Palmoplantar Psoriasis, Nail Psoriasis, Scalp Psoriasis, and Intertriginous Psoriasis. *Indian. J. Dermatol.* **2017**, *62*, 113–122. [CrossRef]
20. Zhang, X.; Xie, B.; He, Y. Efficacy of Systemic Treatments of Nail Psoriasis: A Systemic Literature Review and Meta-Analysis. *Front. Med.* **2021**, *8*, 620562. [CrossRef]
21. Cassell, S.E.; Bieber, J.D.; Rich, P.; Tutuncu, Z.N.; Lee, S.J.; Kalunian, K.C.; Wu, C.W.; Kavanaugh, A. The modified Nail Psoriasis Severity Index: Validation of an instrument to assess psoriatic nail involvement in patients with psoriatic arthritis. *J. Rheumatol.* **2007**, *34*, 123–129.
22. Finlay, A.Y.; Khan, G.K. Dermatology Life Quality Index (DLQI)--a simple practical measure for routine clinical use. *Clin. Exp. Dermatol.* **1994**, *19*, 210–216. [CrossRef] [PubMed]
23. Granieri, G.; Oranges, T.; Morganti, R.; Janowska, A.; Romanelli, M.; Manni, E.; Dini, V. Ultra-high frequency ultrasound detection of the dermo-epidermal junction: Its potential role in dermatology. *Exp. Dermatol.* **2022**, *31*, 1863–1871. [CrossRef] [PubMed]
24. Szymoniak-Lipska, M.; Polańska, A.; Jenerowicz, D.; Lipski, A.; Żaba, R.; Adamski, Z.; Dańczak-Pazdrowska, A. High-Frequency Ultrasonography and Evaporimetry in Non-invasive Evaluation of the Nail Unit. *Front. Med.* **2021**, *8*, 686470. [CrossRef] [PubMed]
25. Agache, M.; Popescu, C.C.; Enache, L.; Dumitrescu, B.M.; Codreanu, C. Nail Ultrasound in Psoriasis and Psoriatic Arthritis-A Narrative Review. *Diagnostics* **2023**, *13*, 2236. [CrossRef] [PubMed]
26. Wortsman, X.; Gutierrez, M.; Saavedra, T.; Honeyman, J. The role of ultrasound in rheumatic skin and nail lesions: A multispecialist approach. *Clin. Rheumatol.* **2011**, *30*, 739–748. [CrossRef] [PubMed]
27. Cecchini, A.; Montella, A.; Ena, P.; Meloni, G.B.; Mazzarello, V. Ultrasound anatomy of normal nails unit with 18 mHz linear transducer. *Ital. J. Anat. Embryol.* **2009**, *114*, 137–144.
28. Gisondi, P.; Idolazzi, L.; Girolomoni, G. Ultrasonography reveals nail thickening in patients with chronic plaque psoriasis. *Arch. Dermatol. Res.* **2012**, *304*, 727–732. [CrossRef]
29. Ally Essayed, S.M.; Al-Shatouri, M.A.; Nasr Allah, Y.S.; Atwa, M.A. Ultrasonographic characterization of the nails in patients with psoriasis and onychomycosis. *Egypt. J. Radiol. Nucl. Med.* **2015**, *46*, 733–739. [CrossRef]
30. Sandobal, C.; Carbó, E.; Iribas, J.; Roverano, S.; Paira, S. Ultrasound nail imaging on patients with psoriasis and psoriatic arthritis compared with rheumatoid arthritis and control subjects. *J. Clin. Rheumatol.* **2014**, *20*, 21–24. [CrossRef]
31. Marina, M.E.; Solomon, C.; Bolboaca, S.D.; Bocsa, C.; Mihu, C.M.; Tătaru, A.D. High-frequency sonography in the evaluation of nail psoriasis. *Med. Ultrason.* **2016**, *18*, 312–317. [CrossRef] [PubMed]
32. Gutierrez-Manjarrez, J.; Gutierrez, M.; Bertolazzi, C.; Afaro-Rodriguez, A.; Pineda, C. Ultrasound as a useful tool to integrate the clinical assessment of nail involvement in psoriatic arthritis. *Reumatologia* **2018**, *56*, 42–44. [CrossRef] [PubMed]
33. Krajewska-Włodarczyk, M.; Owczarczyk-Saczonek, A.; Placek, W.; Wojtkiewicz, M.; Wojtkiewicz, J. Effect of Methotrexate in the Treatment of Distal Interphalangeal Joint Extensor Tendon Enthesopathy in Patients with Nail Psoriasis. *J. Clin. Med.* **2018**, *7*, 546. [CrossRef] [PubMed]
34. Krajewska-Włodarczyk, M.; Zuber, Z.; Owczarczyk-Saczonek, A. Ultrasound Evaluation of the Effectiveness of the Use of Acitretin in the Treatment of Nail Psoriasis. *J. Clin. Med.* **2021**, *10*, 2122. [CrossRef]

35. Krajewska-Włodarczyk, M.; Owczarczyk-Saczonek, A.; Placek, W.; Wojtkiewicz, M.; Wiktorowicz, A.; Wojtkiewicz, J. Ultrasound Assessment of Changes in Nails in Psoriasis and Psoriatic Arthritis. *BioMed Res. Int.* **2018**, *2018*, 8251097. [CrossRef]
36. McGonagle, D. Enthesitis: An autoinflammatory lesion linking nail and joint involvement in psoriatic disease. *J. Eur. Acad. Dermatol. Venereol.* **2009**, *23* (Suppl. S1), 9–13. [CrossRef]

Disclaimer/Publisher's Note: The statements, opinions and data contained in all publications are solely those of the individual author(s) and contributor(s) and not of MDPI and/or the editor(s). MDPI and/or the editor(s) disclaim responsibility for any injury to people or property resulting from any ideas, methods, instructions or products referred to in the content.

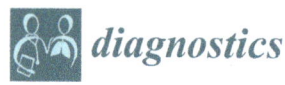

Article

Ultra-High-Frequency Ultrasonography of Labial Glands in Pediatric Sjögren's Disease: A Preliminary Study

Edoardo Marrani [1,*], Giovanni Fulvio [2], Camilla Virgili [1], Rossana Izzetti [3], Valentina Dini [4], Teresa Oranges [5], Chiara Baldini [2] and Gabriele Simonini [1,6]

1. Rheumatology Unit, AOU Meyer IRCCS, 50139 Firenze, Italy
2. Rheumatology Unit, Department of Clinical and Experimental Medicine, University of Pisa, 56126 Pisa, Italy
3. Dentistry and Oral Surgery, AOU Pisana, 56126 Pisa, Italy
4. Dermatology Unit, AOU Pisana, 56126 Pisa, Italy
5. Dermatology Unit, AOU Meyer IRCCS, 50139 Firenze, Italy
6. Neurosciences, Psychology, Drug Research and Child Health (NEUROFARBA) Department, University of Firenze, 50139 Firenze, Italy
* Correspondence: edoardo.marrani@meyer.it; Tel.: +39-0555662924

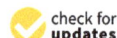

Citation: Marrani, E.; Fulvio, G.; Virgili, C.; Izzetti, R.; Dini, V.; Oranges, T.; Baldini, C.; Simonini, G. Ultra-High-Frequency Ultrasonography of Labial Glands in Pediatric Sjögren's Disease: A Preliminary Study. *Diagnostics* 2023, 13, 2695. https://doi.org/10.3390/diagnostics13162695

Academic Editor: Po-Hsiang Tsui

Received: 23 July 2023
Revised: 14 August 2023
Accepted: 15 August 2023
Published: 16 August 2023

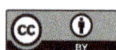

Copyright: © 2023 by the authors. Licensee MDPI, Basel, Switzerland. This article is an open access article distributed under the terms and conditions of the Creative Commons Attribution (CC BY) license (https://creativecommons.org/licenses/by/4.0/).

Abstract: Sjögren's disease (SD) is a chronic autoimmune disease primarily affecting lacrimal and salivary glands. The diagnosis of pediatric SD mostly relies on clinical suspect, resulting in a significant diagnostic delay. Recently, ultrahigh-frequency ultrasound (UHFUS) of labial glands has been proposed as a diagnostic method in adults with suspected SD. Until now, there have been no studies about UHFUS in pediatric diagnostic work-up. The aim of the study was to evaluate the potential role of UHFUS of minor salivary glands in pediatric SD. Consecutive pediatric patients with a diagnosis of pediatric SD seen at AOU Meyer IRCSS were evaluated. Intraoral UHFUS scan of the lip mucosa was performed with Vevo MD equipment, using a 70 MHz probe with a standardized protocol and the images were independently reviewed by two operators. Lip salivary glands were assessed by using a four-grade semiquantitative scoring system for parenchymal alteration and vascularization. Twelve patients were included. When applying UHFUS to this cohort of patients, all patients showed a UHFUS grade of ≥1 with 8/12 showing a mild glandular alteration (i.e., grade 1), 2/12 a moderate glandular alteration (i.e., grade 2) and finally 2/12 a severe glandular alteration (i.e., grade 3). Moderate intraglandular vascularization was seen in 9/12, with only 3/12 showing mild intraglandular vascularization. Due to limited size of the sample, the relationship between histological findings, autoantibodies status and UHFUS grade could not be performed. This preliminary study seems to report UHFUS as feasibility technique to identify salivary gland alterations in children with a clinical suspect of SD.

Keywords: Sjögren's syndrome; pediatric Sjögren's disease; ultrahigh-frequency ultrasound; labial salivary glands; childhood-onset Sjögren's syndrome

1. Introduction

Sjögren's disease (SD) is a chronic autoimmune disease primarily affecting lacrimal and salivary glands. It presents a spectrum of manifestations, ranging from organ-specific autoimmune symptoms to a systemic disorder, and even to an increased risk of B cell lymphoma. Most common symptoms are dry eyes (keratoconjunctivitis sicca) and dry mouth (xerostomia) [1,2].

On the contrary, in children, symptoms of dryness are infrequent due to the low damage burden and the physiological increase in secretory function: recurrent swelling of the parotid glands is commonly reported, but also unspecific symptoms such as arthralgia [1,3,4].

The first official description of a case of pediatric SD was published in 1965 [5], but a description published in 1938 of sicca syndrome and recurrent salivary gland swelling in a 17-year-old girl could represent the first published case of SD in childhood [6].

Nowadays, the diagnosis is established adopting the American College of Rheumatology/European League Against Rheumatism (ACR/EULAR) classification criteria, which are specifically designed for adults [7].

Recently, ultrahigh-frequency ultrasound (UHFUS) of labial glands has been proposed as a novel tool for the noninvasive assessment of labial salivary gland involvement in adults with suspected SD.

Ultrahigh-frequency ultrasound (UHFUS) is a technique, recently introduced, characterized by using ultrasound frequencies in the range between 30 and 100 MHz. Instead, conventional ultrasound techniques involve the use of devices reaching frequencies of 10 to 15 MHz, maximum up to 22 MHz [8,9].

The use of frequencies that are higher than conventional ultrasonography improves spatial resolution at the expense of tissue penetration, which is as low as 10.0 mm from the surface when applying 70 MHz frequencies. However, UHFUS can provide submillimeter image resolution, so it can improve detailed visualizations of superficial anatomical structures [8].

This characteristic has allowed for spreading of the UHFUS technique for the imaging of skin, blood vessels, musculoskeletal anatomy, oral mucosa, and small parts.

In adults, good correlation between ultrasound patterns and histopathologic features of minor salivary glands have been documented, as well as a high negative predictive values of a negative UHFUS in the diagnosis of SD in sicca syndrome in adults [10]. Up to now, no studies have applied UHFUS for the clinical characterization of SD in pediatric patients.

2. Objectives

The aim of the study is to identify the ultrasound patterns at UHFUS of minor salivary glands in a cohort of pediatric patients with SD.

3. Methods

Consecutive pediatric patients with clinical diagnosis of pediatric-onset SD seen at AOU Meyer between April 2021 and April 2022 were included in this study. All these patients underwent a diagnostic workup comprehensive of minor salivary glands UHFUS.

To be eligible, patients should have received a clinical diagnosis of SD before the age of 16 years, according to a combined set of clinical, serological and instrumental findings. Clinical, radiological and histopathological findings were retrospectively collected using a dedicated case report form (CRF). For each patient, we collected demographics data, age of onset, clinical presentation both at the time of the diagnosis and at the last visit, subjective assessment of ocular, oral and vaginal dryness, serological data including blood count, kidney and liver function, C reactive protein, antinuclear antibodies, anti-Ro/SSA, anti-La/SSB, rheumatoid factor, C3 and C4 levels and presence of hypergammaglobulinemia. Tear secretion was evaluated using the Schirmer test, break-up time (BUT) test or both. We considered levels of <10 mm wetting of the paper strip in Schirmer test and levels <10 sec for BUT test as pathological. Indeed, there no validated parameters for these tests in the healthy pediatric population; however, a recent meta-analysis reported a secretion >15 mm as a normal value, and we assume 10 mm as a cutoff for abnormal secretion [11].

Ultrasonography and Biopsy

Intraoral UHFUS scan of the lip mucosa was performed with Vevo MD equipment (Vevo® MD, Fujifilm, Visualsonics) with a standardized protocol. For each patient, a standardized intraoral UHFUS examination of the internal surface of the lower lip (central, left and right compartment) was carried out using a 70 MHz probe with the following characteristics: bandwidth 29–71 MHz, nominal frequency 52 MHz, axial resolution 30 μm, lateral resolution 65 μm, maximum depth 10.0 mm, maximum image width 9.7 mm, maximum image depth 10.0 mm, focal depth 5 mm. For each compartment, axial and longitudinal B-mode acquisitions were obtained. The UHFUS scans were performed using a standardized preset, keeping gain, time gain compensation, dynamic range, mechanical index and thermal index constant. Scan depth and focus position were adjusted to optimize the scan. The scans were saved as DICOM format images and were processed using Horos software (https://horosproject.org). The images were independently reviewed by two operators.

Labial salivary glands (LSG) were assessed by using a four-grade semiquantitative scoring system, similar to the OMERACT scoring system used for major salivary glands [8]. Namely, grade = 0: normal glandular parenchyma; grade = 1: the presence of mild glandular alteration, with fine echogenicity in absence of clear alterations, or slight, diffuse glandular hypoechogenicity; grade = 2: a moderate glandular alteration, with the presence of focal hypoechoic areas, but partial conservation of normal glandular parenchyma; and finally, grade = 3: a severe glandular alteration, with diffuse presence of hypoechoic areas in absence of normal glandular parenchyma, or presence of glandular fibrosis. As a second parameter, we evaluated glandular vascularization, using a consensus-based color Doppler semiquantitative score as suggested by Hočevar et al. [12]. It distinguishes four grades: grade 0: no visible vascular signals; grade 1: focal, dispersed vascular signals; grade 2: diffuse vascular signals detected in <50% of the gland; grade 3: diffuse vascular signals in >50% of the gland.

Finally, histopathological parameters were assessed through LSG biopsy, according to Chisholm and Mason scoring system, which includes 5 grades from 0 to 4, based on the presence of slight or moderate lymphocytic infiltration and/or focus of lymphocytes [13,14]). We considered as a positive biopsy any grade of focal sialadenitis, that is, a focus score > 0 foci/4 mm^2 [3,4,15].

Descriptive statistics were used to summarize the data, including means, medians and standard deviations for continuous variables, and frequencies and percentages for categorical variables.

4. Results

We included a total of twelve patients in the study, followed by our center for pediatric SD (n = 12, 11 females; 10 Caucasian, 2 Asian). They had a median age at the diagnosis of 13.5 years (range 7.75–17) and a median disease duration of 13.5 months (range 1–94).

Concerning comorbidities, 50% of our patients had also other autoimmune diseases (6/12: 1 celiac disease and Hashimoto thyroiditis, 1 celiac disease, 1 Basedow disease upon Hashimoto thyroiditis, 1 universalis alopecias, 1 systemic lupus erythematosus, 1 autoimmune panniculitis). Five patients also had familiar history positive for autoimmune diseases.

The clinical phenotype at the time of the diagnosis was widely heterogeneous. The features of the patients at time of the diagnosis are summarized in Table 1. Four patients complained of sicca syndrome, primarily affecting the eyes, but in three cases also the mouth; one of them presented not only oral and ocular but also vaginal dryness. They all presented sicca syndrome combined with other symptoms, such as Raynaud phenomenon (2/4), arthritis with morning stiffness (2/4), gastrointestinal manifestations as abdominal pain and/or diarrhea (3/4), asthenia (1/4) and cutaneous vasculitis.

Only two of our patients presented the most typical symptom of pediatric SD, recurrent swelling of parotid gland: one of them is the only boy, the other one is the patient who showed the earliest onset of symptoms (6 years old at the first episode of parotitis). Four patients suffered for cutaneous involvement: one of them presented only a cutaneous lipodystrophy; three patients started with photosensitive erythema, two of them as the only symptom, while in the other one it was combined with kidney involvement (renal tubular acidosis and proteinuria). Two patients started with a generic presentation of arthralgias: one of them combined with systemic symptoms (fever and asthenia), the other one with a mucocutaneous involvement (cutaneous vasculitis and recurring aphthous stomatitis). There was also a girl who only presented Raynaud's phenomenon.

Table 1. Clinical and serological features.

Characteristics	Sicca Syndrome (n = 4)	Parotitis (n = 2)	Non-Sicca, Non-Parotitis (n = 6)	Total (n = 12)
Age at diagnosis (median year)	14.25	11.5	13.76	13.5
Age at diagnosis (age range)	9.75–17	9.83–13.08	7.75–16	7.75–17
Female, n (%)	4 (100%)	1 (50%)	6 (100%)	11 (92%)
Other autoimmune diseases	1 (25%)	2 (100%)	3 (50%)	6 (50%)
Familiar history of autoimmune diseases	1 (25%)	1 (50%)	3 (50%)	5 (42%)
Sicca				
- Oral dryness	3 (75%)	0 (0%)		3 (25%)
- Ocular dryness	4 (100%)	0 (0%)		4 (33%)
- Vaginal dryness	1 (25%)	0 (0%)		1/11 (9%)
Parotitis	0 (0%)	2 (100%)		2 (17%)
Arthralgias	0 (0%)	0 (0%)	2 (33%)	2 (17%)
Arthritis	2 (50%)	0 (0%)	0 (0%)	2 (17%)
Asthenia	1 (25%)	0 (0%)	1 (17%)	2 (17%)
Fever	0 (0%)	0 (0%)	2 (33%)	2 (17%)
Raynaud	2 (50%)	0 (0%)	2 (33%)	4 (33%)
Mucocutaneous involvement	1 (25%)	1 (50%)	4 (67%)	6 (50%)
Renal involvement	0 (0%)	0 (0%)	1 (17%)	1 (8%)
Gastrointestinal involvement	3 (75%)	0 (0%)	0 (0%)	3 (25%)
Cytopenia	1 (25%)	0 (0%)	3 (50%)	4 (33%)
Hypergamma	2 (50%)	0 (0%)	3 (50%)	5 (42%)
Hypocomplementemia	0 (0%)	0 (0%)	1 (17%)	1 (8%)
ANA+	4 (100%)	2 (100%)	5 (83%)	11 (92%)
Ro/SSA +	2 (50%)	0 (0%)	4 (67%)	6 (50%)
La/SSB +	1 (25%)	0 (0%)	0 (0%)	1 (8%)

About laboratory exams, 4/12 patients showed blood count alterations (a variable combination of anemia, lymphocytopenia, neutropenia, thrombocytopenia); 4/12 presented a typical hypergammaglobulinemia (defined as >2 SD according to the age) and 1/12 had hypocomplementemia as the only laboratory alteration. Eleven patients were ANA positive; Ro/SSA were positive in 6/12 while just one tested positive for La/SSB. Two patients presented positive Rheumatoid factor, while all of the patients tested for other autoantibodies (anti-dsDNA or anti-Smith antibodies) resulted negative. However, not all of our patients were tested for each of these antibodies (we had 7/12 tested for Rheumatoid factor, 10/12 for anti-Smith and 8/12 for anti-dsDNA).

In our sample population, 10/12 underwent Schirmer test, with positive results in at least one eye in 7/10, and 8/12 underwent break-up time (BUT) test, with positive results in five cases.

Minor salivary gland biopsy was performed in 9/12, showing inflammatory chronic sialadenitis in 8/12. We chose to avoid performing biopsy in 3/12 patients, since they had typical sicca symptoms combined with positive Ro/SSA autoantibodies.

At the moment of the biopsy, treatment with hydroxychloroquine was ongoing in 11/12; only one of our patients did not assume any therapy.

Only two of our patients (2/12, 16%) met ACR/EULAR diagnostic criteria. Among the 10 patients who did not meet ACR/EULAR criteria, 8/10 (80%) did not present any sicca symptoms (first inclusion criteria), while in the other 2/10 we did not perform all examinations included in classification criteria. We cannot exclude that if we performed more diagnostic exams our patients would have fulfilled diagnostic criteria in a higher percentage. We found more adherence to pediatric Bartunkova criteria (5/12; 41%). In this case, 4/7 (57%) of patients did not fulfil criteria due to a negative autoimmune profile, 2/7 (29%) because of compresence of other autoimmune disease and the other one (1/7, 14%) because she did not present any of the symptoms considered in these criteria (sicca syndrome or systemic symptoms, such as fever of unknown origin, noninflammatory arthralgias, hypokalemic paralysis, abdominal pain).

When applying UHFUS to this cohort of patients, all patients showed a UHFUS grade of ≥ 1, with 8/12 showing a mild glandular alteration (i.e., grade 1), 2/12 a moderate glandular alteration (i.e., grade 2) and finally 2/12 a severe glandular alteration (i.e., grade 3). Moderate intraglandular vascularization was seen in 9/12, with only 3/12 showing mild intraglandular vascularization. These features are summarized in Table 2. Figure 1 represents grade 1 of parenchymal involvement and it belongs to a patient who presented at the time of diagnosis only photosensitive erythema combined to hypocomplementemia; Figure 2 represents grade 2 of glandular alteration: this patient did not present sicca syndrome nor recurrent swelling of parotid, but she had arthralgias, mucocutaneous and hematological involvement. Figures 3 and 4 are examples of severe glandular alteration with moderate intraglandular vascularization: they belong to a patient with sicca syndrome, mucocutaneous and hematological involvement and presence of Ro/SSA, La/SSB and Rheumatoid factor.

Due to limited size of the sample, the relationship between histological findings, autoantibodies status and UHFUS grade could not be performed. However, through the data at our disposal, we can suppose a correlation between a higher degree of glandular architecture alteration seen at UHFUS and more clinical signs of B cell activation. Indeed, among the two patients with severe glandular alteration, both presented strong hematologic involvement (anemia and/or lymphocytopenia and hypergammaglobulinemia); one of them also had positive LA/SSB and rheumatoid factor, while the other one was the only patient in our sample who also presented renal involvement (proteinuria).

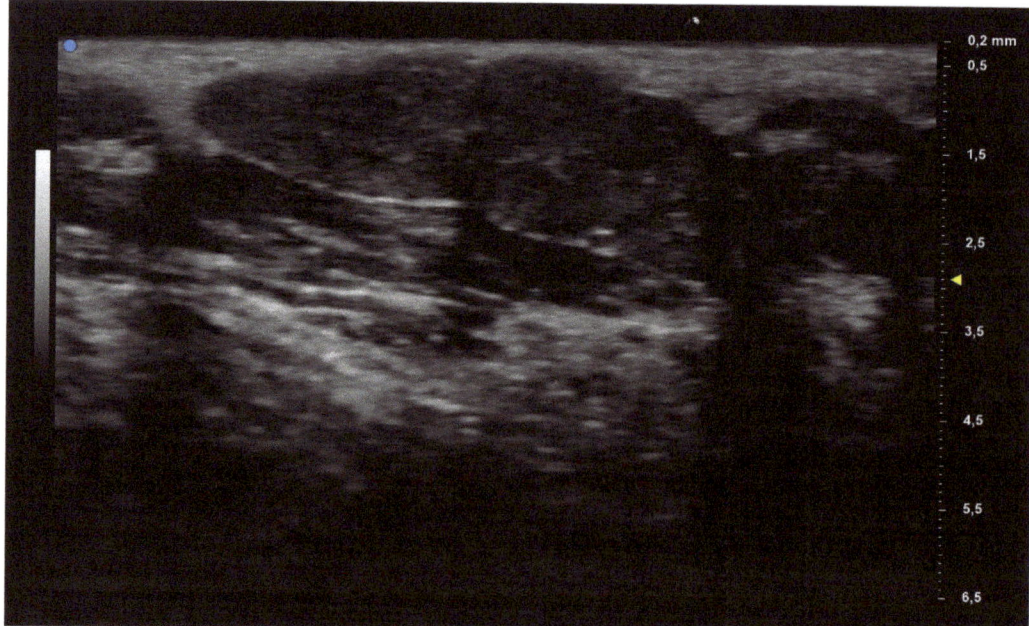

Figure 1. Mild glandular alteration (grade 1).

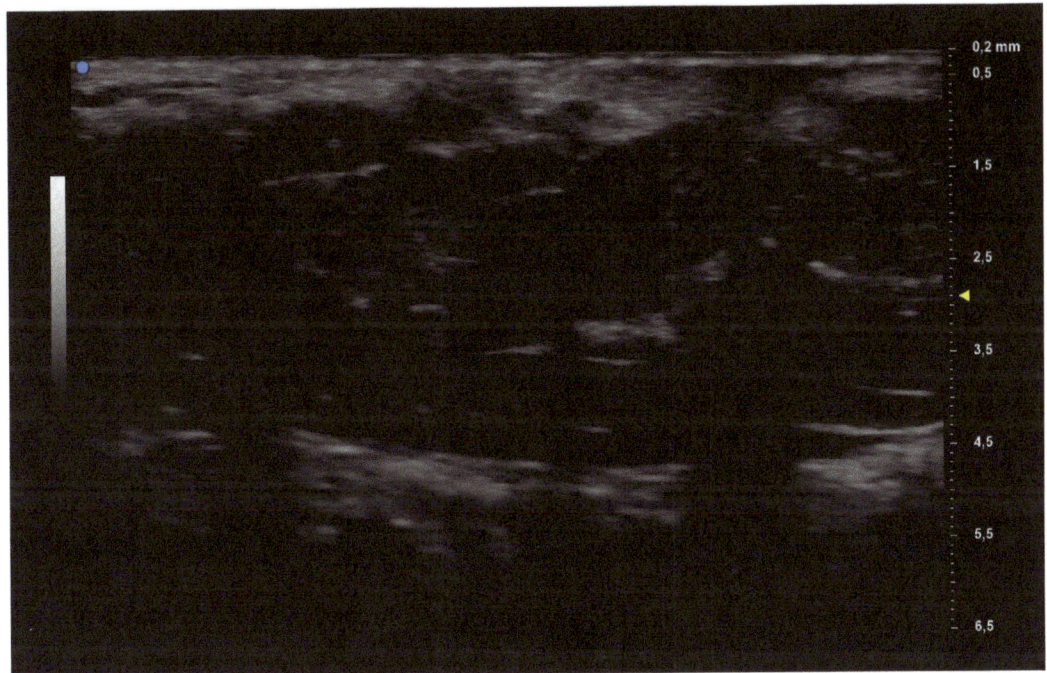

Figure 2. Moderate glandular alteration (grade 2).

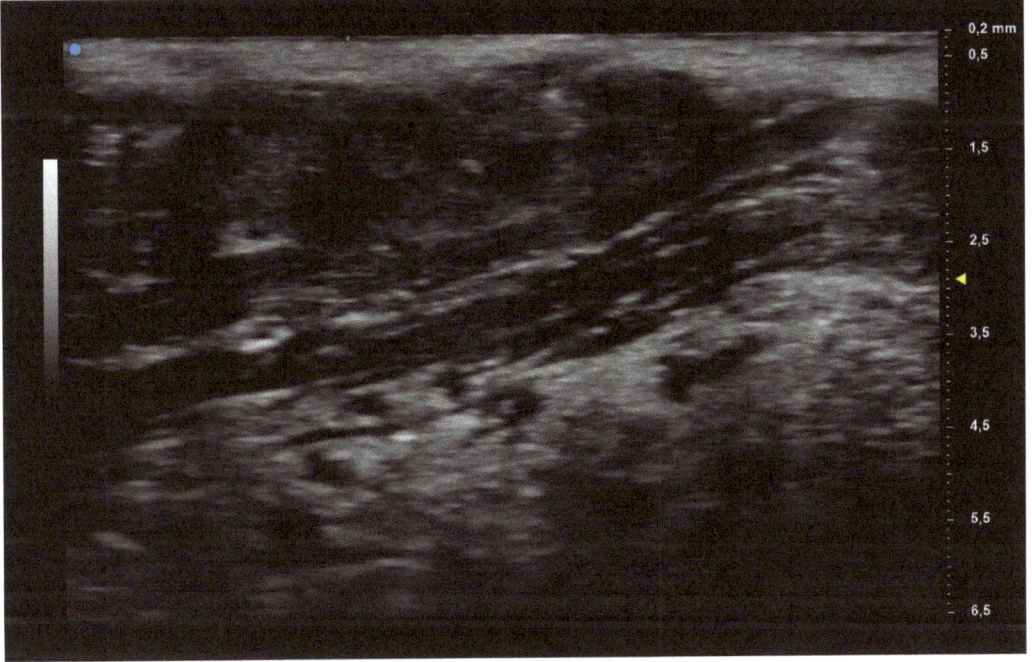

Figure 3. Severe glandular alteration (grade 3).

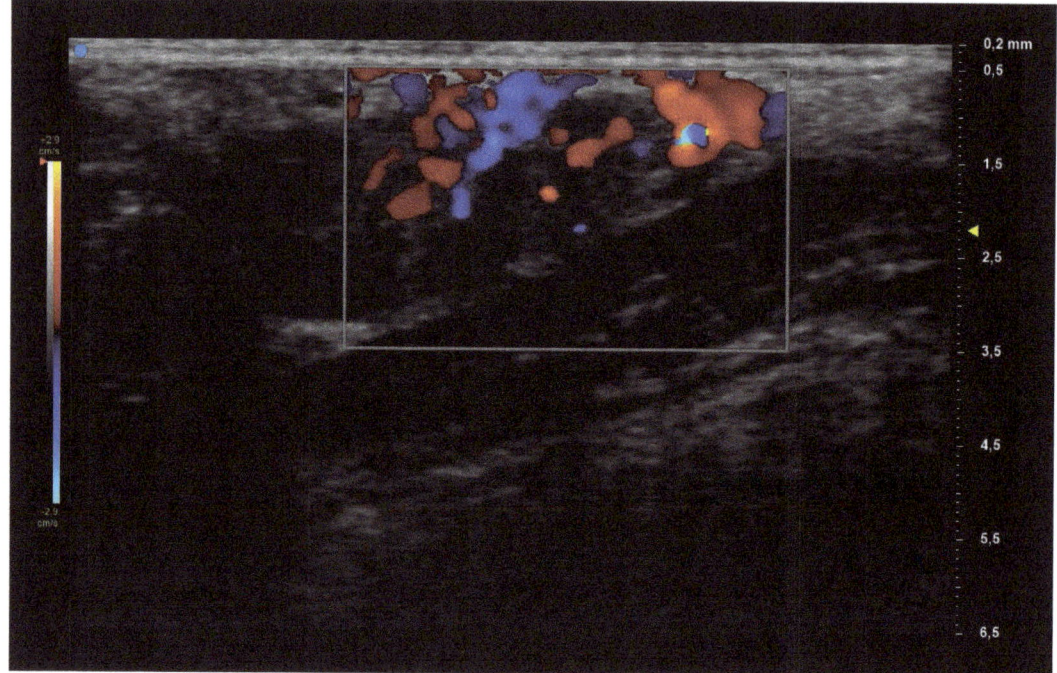

Figure 4. Moderate vascularization.

Table 2. UHFUS characteristics according to clinical features.

UHFUS Characteristics	Sicca Syndrome (n = 4)	Parotitis (n = 2)	Non-Sicca, Non- Parotitis (n = 6)	Total (n = 12)
Grade 1	3 (75%)	1 (50%)	4 (67%)	8 (67%)
Grade 2	0 (0%)	1 (50%)	1 (17%)	2 (17%)
Grade 3	1 (25%)	0 (0%)	1 (17%)	2 (17%)
Mild vascularization	1 (25%)	1 (50%)	1 (17%)	3 (25%)
Moderate vascularization	3 (75%)	1 (50%)	5 (83%)	9 (75%)

5. Discussion

SD is a chronic autoimmune disease characterized clinically by the destruction of the epithelium of the exocrine glands, as a consequence of abnormal B cell and T cell responses to the autoantigens Ro/SSA and La/SSB, among others [16]. One of the main characteristics is the presence of a chronic lymphocytic infiltrate in the glandular parenchyma [9]. The presence of positive autoimmune profile years before diagnosis suggests that the autoimmune process is active years before clinical onset [17]. Due to the multisystem involvement during the course of the disease, clinical heterogeneity in terms of presentation, disease course and outcome is reported for adult patients.

Consequently, there is still no single clinical, laboratory, pathological or radiological feature that could be used as a "gold standard" for its diagnosis and/or classification [2].

The diagnosis of the disease usually is based on objective tests able to quantify patients' ocular or oral dryness, in association with serologic or histopathologic evidence of an underlying autoimmune basis for the exocrine glandular dysfunction and with demonstration of subsequent inflammation [10].

Diagnosis, therefore, usually combines laboratory exams (i.e., autoantibodies or other markers of B cell activation, such as cytopenia, hypergammaglobulinemia and complement factor consumption), functional tests (i.e., unstimulated saliva flow rate, Ocular Staining Score, Schirmer's test) and anatomic evaluations, such as salivary glands ultrasound [2,7].

The test still considered the "gold standard" for SD diagnosis remains the LSG biopsy, which allows for identifying a typical focal lymphocytic sialadenitis (FLS), which is considered the hallmark of SD at tissue level [10,18]. LSG have historically been chosen because they are easily accessible, since they lie above the muscle layer, covered by a thin layer of fibrous connective tissue and oral mucous membrane, and because of the low risk of excessive bleeding [13]. However, the biopsy remains an invasive procedure, especially in a pediatric patient and false negative results due to sampling errors.

There have been several proposals for classification criteria that combine the results of these different tests: for a long period, there have been different proposals from different societies, such as 2002 AECG criteria (American–European Consensus Group) [19] or 2012 SICCA-ACR criteria (Sjogren's International Collaborative Clinical Alliance–American College of Rheumatology) [20], but the SD community recognized the need for an international consensus. Today, the most used is the consensus ACR/EULAR, which results from the overlap of the two previous sets, and it has been recognized by both of the societies [2,7]. However, all of these criteria specifically refer to adult population and they were developed for classification purposes, even though the ACR/EULAR 2016 criteria are also used in clinical practice to establish a diagnosis of SD.

Recently, UFHUS has been proposed as a new method for diagnosis in adults with suspected SD. From the beginning of 2000s, UHFUS was used as a support in dermatologic, vascular, rheumatologic and musculoskeletal fields, mainly in adult populations. There are fewer studies on pediatric populations, mostly concerning vascular morphology [8]. Its importance relies on the capacity to provide a great increase in resolution, that in some case surpasses that of computerized tomography (CT) or magnetic resonance imaging (MRI). The possibility to investigate only the first centimeters of the body surface, which represents the main limit of this method, makes UHFUS particularly suitable for the study of minor salivary glands. Combining its advantages, such as portability, low cost, lack of the need for radiation and sedation and safety, UHFUS can serve as a useful clinical tool in the management of pediatric patients [21].

In patients with suspected SD, minor salivary glands can be imaged with UHFUS by using 70 MHz frequencies, so as to obtain information on parenchymal alterations and on inflammation grade [8]. It can also be used to guide LSG biopsy [9]. According to Ferro et. al, this technique seems to have a higher sensibility than traditional major salivary glands ultrasonography (SGUS) and it is associated with a high negative predictive value. In future, it could be used to avoid biopsy in subject with a low pretest likelihood of being affected by SD, but there is still no defined optimal cutoff [10].

Pediatric SD is a rare condition, and its prevalence is underestimated due to the lack of standardized diagnostic criteria and the subtle early clinical presentation.

Neither the AECG criteria nor the ACR/EULAR criteria are validated for children [3,22]. As already reported, SD has a heterogeneous phenotype, and pediatric subjects have a different clinical presentation. Indeed, they might present reduced prevalence of symptoms related to high disease burden (i.e., symptoms of dryness) as these features are associated with long-lasting inflammation and are more likely to reflect damage accrual more than inflammation itself. Therefore, as the classification criteria are mostly based on features of overt glandular dysfunction, application of these criteria to pediatric patients for a diagnostic purpose might result in underestimation of disease prevalence. Furthermore, tests to assess oral or ocular dryness might be challenging in younger children due to low compliance and due to the lack of normal values for a healthy pediatric population [23]. A proposal for diagnostic criteria in children and adolescents came from Bartunkova et al. [24], but there are still no diagnostic criteria widely accepted for the pediatric population [23].

As suggested by Basiaga et al., lymphocytic infiltration and production of autoantibodies can be interpreted as early features in the pathogenesis that lead to subsequent gland dysfunction and end-organ damage. In line with this hypothesis, children could represent an early stage in the development of SD and the damage accrual over time might result in the adding of clinical features and lead to a full-blown phenotype in later stages of life. This is exemplified by the progressive lymphocytic infiltration of the glands from the pediatric age to adulthood, and so of any focal sialadenitis less than the currently defined cutoff may be sufficient to support diagnosis, as we assumed in our study [3].

Furthermore, a recent study revealed that in pediatric patients with recurrent parotitis, SD diagnosis was very frequent. However, it remains still unclear how to differentiate recurrent juvenile recurrent parotitis from SD, since classification criteria were usually not met [25]. Interestingly, in this setting, SGUS and LSG biopsy were proposed in the workup of recurrent parotitis [25,26]. However, all the patients with parotitis had a positive SGUS and not all the patients had FS higher than 1. Instead, concerning UHFUS, that combine the ultrasonography with the need of labial salivary glands assessment, there are still no studies, but it could represent a complementary tool to differentiate SD patients with or without recurrent parotitis.

All these features make pediatric SD difficult to define, and they cause a significant delay in diagnosis. Improving pediatric diagnosis could not only allow for identifying children with SD prior to gland dysfunction, but also be useful for identifying of classifying adult patients in earlier stages of disease [3].

New approaches to a faster diagnosis are urgently needed in clinical practice. This preliminary pilot study seems to report UHFUS as a feasible technique able to identify salivary gland alterations in children with a clinical suspect of SD. This technique might contribute to driving guided lip biopsy, thus reducing the rate of false negatives.

Limits of our study include the small population sample size, retrospective data collection with some missing data, lack of comparison with healthy patients and the absence of validated parameters in a healthy population for correct understanding of UHFUS results, regarding vascularization in particular. Moreover, we did not perform the UFHUS at a standard time point (i.e., at the diagnosis) and this might thus hamper the possibility of phenotypically stratify these patients; at the same time, the reduced sample size did not allow for making any statistical analysis to correlate UFHUS findings and clinical or histopathological features.

Further studies are currently in progress in our clinics to identify the exact role of UHFUS and its potential predictive role of the various patterns observed in pediatric SD. We would like to primarily define normal patterns of UHFUS in healthy children so as to also establish validated parameters in the pediatric population. Our future studies should include a larger patient sample and comparison with healthy children.

Thanks to this preliminary study, it will be possible to extend the use of a sensible and noninvasive diagnostic method to the pediatric population, thus improving the diagnostic work-up of pediatric SD.

Author Contributions: Conceptualization, G.S., V.D. and C.B.; methodology, C.B. and G.S.; investigation, R.I., E.M., T.O. and G.F.; data curation, E.M. and C.V.; writing—original draft preparation, E.M. and C.V.; writing—review and editing, G.F. and T.O.; visualization, V.D.; supervision, C.B. and G.S. All authors have read and agreed to the published version of the manuscript.

Funding: This research received no external funding.

Institutional Review Board Statement: This study was conducted in accordance with the Declaration of Helsinki and approved by the Regional Pediatric Ethics Committee of the Tuscany Region.

Informed Consent Statement: Informed consent was obtained from all subjects involved in this study.

Data Availability Statement: The data presented in this study are available on request from the corresponding author. The data are not publicly available due to privacy reason.

Conflicts of Interest: The authors declare no conflict of interest.

References

1. Botsios, C.; Furlan, A.; Ostuni, P.; Sfriso, P.; Andretta, M.; Ometto, F.; Raffeiner, B.; Todesco, S.; Punzi, L. Elderly onset of primary Sjögren's syndrome: Clinical manifestations, serological features and oral/ocular diagnostic tests. Comparison with adult and young onset of the disease in a cohort of 336 Italian patients. *Jt. Bone Spine* **2011**, *78*, 171–174. [CrossRef] [PubMed]
2. Jonsson, R.; Brokstad, K.A.; Jonsson, M.V.; Delaleu, N.; Skarstein, K. Current concepts on Sjögren's syndrome—Classification criteria and biomarkers. *Eur. J. Oral. Sci.* **2018**, *126*, 37–48. [CrossRef]
3. Basiaga, M.L.; Stern, S.M.; Mehta, J.J.; Edens, C.; Randell, R.L.; Pomorska, A.; Irga-Jaworska, N.; Ibarra, M.F.; Bracaglia, C.; Nicolai, R.; et al. Childhood Sjögren syndrome: Features of an international cohort and application of the 2016 ACR/EULAR classification criteria. *Rheumatology* **2021**, *60*, 3144–3155. [CrossRef] [PubMed]
4. Yokogawa, N.; Lieberman, S.M.; Sherry, D.D.; Vivino, F.B. Features of childhood Sjögren's syndrome in comparison to adult Sjögren's syndrome: Considerations in establishing child-specific diagnostic criteria. *Clin. Exp. Rheumatol.* **2016**, *34*, 343–351.
5. O'Neill, E.M. Sjogren's syndrome with onset at 10 years of age. *Proc. R. Soc. Med.* **1965**, *58*, 689–690. [CrossRef] [PubMed]
6. Rucker, C.W. KERATITIS SICCA: Report of a Case. *Arch. Ophthalmol.* **1938**, *19*, 584–585. [CrossRef]
7. Shiboski, C.H.; Shiboski, S.C.; Seror, R.; Criswell, L.A.; Labetoulle, M.; Lietman, T.M.; Rasmussen, A.; Scofield, H.; Vitali, C.; Bowman, S.J.; et al. 2016 ACR-EULAR Classification Criteria for primary Sjögren's Syndrome: A Consensus and Data-Driven Methodology Involving Three International Patient Cohorts. *Arthritis Rheumatol.* **2017**, *69*, 35–45. [CrossRef]
8. Izzetti, R.; Vitali, S.; Aringhieri, G.; Nisi, M.; Oranges, T.; Dini, V.; Ferro, F.; Baldini, C.; Romanelli, M.; Caramella, D.; et al. Ultra-High Frequency Ultrasound, A Promising Diagnostic Technique: Review of the Literature and Single-Center Experience. *Can. Assoc. Radiol. J.* **2021**, *72*, 418–431. [CrossRef]
9. Aringhieri, G.; Izzetti, R.; Vitali, S.; Ferro, F.; Gabriele, M.; Baldini, C.; Caramella, D. Ultra-high frequency ultrasound (UHFUS) applications in Sjogren syndrome: Narrative review and current concepts. *Gland. Surg.* **2020**, *9*, 2248–2259. [CrossRef]
10. Ferro, F.; Izzetti, R.; Vitali, S.; Aringhieri, G.; Fonzetti, S.; Donati, V.; Dini, V.; Mosca, M.; Gabriele, M.; Caramella, D.; et al. Ultra-high frequency ultrasonography of labial glands is a highly sensitive tool for the diagnosis of Sjögren's syndrome: A preliminary study. *Clin. Exp. Rheumatol.* **2020**, *38*, 210–215.
11. Chidi-Egboka, N.C.; Briggs, N.E.; Jalbert, I.; Golebiowski, B. The ocular surface in children: A review of current knowledge and meta-analysis of tear film stability and tear secretion in children. *Ocul. Surf.* **2019**, *17*, 28–39. [CrossRef] [PubMed]
12. Hočevar, A.; Bruyn, G.A.; Terslev, L.; De Agustin, J.J.; MacCarter, D.; Chrysidis, S.; Collado, P.; Dejaco, C.; Fana, V.; Filippou, G.; et al. Development of a new ultrasound scoring system to evaluate glandular inflammation in Sjögren's syndrome: An OMERACT reliability exercise. *Rheumatology* **2022**, *61*, 3341–3350. [CrossRef] [PubMed]
13. Chisholm, D.M.; Mason, D.K. Labial salivary gland biopsy in Sjögren's disease. *J. Clin. Pathol.* **1968**, *21*, 656–660. [CrossRef] [PubMed]
14. Bautista-Vargas, M.; Vivas, A.J.; Tobón, G.J. Minor salivary gland biopsy: Its role in the classification and prognosis of Sjögren's syndrome. *Autoimmun. Rev.* **2020**, *19*, 102690. [CrossRef]
15. Randell, R.L.; Lieberman, S.M. Unique Aspects of Pediatric Sjögren Disease. *Rheum. Dis. Clin. N. Am.* **2021**, *47*, 707–723. [CrossRef] [PubMed]
16. Brito-Zerón, P.; Baldini, C.; Bootsma, H.; Bowman, S.J.; Jonsson, R.; Mariette, X.; Sivils, K.; Theander, E.; Tzioufas, A.; Ramos-Casals, M. Sjögren syndrome. *Nat. Rev. Dis. Primer.* **2016**, *2*, 16047. [CrossRef]
17. Theander, E.; Jonsson, R.; Sjöström, B.; Brokstad, K.; Olsson, P.; Henriksson, G. Prediction of Sjögren's Syndrome Years Before Diagnosis and Identification of Patients with Early Onset and Severe Disease Course by Autoantibody Profiling. *Arthritis Rheumatol.* **2015**, *67*, 2427–2436. [CrossRef] [PubMed]
18. Kroese, F.G.M.; Haacke, E.A.; Bombardieri, M. The role of salivary gland histopathology in primary Sjögren's syndrome: Promises and pitfalls. *Clin. Exp. Rheumatol.* **2018**, *36*, 222–233.
19. Vitali, C.; Bombardieri, S.; Jonsson, R.; Moutsopoulos, H.M.; Alexander, E.L.; Carsons, S.E.; Daniels, T.E.; Fox, P.C.; Fox, R.I.; Kassan, S.S.; et al. Classification criteria for Sjögren's syndrome: A revised version of the European criteria proposed by the American-European Consensus Group. *Ann. Rheum. Dis.* **2002**, *61*, 554–558. [CrossRef]
20. Shiboski, S.C.; Shiboski, C.H.; Criswell, L.A.; Baer, A.N.; Challacombe, S.; Lanfranchi, H.; Schiødt, M.; Umehara, H.; Vivino, F.; Zhao, Y.; et al. American College of Rheumatology classification criteria for Sjögren's syndrome: A data-driven, expert consensus approach in the Sjögren's International Collaborative Clinical Alliance cohort. *Arthritis Care Res.* **2012**, *64*, 475–487. [CrossRef]
21. Hwang, M.; Piskunowicz, M.; Darge, K. Advanced Ultrasound Techniques for Pediatric Imaging. *Pediatrics* **2019**, *143*, e20182609. [CrossRef] [PubMed]
22. Hammenfors, D.S.; Valim, V.; Bica, B.E.R.G.; Pasoto, S.G.; Lilleby, V.; Nieto-González, J.C.; Silva, C.A.; Mossel, E.; Pereira, R.M.; Coelho, A.; et al. Juvenile Sjögren's Syndrome: Clinical Characteristics with Focus on Salivary Gland Ultrasonography. *Arthritis Care Res.* **2020**, *72*, 78–87. [CrossRef] [PubMed]
23. Schiffer, B.L.; Stern, S.M.; Park, A.H. Sjögren's syndrome in children with recurrent parotitis. *Int. J. Pediatr. Otorhinolaryngol.* **2020**, *129*, 109768. [CrossRef] [PubMed]
24. Bartůnková, J.; Sedivá, A.; Vencovský, J.; Tesar, V. Primary Sjögren's syndrome in children and adolescents: Proposal for diagnostic criteria. *Clin. Exp. Rheumatol.* **1999**, *17*, 381–386.

25. Pomorska, A.; Świętoń, D.; Lieberman, S.M.; Bryl, E.; Kosiak, W.; Pęksa, R.; Chorążewicz, J.; Kochańska, B.; Kowalska-Skabara, J.; Szumera, M.; et al. Recurrent or persistent salivary gland enlargement in children: When is it Sjögren's? *Semin. Arthritis Rheum.* **2022**, *52*, 151945. [CrossRef]
26. Legger, G.E.; Erdtsieck, M.B.; De Wolff, L.; Stel, A.J.; Los, L.I.; Verstappen, G.M.; Spijkervet, F.K.; Vissink, A.; Van Der Vegt, B.; Kroese, F.G.; et al. Differences in presentation between paediatric- and adult-onset primary Sjögren's syndrome patients. *Clin Exp. Rheumatol.* **2021**, *39*, 85–92. Available online: https://www.clinexprheumatol.org/abstract.asp?a=17694 (accessed on 18 June 2023). [CrossRef]

Disclaimer/Publisher's Note: The statements, opinions and data contained in all publications are solely those of the individual author(s) and contributor(s) and not of MDPI and/or the editor(s). MDPI and/or the editor(s) disclaim responsibility for any injury to people or property resulting from any ideas, methods, instructions or products referred to in the content.

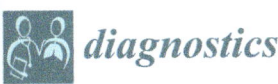

Article

Design of a Pediatric Rectal Ultrasound Probe Intended for Ultra-High Frequency Ultrasound Diagnostics

Maria Evertsson [1,2], Christina Graneli [3,4], Alvina Vernersson [2], Olivia Wiaczek [2], Kristine Hagelsteen [3,4], Tobias Erlöv [2], Magnus Cinthio [2] and Pernilla Stenström [3,4,*]

1. Department of Clinical Sciences, Lund University, 22185 Lund, Sweden
2. Department of Biomedical Engineering, The Faculty of Engineering, Lund University, 22185 Lund, Sweden
3. Department of Pediatrics, Clinical Sciences, Lund University, 22185 Lund, Sweden
4. Department of Pediatric Surgery, Skåne University Hospital Lund, 22185 Lund, Sweden
* Correspondence: pernilla.stenstrom@med.lu.se

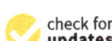

Citation: Evertsson, M.; Graneli, C.; Vernersson, A.; Wiaczek, O.; Hagelsteen, K.; Erlöv, T.; Cinthio, M.; Stenström, P. Design of a Pediatric Rectal Ultrasound Probe Intended for Ultra-High Frequency Ultrasound Diagnostics. *Diagnostics* **2023**, *13*, 1667. https://doi.org/10.3390/diagnostics13101667

Academic Editors: Rossana Izzetti and Marco Nisi

Received: 31 March 2023
Revised: 28 April 2023
Accepted: 28 April 2023
Published: 9 May 2023

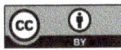

Copyright: © 2023 by the authors. Licensee MDPI, Basel, Switzerland. This article is an open access article distributed under the terms and conditions of the Creative Commons Attribution (CC BY) license (https://creativecommons.org/licenses/by/4.0/).

Abstract: It has been shown that ultra-high frequency (UHF) ultrasound applied to the external bowel wall can delineate the histo-anatomic layers in detail and distinguish normal bowel from aganglionosis. This would potentially reduce or lessen the need for biopsies that are currently mandatory for the diagnosis of Hirschsprung's disease. However, to our knowledge, no suitable rectal probes for such a use are on the market. The aim was to define the specifications of an UHF transrectal ultrasound probe (50 MHz center frequency) suitable for use in infants. Probe requirements according to patient anatomy, clinicians' requests, and biomedical engineering UHF prerequisites were collected within an expert group. Suitable probes on the market and in clinical use were reviewed. The requirements were transferred into the sketching of potential UHF ultrasound transrectal probes followed by their 3D prototype printing. Two prototypes were created and tested by five pediatric surgeons. The larger and straight 8 mm head and shaft probe was preferred as it facilitated stability, ease of anal insertion, and possible UHF technique including 128 piezoelectric elements in a linear array. We hereby present the procedure and considerations behind the development of a proposed new UHF transrectal pediatric probe. Such a device can open new possibilities for the diagnostics of pediatric anorectal conditions.

Keywords: anorectal conditions; diagnosis; Hirschsprung's disease; pediatrics; probe; ultra-high frequency ultrasound

1. Introduction

Hirschsprung's disease (HD) is a congenital disease with an incidence of 1:5000 in newborns [1]. It is characterized by a lack of ganglion cells in the bowel wall (aganglionosis), requiring surgical removal of the affected intestine [2]. Ganglia cells are normally found in the bowel wall's submucosa and myenteric layer [3]. For the diagnostics of HD, a rectal biopsy is taken from the rectum, but there are reports of physical and psychological biopsy-related problems, as well as insufficient accuracy, in up to 50% of cases [4–7]. About 10 times more children than those just with HD, e.g., children with bowel dysmotility, need to undergo investigation by rectal biopsy [7–9]. Finding an instantaneous and secure diagnostic technique for HD to replace rectal biopsy could benefit this patient group enormously.

For replacing biopsy diagnostics, ultra-high frequency (UHF) ultrasound is undergoing research. Histo-anatomic morphometrics have been shown to differentiate between the aganglionic and ganglionic bowel wall [10]. Furthermore, differences have been shown to be replicated on UHF ultrasound (center frequency 50 MHz) imaging of bowel specimens [4]. These studies were performed with the aim of differentiating between aganglionic and ganglionic bowel in children who had already been diagnosed with HD. For primary diagnostics, with the aim of replacing the need for rectal biopsy, transanal and mucosal ultrasound imaging is required. The only UHF ultrasound probes currently available for commercial use today (UHF 48 with bandwidth 20–46 MHz and UHF 70 with bandwidth 29–71 MHz, FUJIFILM VisualSonics, Toronto, Canada) are too large for a child's anus and rectum. A pediatric rectal UHF probe would enable the examination of large cohorts of children. Furthermore, it would facilitate the validation of UHF ultrasound by collecting images of reference bowel wall from healthy children. For other clinical conditions, a pediatric transrectal UHF probe could also facilitate detailed diagnostics of anorectal fistulas, internal and external sphincter injuries and pelvic floor malformations, and aid in the delineation of anorectal tumors.

Our overall aim was to enable diagnostics with UHF ultrasound, but also to open new possibilities for the high-resolution ultrasound imaging of other anorectal and pelvic floor conditions. The specific goal of this study was to establish a requirement specification and suggest prototypes of a rectal UHF ultrasound probe suitable for use in infants. We hereby present the procedure and considerations behind the development of a proposed new pediatric UHF transrectal probe.

2. Materials and Methods

2.1. Settings

The study was performed at a department of pediatric surgery, which was appointed in 2018 as a national center for HD and anorectal malformations. It covers a geographical area of 5 million residents. The process underlying the development of the pediatric UHF probe followed a specific structure and involved an expert study group comprising pediatric surgeons (n = 5) and researchers within biomedical engineering (n = 4). The pediatric surgeons had 8–13 years of specialist experience and were subspecialized within the field of pediatric gastrointestinal surgery. The biomedical engineers and researchers were all specialized in medical ultrasound imaging and had considerable experience in working with UHF ultrasound. One of them also had experience in the life science development of rectal ultrasound probes for adults.

The development procedure was structured according to the following steps:

1. Identification of probe requirements, according to anatomic, clinical and technical considerations;
2. Review of available and, for the purpose, feasible, probes currently on the market and in clinical use;
3. Sketching potential UHF ultrasound transrectal probes;
4. 3D prototype printing;
5. Evaluation of the prototypes.

2.1.1. Anatomic, Clinical and Technological Considerations

Anatomic considerations: The proposed probe was targeted for use in children weighing 3–15 kg. Since rectal ultrasound examinations were intended to be performed without the use of anesthesia or sedatives, patient comfort and safety were key considerations. Therefore, the metrics of pediatric anatomic anorectal anatomy, with regard to anal opening size, rectal diameter and rectum length, were collected from the literature. They were also collected from the medical charts of the last 10 patients treated at the department of pediatric surgery who had undergone anography diagnostics for HD [9]. Close contact between the probe head and the bowel wall to avoid shadowing effects within images was taken into consideration with regard to the proposed probe's anatomic design.

Clinical considerations: Information about clinicians' requirements for a transrectal probe was collected within the expert group and from discussions and clinical observations. Various aspects of patient safety, with regard to movement, environmental circumstances during anal examinations, and the examiner's ergonomics, were taken into consideration when developing the design.

Technological considerations: Technical specifications, based on previous knowledge of UHF ultrasound of the bowel wall, were collected within the expert group. A small-sized pediatric anal probe still needed to include technical prerequisites for encompassing UHF ultrasound technology. The probe center frequency, the number of piezoelectric elements, and the image view were all taken into account. The contact between the probe head and the bowel wall was also contemplated with regard to technical solutions. Electronics requirements were noted for a later evaluation.

2.1.2. Review of Available and Feasible Probes

An analysis of the market was performed to identify currently available probes suitable for use regarding our aim to introduce UHF technology in the form of a pediatric anorectal probe. The overview was intended to cover various probes' physical dimensions, frequency ranges, number of elements and the field of view. Clinical site visits to departments using some small-sized ultrasound alternatives in diagnostics were made in order to provide detailed clinical insights into their use in practice.

2.1.3. Sketching

The identified parameters of the anal tract of importance for the probe's design and size were the diameter of the anal opening, inner diameter of the rectum, and insertion length. All measurements were set to a minimum in order to avoid discomfort for the child, while still enabling the allowance of the identified technical prerequisites. Based on these results, probe prototypes were sketched using a CAD (computer-aided design) program, PTC's Creo Parametric 7.0.2.

2.1.4. 3D Printing of Probe Shell Prototypes

Prototype probe shells were printed using a Formlabs 2 (Formlabs, Somerville, MA, USA) printer and stereolithography. For biocompatibility, BioMed White (Formlabs, USA) was used as a resin polymer. A thickness layer of 50 μm was used, resulting in a total of 3414 layers for each probe prototype. In post-printing processing, the 3D prototypes were placed in isopropanol (75%) for 5 min, cured for 60 min in an ultraviolet oven (Form Cure [Formlabs, USA]) at 60 °C. They were then placed again in a 75% isopropanol bath for 2 min followed by a new cure round at 60 °C in an ultraviolet oven for 20 min. In a final post-processing step, any residuals from the resisting support material were scraped away, and the entire probe was sandpapered.

2.1.5. 3D Prototype Testing

The feasibility of each of the developed 3D-printed prototype probe shells was tested by five pediatric surgeons of both genders. Their preferred grip of the prototype, as well as their opinion on the design and overall handling, were evaluated according to a scheme covering stability, hand movement flexibility and ergonomics in the preferred examination positions.

3. Results

3.1. Anatomic, Clinical and Technological Considerations

Anatomic considerations: Anal opening size: Sizes of anal openings in newborns up to 1-year-olds, with or without malformations or aganglionosis, were reported in the literature to be 12–15 mm [11]. According to the medical charts held by the department of pediatric surgery, anal openings of children with HD undergoing washouts ($n = 10$) or children with anorectal malformations with perineal fistulas ($n = 10$) undergoing calibrations and enemas were 6–10 mm. The diameter of the rectal suction instrument (rbi2®) used for diagnosing HD in children weighing 2.5–7.1 kg was 7 mm, which entered the anus and rectum without any resistance.

Rectal diameter: The rectum width was assessed in anographies in children weighing a median of 4.8 kg (range, 3.1–7.1 kg) undergoing examination for HD ($n = 10$) at the department of pediatric surgery. Five children had rectosigmoid aganglionosis and five had no aganglionosis according to the pathology biopsy report. Their median inner rectal diameter was 14 mm (range 8–25 mm). In the children who underwent pre-operative rectal wash-out prior to surgery for HD, a Foley catheter with a corresponding median size of 7–11 mm was used.

Length of rectum: In order to plan the insertion depth of the proposed probe, the length of the rectum, as measured from the skin as well as 1 cm above the dentate line up to the start of the sigmoid curve, was assessed in the five infants undergoing wash-outs prior to surgery for HD. The length of the rectum, assessed by inserting a soft Foley® catheter, was a median of 50 mm (range, 40–65 mm) before resistance occurred. The length of the rectal suction instrument (rbi2®) in children weighing 2.5–7.1 kg reached up to maximum of 6 cm from the skin verge. A schematic sketch of the anorectal dimensions defined in this study is shown in Figure 1.

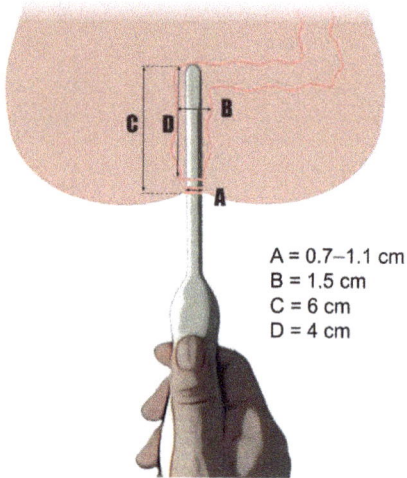

Figure 1. Illustration of a pediatric anorectal probe including both dimensional prerequisites according to clinical measures and the literature, as well as technical feasibility for ultra-high frequency technology. A. Feasible diameter of the probe inserted in the anus without causing any discomfort. B. Size of the rectum's inner diameter. C. Length of the rectum from the skin to the sigmoideum. D. Distance from 1 cm above the linea dentata up to the sigmoideum.

Clinical considerations: With respect to the design of the proposed probe, clinicians' requirements for patient comfort, safety and ergonomics were focused on the size and shape of the probe's head, shaft, and handle. The probe head should be small enough to enter the anus without causing discomfort to the patient. The shaft's length and size should allow flexibility of the probe element direction so that the probe head can reach the mucosa posteriorly, anteriorly and on the lateral sides. The handle should enable the examiner's hand to rest on the underlay in order to eliminate movement when the image is taken. Furthermore, it should fit most surgeons' hands, regardless of their size. The handle and shaft should enable the examination to proceed easily while the examiner stands right in front of the child, as well as on the side of the child. The size and grip of the handle were tested by the surgeons, resulting in a requirement for a handle length of 9–11 cm and a circumference of 4–7 cm (Sketch in Figure 2).

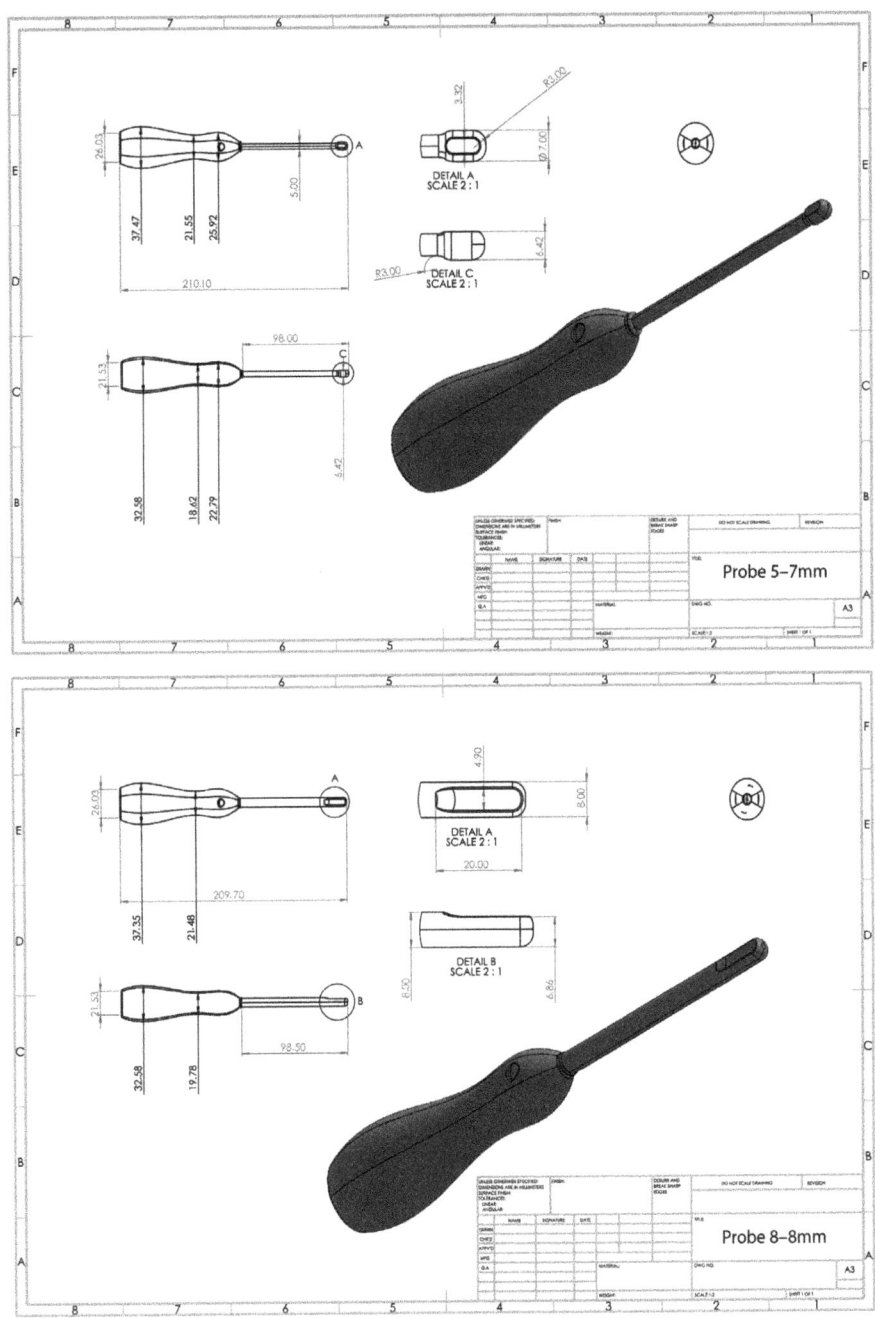

Figure 2. Sketches of two probe prototypes: Probe 5–7 mm with a thinner neck than head and Probe 8–8 mm, i.e., the same diameter for the probe's head and neck Detail A shows where the probe elements would be positioned.

Technological considerations: An ultrasound resolution (frequency) sufficient to replicate all layers of the rectum wall, including the mucosa, submucosa, muscularis interna, muscularis externa and the serosa, was requested.

Center frequencies: Since the rectal wall in children has been shown to be approximately 0.8–2 mm thick and histo-anatomic bowel wall layers extend to 0.2 mm [4,10], the consensus was that visualization of such small anatomy required UHF ultrasound of 30–50 MHz center frequency.

Linear array probe or rotating single-element probe: The probe type used in previous UHF ultrasound studies of examinations of bowel wall ex vivo and in vivo from the serosa was a linear array probe (UHF70, FUJIFILM VisualSonics, Toronto, ON, Canada). A linear array probe produces rectangular images, i.e., field of view, and is often designed to operate at high center frequencies and image superficial structures. It also produces images with both good axial and lateral resolutions. In contrast to this, a rotating single-element probe, as is used in intravascular UHF ultrasound imaging with a circular rotating piezoelectric element probe, has the advantage of creating 360° circumferential images. The downside with a single probe element is diverging ultrasound beams, resulting in poorer lateral resolution compared to a linear array probe, especially at larger depths/distances. Based on these facts, it was decided that a linear array probe was preferable, especially since a higher lateral resolution was favored compared to circumferential imaging.

Longitudinal or transversal imaging: In previous bowel wall examinations using UHF ultrasound, only longitudinal ultrasound imaging with a 256-element linear array probe has been studied (UHF70, FUJIFILM VisualSonics, Toronto, ON, Canada) [4,10]. As a result of this experience, longitudinal imaging was the first choice by the expert group. However, transversal imaging is the most commonly used imaging approach in the clinic. Transversal imaging may be more intuitive to interpret and understand, easier to orient in and, if probe elements are arranged along a curved probe head, a so-called curvilinear array, then it is more beneficial for investigating deeper tissues since a widening image area with depth is obtained. Another approach discussed, enabling both longitudinal and transversal imaging approaches, was a moving element linear array probe delivering a longitudinal image view, collecting 2D images, and turning them into 3D imaging volumes. However, this technique would be sensitive to motion artifacts, which are likely to occur in a baby who is awake during the examination. Since the time span for the elements being in motion is short (approximately 1–3 s for a 90° angle), the possibility of using such a probe was not excluded.

Number of probe elements: More elements deliver a larger field of view but require a larger area on the probe. However, in previous research, where 256 elements were used for diagnostic UHF ultrasound imaging of the bowel wall, only less than half of each available image was required for accurate measurements. Therefore 128 elements were considered to suffice. A smaller number of probe elements, delivering a smaller area, would also increase the likelihood of obtaining good contact between the probe and the mucosa. This, in turn, would reduce the risk of shadowing effects as a result of the presence of air between the probe and the bowel wall. Still, a drawback of a single-element probe is that it must be driven by special motors, which require space and other technology.

Probe contact to bowel wall: To avoid shadowing, air between the probe head and the bowel wall should be limited. Close contact between the probe head and the bowel wall could be obtained by using a larger head in order to fill the rectum's lumen, by the use of a bent, or bendable, probe head. Alternatively, a water-filled balloon surrounding the head could be used, pressing it towards the bowel wall (see endobronchial ultrasound probe, Table 1). It was decided that a straight probe head, without a surrounding balloon, would be both desirable and possible if the stiff shaft could lean against the mucosa in line with the suction biopsy instrument. A smaller area of a linear array probe, including a few elements in combination with an easily maneuverable design, could still enable close contact with the mucosa.

3.2. Review of Available and Feasible Probes

A review of various types of ultrasonography using small probe heads, operating at high center frequencies, was explored in the literature and in manufacturers' product information. This information is collated and presented in Table 1. According to the review, the majority of ultrasound probes in clinical use today are of too large a size for rectal imaging in infants. Alternatively, they deliver too low center frequencies (only around 5–18 MHz) compared to those desired for a pediatric UHF ultrasound probe. Additionally, some of the ultrasound probes identified and observed had very long shafts intended for examinations of tissues at greater distances (such as the heart through the esophagus or the bronchus through the trachea) than the bowel wall anorectally in children. Although the sizes and designs of the heads were of interest, longer probe shafts are not desirable for use in children if they are awake during the examination, because the closer the hand can be to the targeted tissue, the less likelihood there will be of artefacts developing if the patient moves.

Three types of ultrasound probes with specific prerequisites and suitable pediatric dimensions were selected for observation in clinical use. For imaging the lumen of small blood vessels, the high-frequency intravascular ultrasound (IVUS) probe was observed. The IVUS probe is a catheter-based type small enough for use in children, and with a center frequency of 50 MHz, which most likely would be sufficient to view the histo-anatomic layers of the bowel wall. The downside to using a catheter-based ultrasound device in the rectum is that it does not reach to the mucosa circumferentially. Therefore, a large amount of gel will be needed to fil the rectum, in order to avoid air accumulating between the probe and the mucosa.

For imaging cardiac details in small children, the transesophageal probe with linear array elements was inspected, as used prior to cardiac surgery. For imaging details of lung bronchials, the endobronchial ultrasound (EBUS) was observed during bronchoscopy. Both these latter two probes consist of a number of probe elements next to each other (similar to the UHF ultrasound probe used in our project on bowel wall so far) and were also considered to be suitable in size and design for pediatric anorectal use. The observation area was considered to be large enough, but their frequency ranges (3–8 MHz and 5–12 MHz, respectively) were too low for the specified requirements (Table 1).

3.3. Sketches of Probe Shell Prototypes

Suggestions and sketches of two probes were produced, based on the information on suitable size, form, and allowance of a technology including 128-linear elements (Figure 2). The probe heads developed were, according to the collected information, straight and set to sizes of 7 mm and 8 mm, respectively, to suit most infants. To make the probe more maneuverable, a narrowing of the shaft was sketched in one of the suggested prototypes (5 mm shaft diameter). The length between the head and the handle was set to be close to 10 cm. This was in order to allow both flexibility and stability, and for patient comfort and safety. To enable many types of grips and to make the probe easy to handle, the designs of the prototypes' handles were inspired by the shape of a screwdriver but were somewhat larger.

3.4. 3D Printing of Probe Shell Prototypes

Two 3D probes were printed according to the sketches and the methods described above. The proposed 3D probes prototypes are shown in Figure 3.

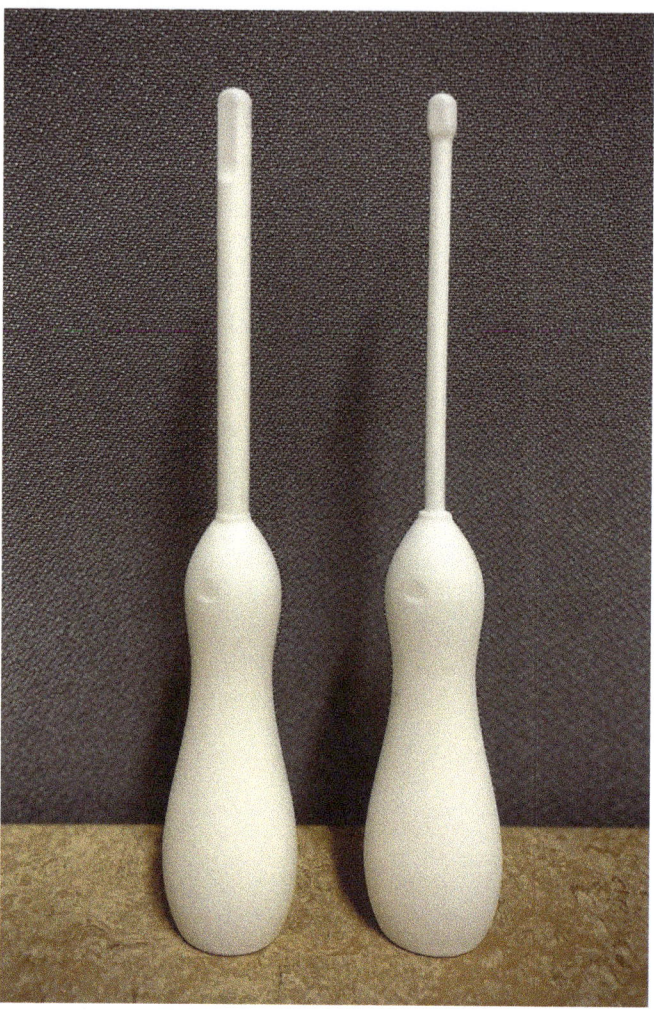

Figure 3. Two prototypes of a pediatric anorectal ultra-high frequency ultrasound probe. The prototype on the left has a head size of 8 mm and a shaft size of 8 mm. The prototype to the right has a head size of 7 mm and a shaft size of 5 mm.

3.5. 3D Prototype Testing

Five pediatric surgeons—three female and two male—tested the two probe prototypes on a baby model. The larger probe, which had a size of 8 mm of both the head and neck, was preferred independently by all surgeons. The reasons stated were that both the design and size facilitated stability and ease of insertion, compared to the somewhat thinner probe prototype with a 7 mm head and a 5 mm shaft (Figure 3). The 8 mm probe prototype allowed the surgeon to hold it comfortably using a one-hand grip. Multiple one-hand grips and working positions for the surgeons were evaluated. Some examiners chose to stand at the feet of the baby during the examination, whereas others preferred to stand by the baby's side. Some preferred to hold the prototype probe very close to the baby, while others preferred to hold it 5–10 cm from the baby's anus. The 8 mm model was also preferred with regard to ergonomics and positioning (Figure 4).

A tactile indicator was printed on the front of the handle of the probe prototype to enable indication of the position of the probe elements. The surgeons' feedback was that this was too small to recognize under the plastic protection wrapped around the probe. The need for enlargement and visibility in updated prototype versions was advocated in order to ensure the correct positioning of the probe.

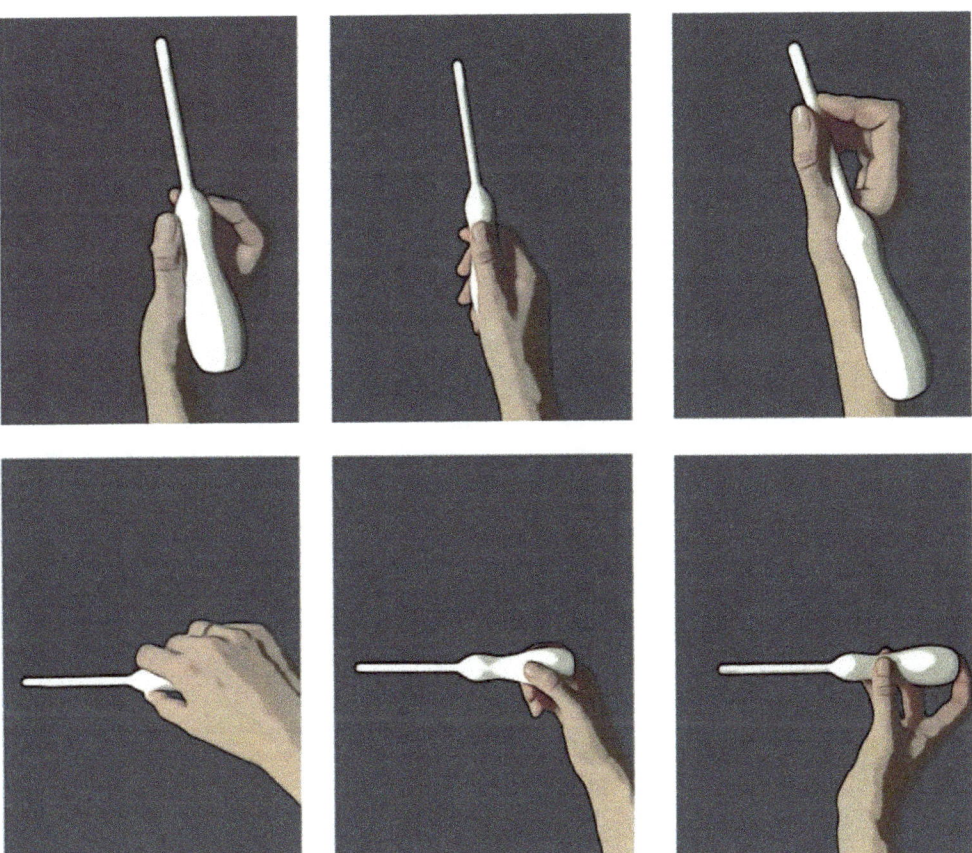

Figure 4. Overview of different grips used by pediatric surgeons of the ultra-high frequency ultrasound probe prototype. The grips shown in the top images were used by surgeons standing at the baby's feet. The grips shown at the bottom were used by surgeons when standing at the side of the baby.

4. Discussion

The aim of this study was to create a geometrically designed requirement specification for a pediatric UHF rectal ultrasound probe in order to enable high-frequency anorectal ultrasound examinations. With information gathered on anorectal measurements and for technology prerequisites, sketches and 3D-printed prototypes were produced and tested. The prototypes selected were reported to be satisfactory with regard to their design and ergonomics. However, some features were missing, such as markings on the handle or neck, to aid the examiner in orientating the probe. During the development process, specific technical uncertainties were raised, especially regarding the type of elements, and the highest center frequency for these, used within a small-diameter probe. The main challenge was to develop a design for a probe that was small and neat, but that still met all technical specification requirements. With this achieved, still bearing in mind that electronic prerequisites need to be considered, this is a first step in the development of a pediatric UHF rectal probe—a product that is urgently required for our pediatric population.

4.1. Design

The pediatric anorectal probe was intended to be used primarily in newborns, since this is the time when the need for an instant diagnostic method for HD and detailed fistula exposure in anorectal malformations is the greatest. As a result of the neonatal consideration, it was decided that the maximum head size should be 7–8 mm. This size was expected to be appropriate, or at least not too large for the majority of patients, since most newborns have an anal opening of a maximum of 12 mm. A small-sized anorectal probe can also be useful in older children. Still, a larger probe head would probably facilitate the connection between the head and the rectal mucosa, which would limit air-induced shadowing effects in the ultrasound images, and the need for gel in the rectal space. Additionally, more advanced technology and electronics could be used if the probe head was larger. However, shadowing effects could be avoided if using only a small area of linear array elements. This is feasible in the examination of a smaller specific area, such as that of the bowel wall instead of aiming for a circular image. In addition to size consideration, and prioritizing comfort for children of low weights, it was decided that the smallest size of probe was preferable. In testing the prototypes, the larger probe with a size of 8 mm of both the head and shaft was preferred by all surgeons in our study, since this design and size facilitated stability and ease of insertion. The bigger geometry could also be more beneficial when accommodating the electronics within. The size of the rectal suction biopsy instrument (rbi2®) is 8 mm, which causes only limited tension at the anal opening for most children. Nevertheless, children with fistulas within anorectal malformations could have anal openings narrower than 8 mm before surgery. With regard to inserting electronics, it might be difficult to create a linear high-frequency probe for anal openings smaller than 8 mm. This remains to be clinically evaluated in the future.

A total probe shaft length was tested by the grip of other instruments and the optimum length was considered to be 10 cm. The length was decided as a trade-off between greater measuring distances provided by longer shafts, e.g., in older children with a longer rectum, and the increased stability given by shorter shafts. The 10 cm shaft length was appreciated by all the surgeons in our study, and no surgeon wished that the length was longer. This shaft length also allowed a stable examination of tissues at a shorter distance from the anus, when holding the probe by the neck, letting the handle rest on the upper side of the hand (Figure 4). The testing revealed satisfaction, especially with regard to grip and a flexible examination, and with being able to hold the probe in a position according to the surgeon's personal preferences, i.e., either standing at the patient's feet or by their side. In particular, the handle's fit in smaller hands was appreciated, allowing easy handling by both genders.

Regarding the angulation of the probe head, this implied the possibility of visualizing specific areas more closely without the need to insert gel into the rectum. However, angulation is not highly desirable, because if the shaft is flexible, then this probably places more demands on technology and electronics. If it is rigid (as in the hockey stick design described in Table 1), then this requires a larger anal opening diameter. During the clinical observation of the transesophageal probe, no angulation of the probe head was required to provide sufficient contact between the probe elements and the esophageal wall. Therefore, a straight probe head–neck was suggested. However, to ensure that a straight head-neck probe with no angulation is the best design for in vivo measurements in the rectum, clinical evaluations are needed.

4.2. Technology

Regarding the probe center frequency, 50 MHz was the level set in this study since this has been shown to be useful in delineating between histo-anatomic layers of the bowel wall. The 50 MHz frequency provides resolution of down to 30–50 μm [12]. However, such high frequencies do not allow imaging of deeper depths and, therefore, not all the layers of the bowel wall. Ultrasound frequencies used clinically today usually exhibit a much lower range (2–15 MHz), resulting in a resolution of a maximum 100 µm [13] and an imaging depth of more than 10 mm. In a pediatric cohort, lower frequencies of 15–20 MHz, corresponding to an imaging depth of approximately 2 cm, are already in use, as for visualizing pelvic floor components. These are, however, not suitable for the detailed diagnosis of pathologies of the bowel wall, e.g., aganglionosis, or for providing in-depth information about the internal sphincter. For such complex investigations, a center frequency of 30–50 MHz is desirable, resulting in an imaging depth of a maximum of 5–10 mm.

To produce a probe with a large bandwidth, covering 25–70 MHz, and which allows imaging at both the lower and higher frequency spans, would be desirable, but it is not currently known if this would be possible. However, the DualproTM IVUS + NIRS probe (Table 1) delivers a frequency span of 30–65 MHz and has a fractional bandwidth of 60%, but its electronics and probe elements differ greatly from those of our ideal array probe.

In conventional ultrasound examinations within the lumen, e.g., rectally and intravascularly, transversal ultrasound images (cross-sectional images) are used most commonly. In contrast to this, in our prior research on the use of UHF ultrasound for discriminating between the aganglionic and ganglionic bowel, a linear array probe producing longitudinal ultrasound images was used [4]. The benefit of longitudinal images is that a larger area of the bowel wall viewed caudally to cranially can be investigated within the same image. A cross-sectional view could, of course, be an option, but investigation as to whether differentiation between ganglionic and aganglionic bowel wall can also be made in cross-sectional images is needed and studies are currently ongoing.

If a transversal imaging approach (cross-sectional images) is preferred, then a curvilinear probe including probe elements arranged along a curved surface would probably be favorable. This is because a curve will allow more elements to be placed in the probe, which would be necessary since a cross-sectional view requires the mounting of elements perpendicular to the shaft, instead of as in the longitudinal case, i.e., in parallel. With such a solution, a decrease in lateral resolution will then be seen, and especially with depth since the ultrasound beams will slightly diverge from each other. A decrease in lateral resolution would, on the other hand, also be the result of a rotating single-element probe. This is since the beamforming will not be able to be performed with a one-element probe because of a diversion of beams. In contrast, a beamforming can be obtained with an array probe. However, if a pediatric rectal probe with circular and cross-sectional UHF imaging is the aim, then a lower lateral resolution might need to be accepted, as long as the resolution of the central image is sufficient. Whether this is good enough to be used for HD diagnosis could be studied, e.g., using the IVUS catheter probe.

A great benefit of using the IVUS technique is that these probes already operate at UHF, which is required for HD diagnostics. Obstacles foreseen with the rectal use of IVUS are the diameter difference between the rectum and probe, and the fact that a stiffer shaft would be desirable to enhance the steering of the probe.

Another option is to rotate a linear array probe within a rigid tube, as in the Endocavity 3D 9038, BK Medical probe (see Table 1). This probe would provide 3D images with high resolution, but the electronics required would most probably not fit into a small-sized pediatric ultrasound probe.

The strengths of this development study are that it followed a participatory design [14] within a high-competence medical center performing unique translational studies of UHF ultrasound of the bowel wall. Additionally, anorectal measurements from radiology reports and clinical observations were collected within a national center with considerable experience in registering pediatric anorectal dimensions. Furthermore, the design specifications presented here are based primarily on patient safety and comfort.

One certain limitation of our study was that all available probes on the market could not be identified. Therefore, some might not have been included in our review, or some that have just been launched onto the market could have been omitted. Another limitation was that the prototype has not yet been tested on a child. The reason for this was that this study was required to be performed in order to be able to obtain ethical approval for testing probes and prototypes anorectally in humans. A serious consideration is that the 8 mm probe head could be too small for manufacturers to choose to invest in financially, as a result of the difficulties and expenses in developing small electronic devices.

4.3. Future Improvements and Work

This study mainly focused on the design aspects and on the technical specifications of a potential pediatric rectal probe. With these considerations now in place, the electronics required for creating an UHF ultrasound probe can begin. One clear improvement of the probe design will be to mark the shaft with depth distances and orientation markings indicating the head's direction up and down. This would facilitate descriptions of examinations and imaging orientation. These indications would preferably be both visual, for example, using colored dots indicating the distance to the tip of the probe, as well as using distinct tactile markings large enough to enable detection through a sterile plastic wrap.

Since existing ultrasound probes have similar designs to our prototypes, such as the Philips S8-3t transesophageal probe, and the endobronchial ultrasound BF-UC190F probe, we believe that the creation of a pediatric UHF rectal probe is feasible. However, we are aware that in order to insert the desired UHF technology into the probe, the demands on its construction and electronics will be high. The results of our study should be widely contemplated with respect to how they can be interpreted from the perspective of previous studies and of the working hypotheses. The findings and their implications should be discussed in the broadest context possible. Future research directions may also be highlighted.

5. Conclusions

This is the first step in developing a novel non-invasive diagnostic method to examine the bowel wall in children—a pediatric anorectal UHF ultrasound probe. We believe that such a device can open new possibilities for diagnosing anorectal conditions in children.

Table 1. Overview of selected probes available on the market and in clinical use for diagnostics.

Probe	Appearance	Applications	Frequency Range (MHz)	Probe Type/Field of View	Number of Elements	Physical Dimensions (mm)	Comments: General and Specifically Regarding Anorectal Use in Children
Transesophageal (TTE) S8-3t, Philips, Amsterdam, The Netherlands [15]		Cardiac imaging from the esophagus. Adapted for use in children.	3–8	Phased array/90° sector.	32	Head: 7.5 × 5.5 × 18.5. Shaft diameter: 5.2. Shaft length: 880.	+ Small-sized probe head + Enables angulation of probe head − Shaft too long to use anorectally in an awake child − Large handle—two hands are needed to rotate the dials on the handle that steer the probe − Too low frequency

Table 1. Cont.

Probe	Appearance	Applications	Frequency Range (MHz)	Probe Type/Field of View	Number of Elements	Physical Dimensions (mm)	Comments: General and Specifically Regarding Anorectal Use in Children
Endobronchial ultrasound, EBUS, BF-UC190F, Olympus Medical Systems, Long Thanh, Vietnam [16]		Pulmonary bronchus imaging.	5–12	Curved linear array/65° sector.		Head diameter: 6.6. Shaft diameter: 6.3. Shaft length: 600.	+ Small-sized probe head + Enables angulation of probe head + Enables taking biopsy + Water-filled balloon around probe head implying better tissue contact in air-filled environment − Shaft too long to use anorectally in an awake child − Too low frequency
Intravascular ultrasound (IVUS), Dualpro™ IVUS + NIRS, Infraredx Inc., Bedford, MA, USA [17]		Imaging from the inside of the lumen of the vessels.	35–65	Rotating single element/360° image.	Single element	Head diameter: 0.8–1.15. Shaft diameter: 1.2. Shaft length: 1600.	+ 360° 3D images + High frequency—high resolution + Extended bandwidth, can transmit both lower and higher frequencies + Near infrared spectroscopy is integrated − Mismatch between rectum and probe diameter, risking insufficient contact and shadowing
Hockey stick L8-18I-RS, GE, Chicago, IL, USA [18]		Shallow imaging, e.g., cardiovascular, musculoskeletal and small parts.	8–18	Linear array/rectangular.			+/− Smaller size than conventional ultrasound probes, but too large to be used anorectally in children − Too short neck − Too low frequency
Laparoscopic L44LA, FujiFilm [19]		Imaging during laparoscopic surgery.	2–13	Linear array/rectangular, maximum width: 36 mm.		Head diameter: 10.	+ Small size of probe head + Angulation of probe head − Shaft too long to use anorectally in an awake child − Too low frequency
Endocavity, 3D 9038, BK Medical, Burlington, MA, USA [20,21]		Transrectal and transvaginal imaging.	4–14	Rotating linear array/360° image.	192	Diameter: 16. Neck length: 155.	+ 360° image created with linear probe + 3D images can be produced − Too large to be used anorectally in children − Too low frequency
Prostate Triplane Transducer, 9018, BK Medical [22,23]		Transrectal probe for prostate imaging.	4–14	Curved linear array/180° sector.	128 + 192	Diameter: 20.	+ Imaging in two perpendicular planes + Enables taking biopsy − Too large to be used in anorectally in children − Too low frequency

Author Contributions: Conceptualization: P.S., M.C. and M.E.; Methodology: P.S., M.C., M.E., A.V., O.W. and T.E.; Analysis: P.S., M.C., M.E., C.G., A.V., O.W. and K.H.; Investigation: M.E., A.V., O.W., P.S. and C.G.; Resources: P.S. and C.G.; Writing—Original Draft Preparation: M.E., P.S., A.V. and O.W.; Writing—review and editing: C.G., T.E., M.C. and K.H.; Visualization: A.V., O.W. and M.E.; Project administration: P.S.; Supervision: M.E., P.S., M.C. and C.G. All authors have read and agreed to the published version of the manuscript.

Funding: Open access funding was provided by Lund University, Sweden. The study was funded by The Swedish Research Council's Starting Grant 2021-01569, The Swedish Regional Research funding (ALF) Region Skåne 43902, Skåne University Hospital's Funding 95911 (SUS Fonder och Stiftelser).

Institutional Review Board Statement: The study was conducted in accordance with the Declaration of Helsinki, and approved by the Local Ethics Committee (DNR 2017/769).

Informed Consent Statement: Parental informed consent was obtained on behalf of all subjects involved in the study.

Data Availability Statement: The data presented in this study are available on reasonable request from the corresponding author.

Acknowledgments: We would like to thank Matthias Götberg, Zahraa Alsafi, Stefan Barath, Misha Bhat and Valeria Perez de Sá for presenting and demonstrating their ultrasound equipment. We would also like to thank Axel Tojo for help with printing the 3D prototypes, and Ros Kenn, Medical Editor, for assistance with editing the manuscript.

Conflicts of Interest: The authors declare no conflict of interest.

References

1. Amandullaevich, A.Y.; Danabaevich, J.K. Ultrasound diagnosis of Hirschsprung's disease in children. *Cent. Asian J. Med. Nat. Sci.* **2022**, *3*, 64–71.
2. Butler Tjaden, N.E.; Trainor, P.A. The developmental etiology and pathogenesis of Hirschsprung disease. *Transl. Res.* **2013**, *162*, 1–15. [CrossRef]
3. Lake, J.I.; Heuckeroth, R.O. Enteric nervous system development: Migration, differentiation, and disease. *Am. J. Physiol. Gastrointest. Liver Physiol.* **2013**, *305*, G1–G24. [CrossRef] [PubMed]
4. Granéli, C.; Erlöv, T.; Mitev, R.M.; Kasselaki, I.; Hagelsteen, K.; Gisselsson, D.; Jansson, T.; Cinthio, M.; Stenström, P. Ultra high frequency ultrasonography to distinguish ganglionic from aganglionic bowel wall in Hirschsprung disease: A first report. *J. Pediatr. Surg.* **2021**, *56*, 2281–2285. [CrossRef] [PubMed]
5. Martucciello, G.; Pini Prato, A.; Puri, P.; Holschneider, A.M.; Meier-Ruge, W.; Jasonni, V.; Tovar, J.A.; Grosfeld, J.L. Controversies concerning diagnostic guidelines for anomalies of the enteric nervous system: A report from the fourth International Symposium on Hirschsprung's disease and related neurocristopathies. *J. Pediatr. Surg.* **2005**, *40*, 1527–1531. [CrossRef] [PubMed]
6. Petchasuwan, C.; Pintong, J. Immunohistochemistry for intestinal ganglion cells and nerve fibers: Aid in the diagnosis of Hirschsprung's disease. *J. Med. Assoc. Thail.* **2000**, *83*, 1402–1409.
7. Fransson, E.; Granéli, C.; Hagelsteen, K.; Tofft, L.; Hambraeus, M.; Munoz Mitev, R.U.; Gisselsson, D.; Stenström, P. Diagnostic efficacy of rectal suction biopsy with regard to weight in children investigated for Hirschsprung's disease. *Children* **2022**, *9*, 124. [CrossRef] [PubMed]
8. Frongia, G.; Günther, P.; Schenk, J.-P.; Strube, K.; Kessler, M.; Mehrabi, A.; Romero, P. Contrast enema for Hirschsprung disease investigation: Diagnostic accuracy and validity for subsequent diagnostic and surgical planning. *Eur. J. Pediatr. Surg.* **2016**, *26*, 207–214. [PubMed]
9. Vult von Steyern, K.; Wingren, P.; Wiklund, M.; Stenström, P.; Arnbjörnsson, E. Visualisation of the rectoanal inhibitory reflex with a modified contrast enema in children with suspected Hirschsprung disease. *Pediatr. Radiol.* **2013**, *43*, 950–957. [CrossRef] [PubMed]
10. Graneli, C.; Patarroyo, S.; Munoz Mitev, R.; Gisselsson, D.; Gottberg, E.; Erlöv, T.; Jansson, T.; Hagelsteen, K.; Cinthio, M.; Stenström, P. Histopathological dimensions differ between aganglionic and ganglionic bowel wall in children with Hirschsprung's disease. *BMC Pediatr.* **2022**, *22*, 723. [CrossRef] [PubMed]
11. Wehrli, L.A.; Reppucci, M.L.; Ketzer, J.; de la Torre, L.; Peña, A.; Bischoff, A. Stricture rate in patients after the repair of anorectal malformation following a standardized dilation protocol. *Pediatr. Surg. Int.* **2022**, *38*, 1717–1721. [CrossRef] [PubMed]
12. Vevo®MD. The World's First Ultra High Frequency Ultrasound Imaging System. Available online: https://www.visualsonics.com/sites/default/files/VisualSonics_VevoMDBrochure_MKT03036_V1.3.pdf (accessed on 30 March 2023).
13. Hoskins, P.; Martin, K.; Thrush, A. (Eds.) *Diagnostic Ultrasound: Physics and Equipment*, 3rd ed.; CRC Press: Boca Raton, FL, USA, 2019.
14. Clemensen, J.; Larsen, S.B.; Kyng, M.; Kirkevold, M. Participatory design in health sciences: Using cooperative experimental methods in developing health services and computer technology. *Qual. Health Res.* **2007**, *17*, 122–130. [CrossRef] [PubMed]

15. S8-3t Sector Array Transducer. Available online: https://www.usa.philips.com/healthcare/product/HC989605431171/s8-3t-sector-array-transducer (accessed on 30 March 2023).
16. EBUS-TBNA_BF-UC190F_Brochures and Flyers (Sellsheets)_EN_E0428389EN_103563. Available online: https://www.olympus-europa.com/medical/en/Products-and-Solutions/Products/Product/BF-UC190F.html (accessed on 30 March 2023).
17. Dualpro IVUS+NIRS. Available online: https://www.infraredx.com/products/dualpro-nirs/ (accessed on 30 March 2023).
18. L8 -18I-RS Probe. Available online: https://services.gehealthcare.co.uk/gehcstorefront/p/5499609 (accessed on 30 March 2023).
19. Transducers. Available online: https://www.fujifilmsurgical.com/transducers/ (accessed on 30 March 2023).
20. 3D X14L4 (9038) Endocavity Transducer. Available online: https://www.bkmedical.com/transducers/endocavity-3d-x14l4/ (accessed on 30 March 2023).
21. *16-01665-00 X14L4 Product Data*; BK Medical: Herlev, Denmark, December 2017.
22. E14C4t (9018) Prostate Triplane Transducer. Available online: https://www.bkmedical.com/transducers/e14c4t-prostate-triplane/ (accessed on 30 March 2023).
23. *16-01257-07 E14C4t Product Data*; BK Medical: Herlev, Denmark, November 2018.

Disclaimer/Publisher's Note: The statements, opinions and data contained in all publications are solely those of the individual author(s) and contributor(s) and not of MDPI and/or the editor(s). MDPI and/or the editor(s) disclaim responsibility for any injury to people or property resulting from any ideas, methods, instructions or products referred to in the content.

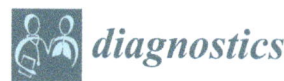

Case Report

High Intensity Focused Ultrasound Ablation for Juvenile Cystic Adenomyosis: Two Case Reports and Literature Review

Xin Liu [1,2,†], Jingxi Wang [2,†], Yanglu Liu [1], Shuang Luo [2,*], Gaowu Yan [3], Huaqi Yang [2], Lili Wan [2] and Guohua Huang [2,*]

[1] School of Medical and Life Science, Chengdu University of Traditional Chinese Medicine, Chengdu 610000, China
[2] Department of Gynecology, Suining Central Hospital, Suining 629000, China; yanghuaqi751@outlook.com (H.Y.)
[3] Department of Radiology and Imaging, Suining Central Hospital, Suining 629000, China
* Correspondence: doctorlsls@sina.com (S.L.); hghyyh@hotmail.com (G.H.)
† These authors contributed equally to this work.

Abstract: Cystic adenomyosis is a rare type of uterine adenomyosis, mainly seen in young women, which is often characterized by severe dysmenorrhea. The quality of life and reproductive function of young women could be affected by misdiagnosis and delayed treatment. At present, there are no universal guidelines and consensus. We report two cases of patients with cystic adenomyosis in juveniles treated with high-intensity focused ultrasound (HIFU) ablation. In the first case, magnetic resonance imaging (MRI) indicated a cystic mass of 2.0 cm × 3.1 cm × 2.4 cm in the uterus. After she underwent HIFU treatment, her pelvic MRI showed a mass of 1.1 × 2.4 cm in size, and her dysmenorrhea symptoms gradually disappeared. In the second case, a pelvic MRI indicated a 5.1 cm × 3.3 cm × 4.7 cm cystic mass in the uterus. After she underwent HIFU and combined four consecutive cycles of GnRH-a treatment, the lesion shrunk 1.2 cm × 1.4 cm × 1.6 cm, without dysmenorrhea. Simultaneously, the report reviewed 14 cases of juvenile cystic adenomyosis over the last ten years. HIFU or HIFU-combined drugs were safe and effective in treating juvenile cystic adenomyosis, but multicenter and prospective studies may be necessary to validate this in the future.

Keywords: juvenile cystic adenomyosis; high-intensity focused ultrasound (HIFU); adolescent; dysmenorrhea

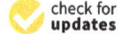

Citation: Liu, X.; Wang, J.; Liu, Y.; Luo, S.; Yan, G.; Yang, H.; Wan, L.; Huang, G. High Intensity Focused Ultrasound Ablation for Juvenile Cystic Adenomyosis: Two Case Reports and Literature Review. *Diagnostics* 2023, *13*, 1608. https://doi.org/10.3390/diagnostics13091608

Academic Editor: Paolo Ivo Cavoretto

Received: 6 March 2023
Revised: 5 April 2023
Accepted: 25 April 2023
Published: 1 May 2023

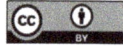

Copyright: © 2023 by the authors. Licensee MDPI, Basel, Switzerland. This article is an open access article distributed under the terms and conditions of the Creative Commons Attribution (CC BY) license (https://creativecommons.org/licenses/by/4.0/).

1. Introduction

Adenomyosis is a common gynecologic disease that mainly occurs in women aged thirty to fifty years and is characterized by the invasion of ectopic endometrial tissue into the myometrium. Myometrial cysts of any size are the direct ultrasonographic features of adenomyosis, and transvaginal 2D ultrasound is the most accurate way to observe this sign [1,2]. However, the lesions of the rare cystic adenomyosis have a diameter of more than 1 cm and are filled with ectopic endometrial tissue and bloody fluid [3]. According to literature reports, the disease has increased in adolescent patients in recent years. We reviewed 14 cases of adolescent cystic adenomyosis in the past decade (Table A1) and found that there was no unified expert consensus on the treatment of adolescent cystic adenomyosis, and the choice of treatment was difficult. Currently, the effect of medication is limited in patients with juvenile cystic adenomyosis. Surgical treatment is a mainly conservative operation with reproductive function preservation, which causes side effects such as adhesion, iatrogenic endometriosis, and a high recurrence rate [4]. Because juvenile cystic adenomyosis patients have fertility requirements, minimally invasive or noninvasive treatments are acceptable. Noninvasive treatment has been of gradually increased in the treatment of cystic adenomyosis. In this report, our center carried out two cases of juvenile cystic adenomyosis treatments using HIFU and HIFU combined with medication.

1.1. Case 1

The patient was 16 years old, without a sexual life history, and was admitted to the hospital with dysmenorrhea for 1 year, uterine occupation for half a year, and abdominal pain for 4 days. The patient had regular menstruation with severe dysmenorrhea. Four days earlier, she developed severe paroxysmal abdominal pain without an obvious trigger, and the VAS score was 7, without any other discomfort (Table 1). She denied having a history of hypertension, diabetes, heart disease, malignancy, and surgery. A physical examination revealed an anterior uterus of normal size and medium texture that was movable and painful pressure. Routine blood tests were normal, and serum tumor markers were CA125: 127.6 U/mL, CA199: 14.5 U/mL, and CEA: 0.3 ng/mL. A transabdominal ultrasound (Philips IU22, Philips) revealed an abnormal uterine development and a bicorned uterus. A posterior pelvic MRI showed a round cystic mass with a size of about 2.0 cm × 3.1 cm × 2.4 cm between the muscle walls of the right lateral wall of the uterus, showing short T1 and long T2 signals. The lesion was significantly enhanced on enhanced scanning, with clear boundaries and uterine cavity compression, which was considered to be cystic adenomyosis (Figure 1). Combining the patient's clinical symptoms and MRI, the patient was diagnosed with juvenile cystic adenomyosis. Because of a strong desire for conservative treatment, she opted for HIFU treatment on 22 November 2017. A focused ultrasonic ablation was performed under sedation and analgesia, and compound polyethylene glycol electrolyte powder was used to induce diarrhea 3 days before treatment. Before the operation, routine skin preparation, degreasing, degassing, catheterization, and indwelling catheter were performed to fill the bladder and establish a safe acoustic channel. The patient was placed in a prone position and given fentanyl citrate and midazolam for sedation and analgesia. The location of the lesion was determined using ultrasound, and the therapeutic power was 200 W. The range of gray change in the lesion was satisfactory at 250 s after irradiation. The ultrasound showed no obvious blood flow signal in the lesion, and ultrasound angiography showed no blood perfusion in the lesion (Figure 2). The details of the procedure were treatment time: 49 min, irradiation time: 250 s, treatment power: 200 W, treatment intensity: 306/s, and an ablation volume evaluation of 80% (Table 2). During the treatment, the patient complained of pain in the treatment area and sacrococcygeal pain, which was relieved after rest. After the operation, the patient's vital signs were stable, and she was advised to rest in a prone position for 2 h and fast from food and drink for 2 h. For the follow-up: the first month after treatment, the pelvic MRI showed a mass of 1.2 cm × 1.9 cm × 1.7 cm (Figure 3), with a reduction rate of 73%. The patient's menstrual volume was the same as before, and her dysmenorrhea symptoms were significantly relieved with a VAS score of 2. Since then, irregular reexamination with ultrasound indicated that the size of the mass was 3–5 cm. The fifth year after treatment, pelvic MRI indicated that the mass was 1.1 cm × 2.4 cm × 1.0 cm (Figure 4), and the volume reduction rate was 69%. However, her menstruation was normal, her dysmenorrhea disappeared, and her VAS score was 0 (Table 1).

Table 1. Pre- and post-treatment parameters in two patients.

Subject	Before HIFU Treatment			After HIFU Treatment			Combined with Drugs
	Lesion Size	Symptoms	VAS Score	Lesion Size (cm)	Symptoms	VAS Score	
Case 1	2.0 cm × 3.1 cm × 2.4 cm	dysmenorrhea	7	1.1 cm × 2.4 cm × 1.0 cm [1]	recovery	0	no
Case 2	5.1 cm × 3.3 cm × 4.7 cm	dysmenorrhea	8	1.2 cm × 1.4 cm × 1.6 cm [2]	recovery	0	yes [3]

[1] Pelvic MRI shows lesions after HIFU treatment (5th year); [2] Pelvic MRI shows lesions after HIFU treatment (8th month); [3] Combined with GnRH-a injection for 4 period.

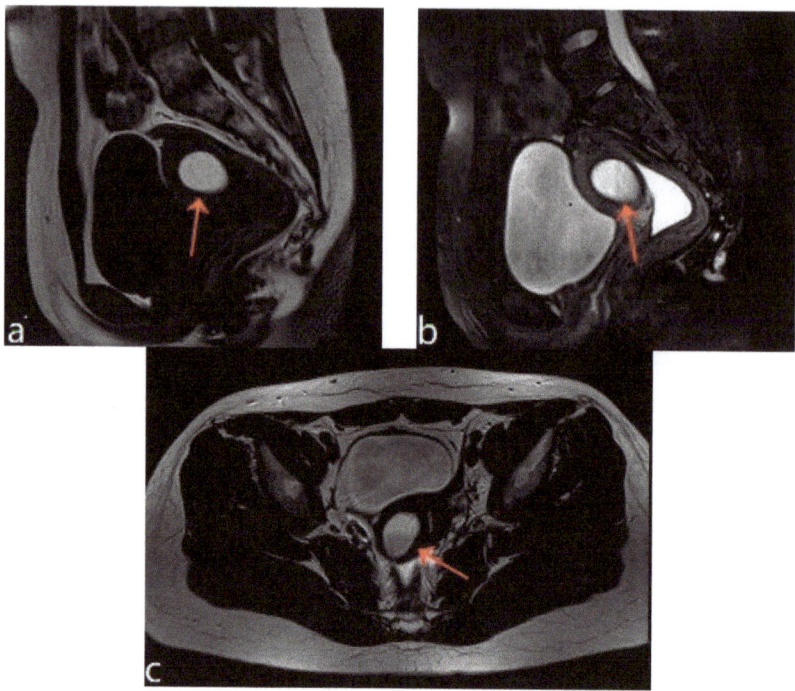

Figure 1. (**a–c**) Pelvic MRI: sagittal T1WI sequence (**a**), sagittal T2WI fat suppression sequence (**b**), and axial T2WI non-fat suppression (**c**) showing a cystic lesion in the right posterior wall of the uterus with regular morphology, oval shape, and clear border (red arrows).

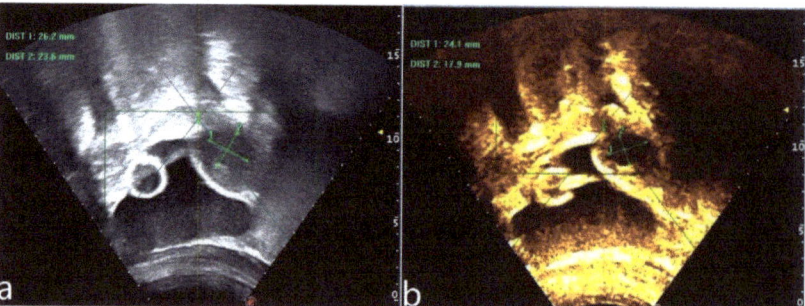

Figure 2. Ultrasound image of the lesion before HIFU treatment (**a**). Ultrasonography after HIFU treatment shows no perfusion of the lesion (**b**).

Table 2. Parameters associated with HIFU treatment in both patients.

Subject	Treatment Time	Irradiation Time	Treatment Power	Treatment Intensity	Ablation Volume Evaluation
Case 1	49 min	250 s	200 W	306/s	80%
Case 2	75 min	650 s	300 W	517/s	90%

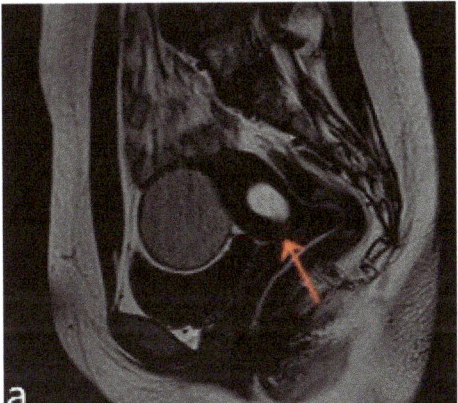
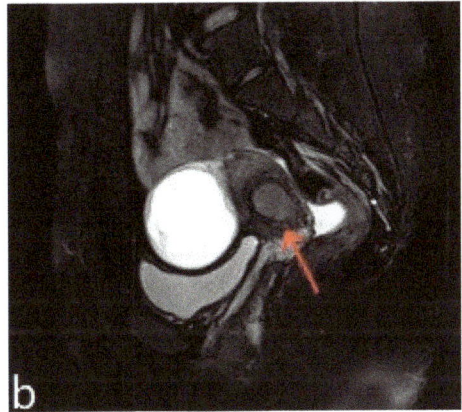

Figure 3. (a,b) Pelvic MRI shows lesions after HIFU treatment (1st month)(red arrows).

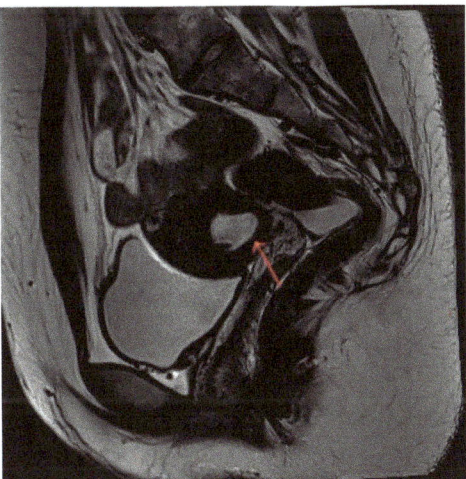

Figure 4. Pelvic MRI shows lesions after HIFU treatment (5th year) (red arrows).

1.2. Case 2

The patient was 20 years old, without a sexual life history. She had normal menstrual cycles with menometrorrhagia and severe dysmenorrhea. She was admitted to the hospital with dysmenorrhea with a progressive aggravation over 5 years. The patient developed dysmenorrhea with progressive aggravation 5 years previously without obvious triggers, and the VAS score was 8 (Table 1). She had been treated with ibuprofen without relief in symptoms. The patient denied a history of hypertension, diabetes, heart disease, malignant tumor, and surgery. A physical examination revealed an enlarged uterus with a medium texture and pressure pain. Routine blood tests and serum tumor markers were normal. A transabdominal ultrasound (Voluson E10, GE Healthcare, Zipf, Austria) revealed a cystic lesion measuring 1.7 cm × 0.9 cm × 1.8 cm in the myometrium. The results of the CDFI: punctate and obvious strip blood flow signals. However, MRI clearly revealed a cystic lesion measuring 5.1 cm × 3.3 cm × 4.7 cm in the myometrium. The enhanced scan indicated a stale haemorrhage in the cystic lesion (Figure 5). According to the patient's history and an auxiliary examination, the patient was diagnosed with juvenile cystic adenomyosis. Because of a strong desire for conservative treatment, she opted for HIFU treatment on

8 April 2022, under sedation and analgesia. The treatment power was 300 W, the irradiation time was 750 s, the treatment intensity was 517/s, and the treatment time was 75 min (Table 2). After the treatment, an ultrasound revealed an overall grayscale change in the lesion, and ultrasound angiography indicated a satisfactory ablation. The ablation volume was evaluated at 90%. The patient's vital signs were stable after treatment. For the follow-up: the pelvic MRI on the first day after treatment showed a uterine cyst of 3.8 cm × 2.6 cm × 3.9 cm (Figure 6), with a reduction rate of 51% in mass volume. One month later, the patient had a menstrual flow of the same volume as before, with relief of dysmenorrhea symptoms and a VAS score of 4. In the second month after treatment, GnRH-a therapy was started for four cycles (28 days for one cycle). Eight months after treatment, a pelvic MRI showed a cystic mass of about 1.2 cm × 1.4 cm × 1.6 cm in size (Figure 7), and the volume reduction rate was 97%. Meanwhile, the patient had normal menstruation without dysmenorrhea, with a VAS score of 0 (Table 1).

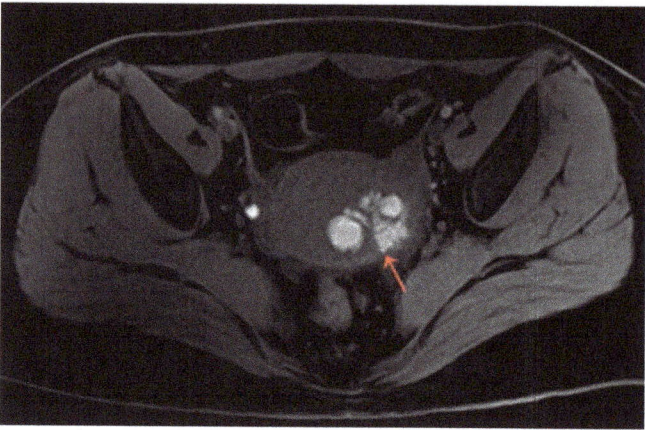

Figure 5. Pelvic MRI shows a cystic lesion with irregular morphology in myometrium (red arrow).

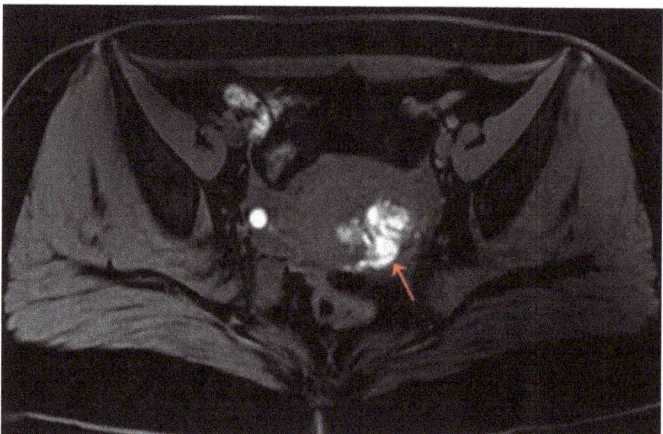

Figure 6. Pelvic MRI shows lesions after HIFU treatment (1st day) (red arrow).

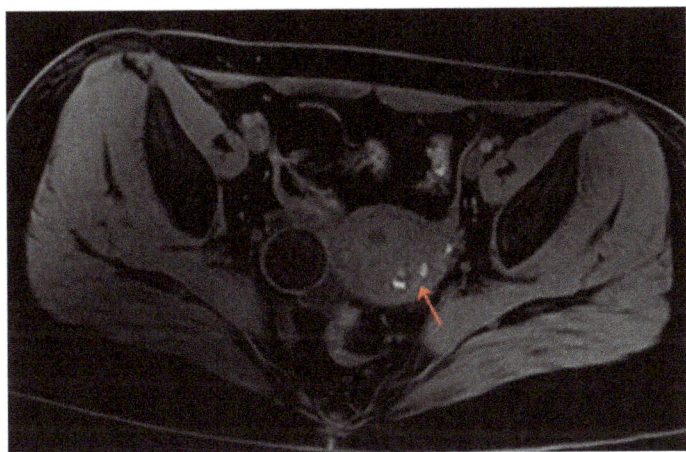

Figure 7. Pelvic MRI shows lesions HIFU treatment (8th month) (red arrow).

2. Discussion

In 1990, Parulekar [5] reported the cystic transformation of uterine adenomyoma, and then in 1996, Tamura [6] et al. first reported a case of cystic adenomyosis in a 16-year-old woman. The incidence of cystic adenomyosis is now reported in the literature to be 5–70%. Currently, there is an increasing and younger trend, with 65–75% of women aged ≤30 years having cystic adenomyosis [7]. The main feature of cystic adenomyosis is the presence of one or more cystic cavities within the myometrium. This cystic cavity contains brownish, stale bloody fluid, and it does not communicate with the uterine cavity [8], while the cyst wall consists of endometrial glands and epithelium of the mesenchyme, surrounded by myometrial tissue. The clinical manifestations are mainly progressive and unbearable dysmenorrhea, menometrorrhagia, menostaxis, pelvic pain, infertility, etc. A few patients may be asymptomatic. A review of the relevant literature in the past 10 years showed that there were a total of 14 cases of adolescent uterine cystic adenomyosis with an average onset age of about 14 years, among which 13 cases had severe dysmenorrhea as the starting symptom. Thus, this progressive and aggravated dysmenorrhea is the main symptom of adolescent uterine cystic adenomyosis. The two patients in this study also fit this characteristic.

Juvenile cystic adenomyosis is rare, with dysmenorrhea as the primary symptom, and is highly misdiagnosed as female obstructive genital tract malformations and uterine myomatous cystic degeneration [7]. Imaging is an effective method for diagnosing the disease, especially MRI, which enables most patients to be diagnosed in early adolescence [9]. MRI not only reflects the characteristic signal of the mass and clarifies the location and size of the mass but also identifies complex uterine malformations, which is the best diagnostic modality for this disease. Its sensitivity can reach 78–88% and specificity 67–93% [10]. Because most patients are adolescents with no sexual history, the application of the transvaginal ultrasound is limited. Transabdominal ultrasound is also often misdiagnosed because of the thickness of the abdominal fat and intra-abdominal gas interference. The first patient in this study had an abdominal ultrasound suggestive of a bicornuate uterus, suggesting that cystic adenomyosis needs to be differentiated from uterine anomalies and is easily misdiagnosed as such. MRI can be used for further identification; reviewing the relevant literature from the last decade, all patients with juvenile cystic adenomyosis were easily diagnosed using MRI. Both patients in this study were also clearly diagnosed using MRI combined with clinical symptoms.

Juvenile cystic adenomyosis differs from adult cystic adenomyosis. Kriplani et al. [11] noted that adult patients with an age of onset older than 30 years, with symptoms resembling typical adenomyosis, mostly had a history of surgical trauma to the uterus. In contrast, Takeuchi et al. [8] stated the diagnostic criteria for juvenile cystic adenomyosis: (1) an age ≤ 30 years; (2) the cyst ≥ 1 cm, with the cavity independent of the uterine cavity and surrounded by hyperplastic smooth muscle tissue; and (3) an early onset of severe dysmenorrhea. However, Chun et al. [12] concluded that the older age of onset defined by Takeuchi could lead to inaccurate typing in some cases and proposed new diagnostic criteria for the adolescent type: (1) an age of onset ≤ 18 years or severe dysmenorrhea within 5 years of menarche; (2) those without a history of uterine surgical operation; and (3) those with a cystic cavity diameter ≥ 5 mm. Both patients in this study presented with severe dysmenorrhea at the age of 15 years and had no previous history of uterine operation. Therefore, they accord with the new diagnostic criteria for adolescents proposed by Chun. This criterion clearly indicates the difference between adolescent and adult forms and improves the diagnostic acuity of clinical workers in juvenile cystic adenomyosis.

Currently, there are no unified guidelines and expert consensus on the diagnosis and treatment of adolescent uterine cystic adenomyosis. Clinical treatment principles focus on symptom relief, lesion size control, and fertility protection. We analyzed the treatment of fourteen cases of adolescent uterine cystic adenomyosis in the past 10 years and found that surgery or combined drug therapy was the primary treatment. Five of the patients were unsatisfactory after pharmacological treatment. The other nine patients were mainly treated with laparoscopic cyst resection or postoperative combined drug therapy, and their symptoms were relieved after surgery. Surgical treatment is an effective way to treat uterine cystic adenomyosis. However, surgery may damage the normal muscle tissue surrounding isolated cystic adenomyosis lesions. For young women with childbearing needs, surgery may increase the risk of uterine rupture during pregnancy and may cause iatrogenic endometriosis during the procedure [13–15]. Therefore, surgical treatment is not well accepted by women who are nullipara. In the two patients reported in this study, the lesions were located between the myometrium, and surgical excision of the cysts was highly likely to damage the normal uterine physiological structure. Therefore, they preferred a non-invasive treatment. In a review of the literature in the past 10 years, only one patient received ethanol injection sclerotherapy, and the symptoms still existed after 5 months of follow-up. Therefore, ethanol injection sclerotherapy has poor clinical efficacy for this disease. Ryo et al. [16] reported a case of cystic adenomyosis with symptom relief after radiofrequency ablation. However, the safe and effective dose of radiofrequency ablation and ethanol is not clear, and pathological diagnosis is not available, which may lead to intrauterine adhesiveness and should be used with caution in patients with childbearing needs [17]. In recent years, the literature on the treatment of juvenile cystic adenomyosis has gradually tended toward minimally invasive or noninvasive treatment, among which HIFU has received much attention for its good safety and effectiveness in the treatment of uterine fibroids and adenomyosis [18]. It principally uses the physical characteristics of tissue penetration and the focusing and energy deposition of the ultrasound to focus in vitro ultrasound on the area of interest in the lesion to produce a thermal effect (instant temperature up to 65~100 °C), cavitation effect, and immune effect to cause irreversible changes in the lesion site, instantaneous protein degeneration, and tissue coagulation necrosis. Finally, by activating the body's own immune mechanism, the necrotic tissue of the lesion is absorbed [19]. HIFU treatment as a new non-invasive treatment method has been reported in cases with good clinical efficacy. Zhou et al. [20] reported three cases of juvenile cystic adenomyosis with complete symptomatic remission with HIFU treatment, but with only 3–6 months of follow-up and without combined drug therapy, and whether there were subsequent fertility implications was not elaborated. Combined with the two patient's histories, physical examinations, and auxiliary examinations, the final clinical diagnosis was juvenile cystic adenomyosis. Both patients underwent ultrasound before HIFU treatment; the ultrasonography showed a rich blood supply in the lesion. After HIFU treatment, ultrasonography showed that the lesion was reduced in size, with satisfactory grayscale changes and no blood perfusion in the lesion area. Neither of the patients had complications such as skin damage, intestinal perforation, or nerve damage during the treatment. Their dysmenorrhea symptoms were significantly relieved or even disappeared after HIFU treatment, and the lesions gradually shrank.

According to the literature, the use of GnRH-a drugs after treatment is mostly recommended to prevent recurrence [21]. The first patient reported in this study was treated with HIFU only and without combined drug therapy, and the follow-up suggested that the mass was not significantly reduced after HIFU treatment, but the dysmenorrhea symptoms were significantly relieved. The second patient was treated with HIFU that was combined with GnRH-a postoperatively, and the follow-up showed a significant reduction of the lesion, with a 97% reduction of the mass volume. Her dysmenorrhea symptoms were completely relieved and have not recurred since the follow-up. Therefore, it is worth noting that in the treatment of juvenile cystic adenomyosis, HIFU combined with drug therapy is significantly better than HIFU therapy alone for lesion size control. A study found that HIFU treatment for adenomyosis does not increase the risk of uterine rupture [22]. We reviewed the literature and found only two patients who had uterine rupture during delivery after HIFU treatment [23,24]. However, the correlation between HIFU treatment for adenomyosis and uterine rupture cannot be explained. The two patients in this study were nullipara, and close observation and follow-up were required before pregnancy, during pregnancy, and during delivery.

3. Conclusions

Juvenile cystic adenomyosis is a specific type of uterine adenomyosis that is rare and very easy to misdiagnose. MRI is of great value for diagnosis. Non-invasive treatment can effectively relieve symptoms, control lesions, and preserve fertility. In this report, follow-ups revealed that HIFU therapy, or HIFU combined with pharmacological therapy, can safely and effectively treat adolescent patients with cystic adenomyosis. However, there is a lack of clinical data supporting a large sample of HIFU treatments for juvenile cystic adenomyosis, and its effects on fertility remain to be further studied.

Author Contributions: Conceptualization, X.L., G.H. and J.W.; methodology, S.L. and X.L.; software, G.Y.; investigation, L.W., and Y.L.; resources, J.W. and X.L.; writing—original draft preparation, X.L. and J.W.; writing—review and editing, S.L. and Y.L.; visualization, G.Y.; supervision, H.Y.; project administration, S.L., G.H. and H.Y.; All authors have read and agreed to the published version of the manuscript.

Funding: This research was funded by [State Key Laboratory of Ultrasound in Medicine and Engineering] grant number [2020KFKT009] and The APC was funded by [State Key Laboratory of Ultrasound in Medicine and Engineering].

Institutional Review Board Statement: All subjects gave their informed consent for inclusion before they participated in the study. The study was conducted according to the guidelines of the Declaration of Helsinki, and approved by the Medical Research Ethics Review Committee of Suining Central Hospital (protocol code KYLLKS20230047 and date of approval: 23 March 2023).

Informed Consent Statement: Informed consent was obtained from all subjects involved in the study.

Data Availability Statement: The data presented in this study are available on request from the corresponding author.

Conflicts of Interest: The authors declare no conflict of interest.

Appendix A

Table A1. Fourteen cases of adolescent uterine cystic adenomyosis in the last decade.

References	Age (years)	Age of Onset	Imagine	Lesion Size (cm)	Menstrual Cycle	Symptoms	SerumCA125 (<35 U/mL)	Treatment	Pathological Diagnosis	Combination	Outcome	Note
Sushila Arya et al. [25]	18	14	US, MRI	3×3 cm^2	Regular	Severe dysmenorrhea, Chronic pelvic pain	Not mentioned	Laparoscopic excision of the mass	Cystic uterine adenomyosis	Postoperative oral contraceptive	Recovery	unicornuate uterus, Follow up for 3 years
Sushila Arya et al. [25]	16	14	US, CT	$5.1 \times 3.6 \times 4.8$ cm^3	Regular	Severe dysmenorrhea, Chronic pelvic pain	Not mentioned	Laparoscopic excision of the mass	Cystic uterine adenomyosis	Postoperative oral contraceptive	Recovery	
Maryjo Marques Branquinho et al. [26]	17	15	US, MRI	$3.3 \times 3.2 \times 2.9$ cm^3	Regular	Severe dysmenorrhea, Chronic pelvic pain	Not mentioned	oral contraceptive	-	-	Recovery	One-year follow-up lesion reduction to 1.5 cm
Athanasios Protopapas et al. [27]	14	13	MRI	$3.8 \times 3.4 \times 3.1$ cm^3	Regular	Severe dysmenorrhea	Not mentioned	Laparoscopic excision of the mass	Cystic uterine adenomyosis	-	Recovery	One year follow-up
F.Minelli et al. [28]	19	18	MRI	$2.6 \times 2.5 \times 2.7$ cm^3	Regular	Severe dysmenorrhea	Not mentioned	Ethanol injection sclerotherapy	Cystic uterine adenomyosis	Postoperative oral contraceptive	Unrelieved	Lesion reduced to 1.1 cm after 5 months of follow-up
Mihajlo Strelec et al. [29]	14	11	US	2 cm	Regular	Severe dysmenorrhea	Not mentioned	Laparoscopic excision of the mass	Cystic uterine adenomyosis	-	Recovery	-
Lieselot Deblaere et al. [30]	16	14	US, MRI	$1.9 \times 1.7 \times 2.0$ cm^3	Regular	Severe dysmenorrhea, Chronic pelvic pain	Not mentioned	Laparoscopic excision of the mass	Cystic uterine adenomyosis	-	Recovery	Ethanol injection sclerotherapy and oral progesterone are ineffective; 3 months follow-up

Table A1. Cont.

References	Age (years)	Age of Onset	Imagine	Lesion Size (cm)	Menstrual Cycle	Symptoms	SerumCA125 (<35 U/mL)	Treatment	Pathological Diagnosis	Combination	Outcome	Note
Annemieke Wilcox et al. [31]	18	13	US, MRI	1.8×2.0 cm^2	Regular	Severe dysmenorrhea, Chronic pelvic pain	Not mentioned	Laparoscopic excision of the mass	Cystic uterine adenomyosis	-	Recovery	Oral contraceptives and IUDs are ineffective; 6 months follow-up
Annemieke Wilcox et al. [31]	18	18	US, MRI	3.5×3.6 cm^2	Regular	Chronic pelvic pain	Not mentioned	Laparoscopic excision of the mass	Cystic uterine adenomyosis	-	Recovery	Oral contraceptives are ineffective
Gaspare Cucinella et al. [32]	25	12	US, MRI	$3.2 \times 4.5 \times 4.1$ cm^3	Regular	Severe dysmenorrhea	38U/mL	Laparoscopic excision of the mass	Cystic uterine adenomyosis	Postoperative GnRH-a for 3 months	Recovery	Medication is ineffective
Jun Kumakiri et al. [33]	20	15	US, MRI	3 cm	Regular	Severe dysmenorrhea	Not mentioned	Laparoscopic excision of the mass	Cystic uterine adenomyosis	-	Recovery	Dysmenorrhea becomes amenorrhea after taking oral denogestrel, and the symptoms persist
Zhou et al. [20]	29	17	US, MRI	$2.5 \times 2.0 \times 2.2$ cm^3	Not mentioned	Severe dysmenorrhea	Not mentioned	HIFU	-	-	Recovery	6 months follow-up
Zhou et al. [20]	20	15	US, MRI	$3.6 \times 4.0 \times 3.0$ cm^3	Not mentioned	Severe dysmenorrhea	Not mentioned	HIFU	-	-	Recovery	6 months follow-up
Zhou et al. [20]	22	13	US, MRI	$2.0 \times 2.0 \times 2.0$ cm^3	Not mentioned	Severe dysmenorrhea	Not mentioned	HIFU	-	-	Recovery	6 months follow-up

References

1. Harmsen, M.J.; Van den Bosch, T.; De Leeuw, R.A.; Dueholm, M.; Exacoustos, C.; Valentin, L.; Hehenkamp, W.J.K.; Groenman, F.; De Bruyn, C.; Rasmussen, C.; et al. Consensus on revised definitions of Morphological Uterus Sonographic Assessment (MUSA) features of adenomyosis: Results of modified Delphi procedure. *Ultrasound Obstet. Gynecol.* **2022**, *60*, 118–131. [CrossRef]
2. Krentel, H.; Keckstein, J.; Füger, T.; Hornung, D.; Theben, J.; Salehin, D.; Buchweitz, O.; Mueller, A.; Schaefer, S.D.; Sillem, M.; et al. Accuracy of ultrasound signs in two-dimensional transvaginal ultrasound for the prediction of adenomyosis: Prospective multicenter study. *Ultrasound Obstet. Gynecol.* **2023**. [CrossRef] [PubMed]
3. Brosens, I.; Gordts, S.; Habiba, M.; Benagiano, G. Uterine Cystic Adenomyosis: A Disease of Younger Women. *J. Pediatr. Adolesc. Gynecol.* **2015**, *28*, 420–426. [CrossRef] [PubMed]
4. Nie, J.C.; Liu, X.S. Precautions in diagnosis and treatment of adolescent adenomyosis. *Chin. J. Fam. Plan. Gynecotokology* **2019**, *11*, 21–23, 44.
5. Parulekar, S.V. Cystic degeneration in an adenomyoma (a case report). *J. Postgrad. Med.* **1990**, *36*, 46–47.
6. Tamura, M.; Fukaya, T.; Takaya, R.; Ip, C.W.; Yajima, A. Juvenile adenomyotic cyst of the corpus uteri with dysmenorrhea. *Tohoku J. Exp. Med.* **1996**, *178*, 339–344. [CrossRef]
7. Liu, X.; Liu, H.Y.; Shi, H.H.; Fan, Q.B.; Yu, X. Advances in diagnosis treatment of cystic adenomyosis. *J. Reprod. Med.* **2015**, *24*, 873–876.
8. Takeuchi, H.; Kitade, M.; Kikuchi, I.; Kumakiri, J.; Kuroda, K.; Jinushi, M. Diagnosis, laparoscopic management, and histopathologic findings of juvenile cystic adenomyoma: A review of nine cases. *Fertil. Steril.* **2010**, *94*, 862–868. [CrossRef]
9. Li, D.L.; Liang, W.T. Diagnosis and treatment of the special types and malignant transformation of adenomyosis. *Chin. J. Pract. Gynecol. Obstet.* **2017**, *33*, 160–163.
10. Ryan, G.L.; Stolpen, A.; Van Voorhis, B.J. An Unusual Cause of Adolescent Dysmenorrhea. *Obstet. Gynecol.* **2006**, *108*, 1017–1022.
11. Kriplani, A.; Mahey, R.; Agarwal, N.; Bhatla, N.; Yadav, R.; Singh, M.K. Laparoscopic Management of Juvenile Cystic Adenomyoma: Four Cases. *J. Minim. Invasive Gynecol.* **2011**, *18*, 343–348. [CrossRef] [PubMed]
12. Chun, S.S.; Hong, D.G.; Seong, W.J.; Choi, M.H.; Lee, T.H. Juvenile Cystic Adenomyoma in a 19-Year-Old Woman: A Case Report with a Proposal for New Diagnostic Criteria. *J. Laparoendosc. Adv. Surg. Tech.* **2011**, *21*, 771–774. [CrossRef]
13. Osada, H. Uterine adenomyosis and adenomyoma: The surgical approach. *Fertil. Steril.* **2018**, *109*, 406–417. [CrossRef] [PubMed]
14. Stratopoulou, C.A.; Donnez, J.; Dolmans, M.-M. Conservative Management of Uterine Adenomyosis: Medical vs. Surgical Approach. *J. Clin. Med.* **2021**, *10*, 4878. [CrossRef]
15. Zhao, X.; Yang, Y. Ultrasound-Guided Transvaginal Aspiration and Sclerotherapy for Uterine Cystic Adenomyosis: Case Report and Literature Review. *Front. Med.* **2022**, *9*, 764523. [CrossRef] [PubMed]
16. Ryo, E.; Takeshita, S.; Shiba, M.; Ayabe, T. Radiofrequency ablation for cystic adenomyosis: A case report. *J. Reprod. Med.* **2006**, *51*, 427–430.
17. Wang, Z.L.; Wang, W.J.; Hao, M. New advances in the diagnosis and treatment of cystic adenomyosis. *Chin. J. Fam. Plan. Gynecotokology* **2019**, *11*, 24–26.
18. Wei, Y.R.; Li, K.Q.; Huang, G.H.; Wang, D.P.; Zhou, L.R. Clinical efficacy of high intensity focused ultrasound ablation for uterine fibroids and adenomyosis. *Chin. J. Ultrasound Med.* **2010**, *26*, 1133–1136.
19. Aili, X.Z.; Guo, Z.Y.; Zhang, X.F. Latest research advances of high intensity focused ultrasound treatment for adenomyosis. *J. ShanDong Univ. (Health Sci.)* **2022**, *60*, 36–42.
20. Zhou, X.-J.; Zhao, Z.-M.; Liu, P.; Zhao, C.-Y.; Lin, Y.-J.; Liu, Y.; Wang, M.; Tian, C.; Li, H.-Y.; Hou, C.-X.; et al. Efficacy of high intensity focused ultrasound treatment for cystic adenomyosis: A report of four cases. *Ann. Palliat. Med.* **2020**, *9*, 3742–3749. [CrossRef]
21. Koukoura, O.; Kapsalaki, E.; Daponte, A.; Pistofidis, G. Laparoscopic treatment of a large uterine cystic adenomyosis in a young patient. *BMJ Case Rep.* **2015**, *2015*, bcr2015210358. [CrossRef] [PubMed]
22. Zhou, C.Y.; Xu, X.J.; He, J. Pregnancy outcomes and symptom improvement of patients with adenomyosis treated with high intensity focused ultrasound ablation. *Zhonghua Fu Chan Ke Za Zhi* **2016**, *51*, 845–849. (In Chinese)
23. Lai, T.H.T.; Seto, M.T.Y.; Cheung, V.Y.T. Intrapartum uterine rupture following ultrasound-guided high-intensity focused ultrasound ablation of uterine fibroid and adenomyosis. *Ultrasound Obstet. Gynecol.* **2022**, *60*, 816–817. [CrossRef]
24. Wu, S.; Liu, J.; Jiang, L.; Yang, L.; Han, Y. Spontaneous rupture of the uterus in the third trimester after high-intensity ultrasound ablation in adenomyosis: A case report. *Front. Med.* **2022**, *9*, 966620. [CrossRef]
25. Arya, S.; Burks, H.R. Juvenile cystic adenomyoma, a rare diagnostic challenge: Case Reports and literature review. *F S Rep.* **2021**, *2*, 166–171.
26. Branquinho, M.M.; Marques, A.L.; Leite, H.B.; Silva, I.S. Juvenile cystic adenomyoma. *BMJ Case Rep.* **2012**, *2012*, bcr2012007006. [CrossRef] [PubMed]
27. Protopapas, A.; Kypriotis, K.; Chatzipapas, I.; Kathopoulis, N.; Sotiropoulou, M.; Michala, L. Juvenile Cystic Adenomyoma vs. Blind Uterine Horn: Challenges in the Diagnosis and Surgical Management. *J. Pediatr. Adolesc. Gynecol.* **2020**, *33*, 735–738. [CrossRef] [PubMed]
28. Minelli, F.; Agostini, A.; Siles, P.; Gnisci, A.; Pivano, A. Treatment of juvenile cystic adenomyoma by sclerotherapy with alcohol instillation: A case report. *J. Gynecol. Obstet. Hum. Reprod.* **2021**, *50*, 102081. [CrossRef] [PubMed]

29. Strelec, M.; Banović, M.; Banović, V.; Sirovec, A. Juvenile cystic adenomyoma mimicking a Mullerian uterine anomaly successfully treated by laparoscopic excision. *Int. J. Gynecol. Obstet.* **2019**, *146*, 265–266. [CrossRef]
30. Deblaere, L.; Froyman, W.; Bosch, T.V.D.; Van Rompuy, A.; Kaijser, J.; Deprest, J.; Timmerman, D. Juvenile cystic adenomyosis: A case report and review of the literature. *Australas. J. Ultrasound Med.* **2019**, *22*, 295–300. [CrossRef]
31. Wilcox, A.; Schmidt, M.; Luciano, D. Identification of Juvenile Cystic Adenomyoma Using High-Resolution Imaging. *Obstet. Gynecol.* **2020**, *136*, 1021–1024. [CrossRef] [PubMed]
32. Cucinella, G.; Billone, V.; Pitruzzella, I.; Monte, A.I.L.; Palumbo, V.D.; Perino, A. Adenomyotic Cyst in a 25-Year-Old Woman: Case Report. *J. Minim. Invasive Gynecol.* **2013**, *20*, 894–898. [CrossRef] [PubMed]
33. Kumakiri, J.; Kikuchi, I.; Sogawa, Y.; Jinushi, M.; Aoki, Y.; Kitade, M.; Takeda, S. Single-incision laparoscopic surgery using an articulating monopolar for juvenile cystic adenomyoma. *Minim. Invasive Ther. Allied Technol.* **2013**, *22*, 312–315. [CrossRef] [PubMed]

Disclaimer/Publisher's Note: The statements, opinions and data contained in all publications are solely those of the individual author(s) and contributor(s) and not of MDPI and/or the editor(s). MDPI and/or the editor(s) disclaim responsibility for any injury to people or property resulting from any ideas, methods, instructions or products referred to in the content.

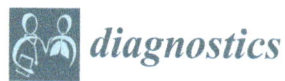

Article

A Hypothesis on the Progression of Insulin-Induced Lipohypertrophy: An Integrated Result of High-Frequency Ultrasound Imaging and Blood Glucose Control of Patients

Jian Yu [1,†], Hong Wang [1,†], Meijing Zhou [1,†], Min Zhu [1], Jing Hang [2], Min Shen [1], Xin Jin [3,*], Yun Shi [1,*], Jingjing Xu [1,4,*] and Tao Yang [1]

1. Department of Endocrinology, The First Affiliated Hospital with Nanjing Medical University (Jiangsu Province Hospital), Nanjing 210029, China
2. Department of Ultrasound, The First Affiliated Hospital with Nanjing Medical University (Jiangsu Province Hospital), Nanjing 210029, China
3. Department of Hospital Pharmacy, The Affiliated Suqian First People's Hospital of Nanjing Medical University, Suqian 223800, China
4. Department of Nursing, The First Affiliated Hospital with Nanjing Medical University (Jiangsu Province Hospital), Nanjing 210029, China
* Correspondence: jinxin871211@163.com (X.J.); drshiyun@163.com (Y.S.); dsnxjj@njmu.edu.cn (J.X.)
† These authors contributed equally to this work.

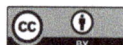

Citation: Yu, J.; Wang, H.; Zhou, M.; Zhu, M.; Hang, J.; Shen, M.; Jin, X.; Shi, Y.; Xu, J.; Yang, T. A Hypothesis on the Progression of Insulin-Induced Lipohypertrophy: An Integrated Result of High-Frequency Ultrasound Imaging and Blood Glucose Control of Patients. *Diagnostics* 2023, 13, 1515. https://doi.org/10.3390/diagnostics13091515

Academic Editors: Rossana Izzetti and Marco Nisi

Received: 6 March 2023
Revised: 26 March 2023
Accepted: 29 March 2023
Published: 23 April 2023

Copyright: © 2023 by the authors. Licensee MDPI, Basel, Switzerland. This article is an open access article distributed under the terms and conditions of the Creative Commons Attribution (CC BY) license (https://creativecommons.org/licenses/by/4.0/).

Abstract: Aims: To put forward a scientific hypothesis about the progression of insulin-injection-induced lipohypertrophy (LH) according to the high-frequency ultrasonic imaging of insulin injection sites and the blood glucose control of patients. Methods: A total of 344 patients were screened for LH by means of high-frequency ultrasound scanning. The results of their ultrasound examination were described in detail and categorized into several subtypes. Seventeen patients with different subtypes of LH were followed up to predict the progression of LH. To further verify our hypothesis, the effects of different types of LH on glycemic control of patients were observed by comparing glycated hemoglobin A1c (HbA$_{1C}$) and other glycemic-related indicators. Results: LH was found in 255 (74.1%) patients. According to the high-frequency ultrasonic imaging characteristics, LH can be categorized into three subtypes in general. Among all the LHs, the most common type observed was nodular hyperechoic LH (n = 167, 65.5%), followed by diffuse hyperechoic LH (n = 70, 27.5%), then hypoechoic LH (n = 18, 7.0%). At the follow-up after six months, all 10 patients with nodular hyperechoic LH had LH faded away. Of the five patients with diffuse hyperechoic LH, two had inapparent LH, and three had diffuse hyperechoic parts which had shrunk under ultrasound. No obvious changes were observed in the two cases of hypoechoic LH. Compared with the LH-free group, the mean HbA$_{1C}$ of the nodular hyperechoic LH group increased by 0.8% (9 mmol/mol) (95% CI:−1.394~−0.168, p = 0.005), that of the diffuse hyperechoic LH group increased by 2.0% (21 mmol/mol) (95% CI: −2.696~−1.20, p < 0.001), and that of the hypoechoic LH group increased by 1.5% (16 mmol/mol) (95% CI: −2.689~−0.275, p = 0.007). Conclusions: It was hypothesized that the earlier stage of LH is nodular hyperechoic LH. If nodular LH is not found in time and the patient continues to inject insulin at the LH site and/or reuse needles, LH will develop into a diffuse type or, even worse, a hypoechoic one. Different subtypes of LH may represent differences in severity when blood glucose control is considered as an important resolution indicator. Further studies are needed to confirm our hypothesis on the progression and reversion of insulin-induced lipohypertrophy.

Keywords: lipohypertrophy (LH); glycated hemoglobin (HbA$_{1C}$); ultrasound; insulin injection

1. Introduction

The number of patients with diabetes worldwide is estimated to reach 783 million by 2045 [1]. All patients with type 1 diabetes and type 2 diabetes who are not effective at controlling their blood glucose with oral medications will have to initiate insulin injection therapy eventually. So, a considerable number of patients with diabetes need insulin therapy to maintain their glucose at a near-normal level. Lipohypertrophy (LH) is the most common local complication caused by multiple overlapping insulin injections, and it is one of the most prominent contributors to poor metabolic control [2]. Moreover, LH is associated with nearly one-third greater insulin consumption, with large cost implications [3].

The existing methods for detecting insulin injection-related lipohypertrophy (LH) mainly include two techniques—clinical examination (inspection and palpation) and high-frequency ultrasound scanning. Clinical examination tends to be more convenient and cost-effective, whereas ultrasonography can provide us with a further understanding of LH, especially in terms of different pathological changes related to LH. After the concept of subclinical LH was proposed [4,5], ultrasound scanning was proposed as a potentially more advanced and objective method for detecting LH because ultrasound can better describe the characteristics and morphology of LH induced by insulin injection [6,7] and can rather effectively reduce the rate of missed diagnosis of LH [8,9].

LH has received much attention in the past decade because it has previously been observed that the occurrence of LH is associated with poorer glycemic control in patients, regardless of whether the diagnosis of LH in these studies was based on clinical examination or ultrasound screening [8,10–12]. Moreover, Volkova [4] confirmed that LH detected by ultrasonography without visual and palpable changes could also worsen the compensation of glycemic control, which further emphasizes the importance of using ultrasound scanning in detecting LH.

Overall, these studies focused on identifying the presence or absence of LH and evaluating the relationship between the occurrence of LH and glycemic control. To go further, there is little discussion about whether there are different types of LH and whether the presence of LH (no matter which type) will definitely affect the control of blood glucose of patients.

Currently, our understanding of LH is still far from comprehensive, especially regarding the classification or development process of LH. We firmly believe that, like all other diabetes-related complications, we need to explore the progression of LH in depth and try to grade LH scientifically, so that more targeted treatment or prevention measures can be taken.

Clinically, ultrasound has been of great value in assessing the severity of many diseases for a long time [13,14]. Therefore, the main purpose of this study is to screen all insulin injection sites of patients by means of high-frequency ultrasound and to find out whether patients have LH and summarize the type of LH. The changes in the ultrasound images of those existing LHs after stopping the injection at the lesion site were followed up. Then, we propose a scientific hypothesis about the progression of LH. On this basis, glycated hemoglobin (HbA1c), TIR (time in range) and CV (coefficient of variation), as the key indicators of blood glucose control of patients with different subtypes of LH, are compared to verify our hypothesis.

2. Research Design and Methods

2.1. Study Participants

Participants were recruited in sequence at the National Endocrinology and Metabolism Center (Level iii) of a University Hospital in Nanjing, China, from March 2021 to February 2022. The study inclusion criteria were: a diagnosis of type 1 or type 2 diabetes mellitus; having been treated with insulin injections for at least the last 6 months; and no extended cutaneous diseases. The exclusion criteria were: being prescribed a glucagon-like peptide-1 agonist; having dermatitis or any other cutaneous disease; and having other diseases that may affect HbA1c, such as anemia. This study was conducted in accordance with the Declaration of Helsinki. Approval for the study protocol was granted by the research ethics committee of the First Affiliated Hospital of Nanjing Medical University (2019-SR-268). Patients were informed about the aim and methods of the study verbally and in written form. We obtained written informed consent from all participants before enrollment in the study.

2.2. Data Collection

In this study, trained medical professionals consulted the medical records of enrolled patients, and extracted the following information: age, gender, body mass index, type of diabetes, diabetes duration, insulin injection duration. After that, all the extracted information was verified again by the professional with the patient to ensure the accuracy of the data. All of the personal information was recorded and kept confidential.

Assessment of LHs: All participants underwent ultrasound scanning conducted by two qualified radiologists, respectively, following the unified protocol which has been reported elsewhere [5,15]. An Esaote My Lab60 linear multifrequency probe (6–18 MHz) was used for ultrasound scanning. Each patient underwent an additional examination at one centimeter above the navel (where insulin has never been injected) as their self-control. At each site, thickness, echo, the blood flow of subcutaneous tissue, and the boundary between the subcutaneous tissue and the dermis were examined and recorded carefully to find out whether the patients had LH according to the criteria described by Kapeluto et al. [6,16]. If the results of the two radiologists were inconsistent, a third radiologist helped to make the final judgment. The inter-examiner agreement was high, with a Cohen's kappa coefficient of 0.95.

If different types of LH were found in a same patient, we later classified the patient into the subgroup of the most serious type of LH found by the patient.

LHs follow-up at six months: In order to observe the ultrasonic changes of LHs, 10 patients with nodular LH, 5 with diffuse LH, and 2 with hypoechoic LH were randomly selected for follow-up 6 months later. The LH sites of these patients were specifically marked and photographed. The researchers and patients kept the body surface photo of the lesion part, respectively. The patient was told to refer to the photo before each insulin injection to make sure that the lesion site was not injected any more. Meanwhile, the researchers needed to ensure that the previous LH locations were correctly identified at follow-up according to the detailed records and photographs.

Assessment of HbA_{1C}: Two milliliters of whole blood was taken from all patients and placed in an anticoagulant EDTA test tube, and HbA1c was detected via a Clover A1c analyzer (D10 hemoglobin detection system Specifications).

All participants diagnosed with LH by ultrasound were informed of the specific extent and location of any LH areas and advised to avoid further insulin injections into these areas. Doctors were also advised to adjust insulin doses to reduce the risk of hypoglycemia when injected at sites without LH.

2.3. Statistical Analysis

Continuous variables were reported as mean $\pm$ SD or M (Q1,Q3), and categorical variables were summarized as rate or percentage. Independent sample t-tests and one-way ANOVA were used to compare the data between groups. Odds ratios (ORs) with 95% confidence intervals (CIs) were used to report results. All data were analyzed using SPSS (version 26.0; SPSS Inc., Chicago, IL, USA). A p-value below 0.05 ($p < 0.05$) was considered statistically significant.

3. Results

3.1. Sample Characteristics

In total, 344 patients were enrolled in this study. Among them, 195 patients (56.7%) were male. The study population had a median age of 57 (30, 66) years. Of the 344 participants, 136 had type 1 diabetes and 208 had type 2 diabetes. The median insulin exposure duration is 6.2 (2.8, 11.0) years. Their average BMI was 23.3 $\pm$ 4.0 kg/m^2.

3.2. Lipohypertrophy Findings and Characteristics

Of all 344 patients, 255 (76.1%) were found to have LH via ultrasound. The LH imaging manifestations of these 255 patients were mainly classified into two types, hyperechoic LH (237 cases) and hypoechogenic LH (18 cases). Of all patients with hyperechoic LH, 167 showed nodular hyperechoic LH, and 70 showed diffuse hyperechoic LH. (Figure 1).

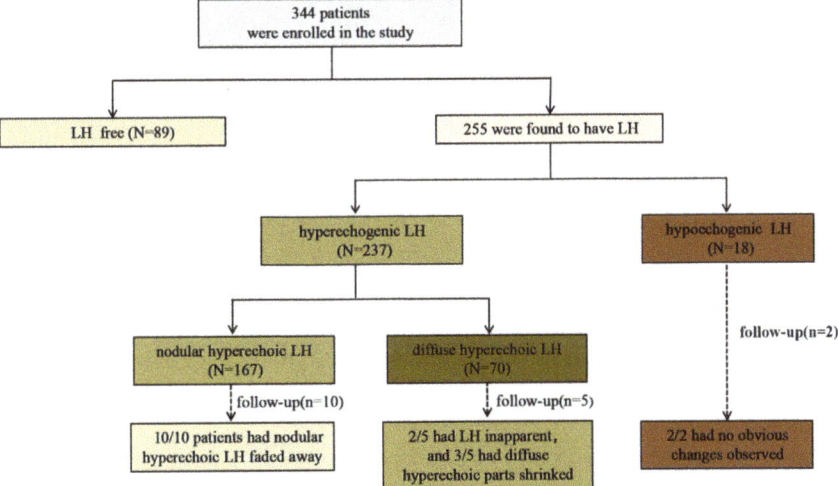

Figure 1. Lipohypertrophy findings in this study.

Features of different types of LH examined via ultrasound are shown in Figure 2. The layers of skin and muscle are clearly demarcated in areas where insulin has never been injected, and the ultrasound heterogeneity in each layer is small (Figure 2a). Nodular hyperechoic LH refers to the nodular region with an abnormally increased echo in the subcutaneous fat layer in the insulin injection area, with relatively clear and measurable boundaries and no obvious envelope (Figure 2b). In contrast to nodular LH, diffuse hyperechoic LH is an abnormally hyperechoic region with no distinct boundaries in length and/or width (usually more than the field of view of one probe—the probe in this study provides a 40 mm diameter field of view), and in general, their depth can be measured (Figure 2c). Hypoechoic LH is characterized by extremely low echo or even no echo in the subcutaneous adipose tissue, and the fibrotic tissue within this area is almost invisible compared to the normal area (Figure 2d).

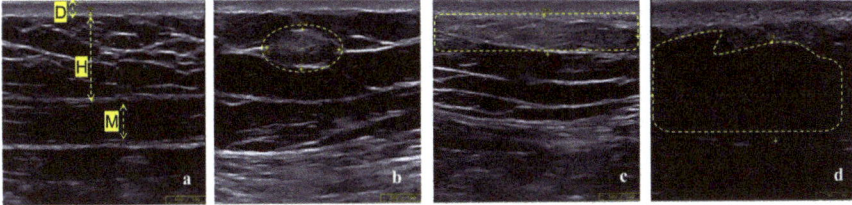

Figure 2. Imaging features of normal tissue and LH under ultrasound. (**a**) D, dermis; H, hypodermis (mainly adipose tissue); M, muscular layer. Each layer is clearly demarcated. (**b**) Nodular hyperechoic LH with obvious space occupying sensation. (**c**) Diffuse hyperechoic LH presented with no clear demarcation from the dermis. (**d**) Hypoechoic LH with irregular boundary, which is similar to adipose tissue liquefaction.

3.3. LH Follow-Up by Ultrasound Assessment

All 17 patients selected for follow-up reconfirmed that they had avoided the LH site for insulin injection in the past 6 months and had adopted the correct injection method. No newly emerged LH was found. At the follow-up after six months, obvious changes were observed in LHs of both hyperechoic types. All 10 patients with nodular hyperechoic LH displayed LH which had faded away. Of the five patients with diffuse hyperechoic LH, two had inapparent LH, and three had diffuse hyperechoic parts which shrank to nodular hyperechoic LH and then regressed. (Figure 3). The shrunken parts looked similar to the nodular LHs, with a slightly less regular boundary. No obvious changes were observed in two cases of hypoechoic LH. One patient ultimately chose minimally invasive surgery to remove the lesion (Figure 4).

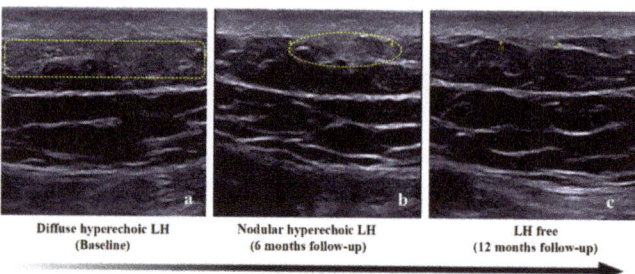

Figure 3. Examples of the changes in hyperechoic LH under ultrasound at follow-up. Diffuse hyperechoic LH at baseline (**a**) had obviously shrunk to nodular LH at 6 months follow-up (**b**). Additionally, the hyperechoic area could not be observed at 12 months follow-up (**c**) in the same patient (patient NO. 14).

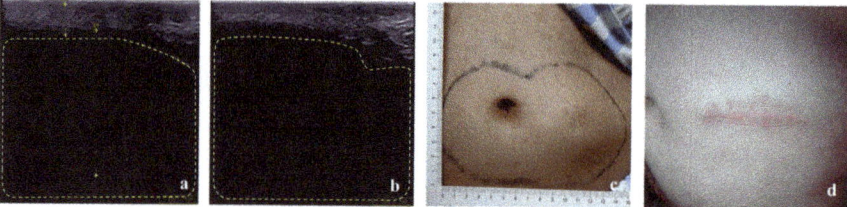

Figure 4. No obvious hints of improvement were observed in the case with hypoechoic LH at 6 months follow-up (**b** vs. **a**). The patient finally had his lesion removed by surgery (**d** vs. **c**). After stopping insulin injection at the LH lesion site, his required daily dosage of insulin decreased significantly (60 U vs. 20 U).

3.4. Hypothesis on the Progression of Insulin Induced Lipohypertrophy

It is certain that the layering of normal skin should be very clear (Figure 5a). Insulin needs to be injected into the normal hypodermis layer to exert its full effect on lowering blood sugar. Based on our clinical observations and the findings from this study, it could be hypothesized that the earlier stage of LH is nodular hyperechoic LH (Figure 5b). If nodular LH is not found in time and the patient continues to inject insulin at the LH site and/or reuse needles, LH will develop into a diffuse type (Figure 5c) or, even worse, a hypoechoic one (Figure 5d). Usually at this time, the dermis layer will also have obvious thickness changes. By strengthening the intervention of correct injection behavior, hyperechoic LH can gradually be repaired, but hypoechoic LH cannot easily heal by itself.

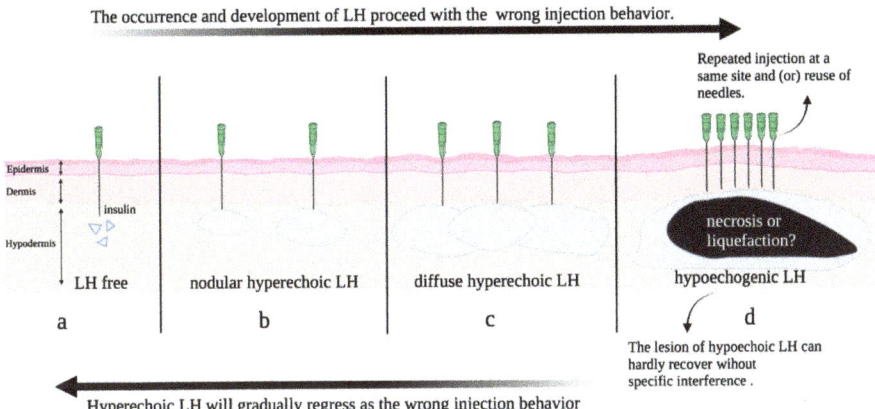

Figure 5. A hypothesis on the progression and revision of insulin induced lipohypertrophy.

3.5. Differences of Blood Glucose Control in Patients with Different Types of LH

In order to further understand the effects of different types of LH on blood glucose and verify our hypothesis, all patients were tested for HbA1c at the same time of LH examination. Of all the patients, the most common type of LH observed was nodular hyperechoic LH (with mean HbA_{1C} 8.4 ± 1.9% (68 ± 20 mmol/mol)), followed by diffuse hyperechoic LH (with mean HbA_{1C} 9.6 ± 2.0% (81 ± 21 mmol/mol)), then hypoechoic LH (with mean HbA_{1C} 9.1 ± 1.3% (75 ± 14 mmol/mol)) (Figure 6). Patients with LH had significantly higher HbA_{1C} than those without (8.7 ± 1.9% vs. 7.6 ± 1.5% (72 ± 21 mmol/mol vs. 60 ± 17 mmol/mol), $p < 0.001$). On this basis, further group differences were detected using one-way ANOVA with Bonferroni post hoc tests. The test results showed that compared with the LH-free group, the mean HbA_{1C} of the nodular hyperechoic LH group increased by 0.8% (9 mmol/mol) (95% CI: −1.394~−0.168, $p = 0.005$), that of the diffuse hyperechoic LH group increased by 2.0% (21 mmol/mol) (95% CI: −2.696~−1.20, $p < 0.001$), and that of the hypoechoic LH group increased by 1.5% (16 mmol/mol) (95% CI: −2.689~−0.275, $p = 0.007$); compared with the diffuse LH hyperechoic LH group, the mean HbA_{1C} of the nodular hyperechoic LH group decreased by 1.2% (13 mmol/mol) ($p < 0.001$).

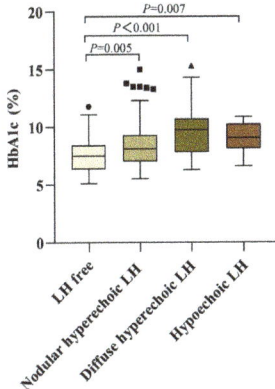

Figure 6. Comparison of HbA1c in different subtypes of LH ($N = 344$).

In addition, there were 34 patients with type 1 diabetes (T1DM) who had been wearing their flash glucose monitoring system (FGM) for more than 1 week when they were recruited to this study. After obtaining their consent, the original blood glucose values recorded by the system were derived. TIR and CV, as the two key indicators of blood glucose control, were calculated by using the calculation software Easy GV version 9.0 R from Oxford University (the data for the first 3 days were excluded considering the possible errors during the initialization of FGM). Ten of these 34 patients with type 1 diabetes were LH-free, 15 were with nodular hyperechoic LH, 9 had diffuse hyperechoic LH, and none had hypoechoic LH. Group differences of TIR and CV were detected using one-way ANOVA with Bonferroni post hoc tests. The results showed that the LH-free group had the highest TIR and the lowest CV, whilst diffuse hyperechoic LH had the lowest TIR and the highest CV among the three groups (Figure 7).

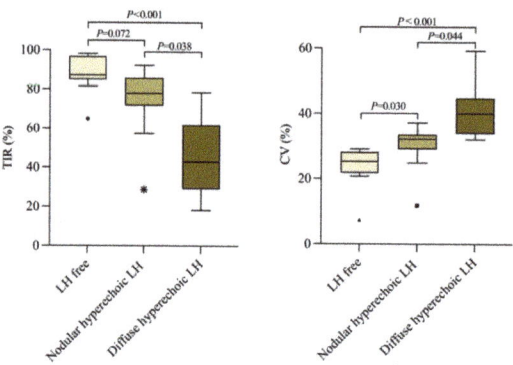

Figure 7. Comparison of TIR and CV in different subtypes of LH in T1DM patients (N = 34) * indicates abnormal values.

4. Discussion

Ultrasonography has been widely used in different clinical areas, especially in intensive care units [17]. At the same time, ultrasound technology has certain advantages in the differential diagnosis of certain diseases [18]. LH is typically diagnosed via visual inspection and palpation in clinical practice because of its operability and convenience. With the widespread use of ultrasonography, specialists have placed high-frequency ultrasound scanning in a more advanced position in identifying LH. The incidence of LH based on ultrasound diagnosis is 14.5–86.5%, and the median incidence is 56.6% [19]. In our study, the incidence of LH was 74.1% (255/344), which was consistent with previous reports, indicating that LH is a fairly common complication in patients with insulin injections, which attracts our attention.

One advantage of using ultrasound scanning to diagnose LH is that it cannot only judge whether the patient has LH or not but can also further provide a more objective presentation, especially in that ultrasound can clarify the nature, characteristics, and size of lesion sites. Previous studies have described the ultrasound features of LH and proposed specific, reproducible criteria for the detection of LH [16]. It must be noted that due to repeated injections and inflammatory reactions, a hyperechogenic area might be a sign of fibrotic tissue, so careful discrimination is necessary. Our study screened 344 subjects for LH using the same diagnostic criteria and found that the most common type of LH was hyperechoic. Which can be divided into the nodular hyperechoic type and diffuse hyperechoic type. Additionally, the incidence of hypoechoic type was lowest in the Chinese population. As far as we know, this classification and the associated manifestations of LH have not been previously summarized and described in detail. Meanwhile, the incidence of different types of LH has not been reported before. We firmly believe that the different types, characteristics, and incidence of each type of LH described in this paper are an important supplement to previous studies.

On the one hand, the staging of many diseases is based on the imaging of ultrasound examination, so we also try to classify LH based on different imaging manifestations. According to our follow-up, nodular hyperechoic LHs are the easiest to regress, diffuse hyperechoic LHs will gradually shrink to nodular hyperechoic LHs and then regress, while hypoechoic LHs are the most difficult to heal. So, we firmly believe that the earlier stage of LH is nodular hyperechoic LH. As time goes on, LH will develop into a diffuse type or, even worse, a hypoechoic one.

On the other hand, it is also an important prerequisite to combine different types of LH with patients' metabolic indicators for classification. HbA_{1C} is the most commonly used indicator to measure blood glucose control in patients, because it is believed to reflect average blood glucose levels over several months and has a strong predictive value for diabetes complications [20]. To our knowledge, there is no study comparing HbA_{1C} in patients with different types of LH. Our results showed that patients with diffuse hyperechoic LH had worse blood glucose control than nodular hyperechoic LH. A possible explanation for this might be that diffuse LH is more serious than the nodular type regarding the effect on blood glucose. Similarly, our TIR and CV data of 34 type 1 patients with FGM also proved this.

Since the number of patients with hypoechoic type LH was small in this study, we could not confidently confirm the relationship between this type of LH and patients' glycemic control, and we need to further increase the sample size to clarify this point. According to our clinical experience, the hypoechoic type is the most serious type, causing large glycemic variability and frequent hypoglycemia in patients, which is in accordance with the case report of Gentile S [21]. Additionally, this is consistent with our observation that patients with hypoechoic LH do not have the highest HbA_{1C} among all of the participants. This may be because more frequent episodes of hypoglycemia lead to false-negative HbA1c results.

Some studies have paid attention to the grading of LH. Demir G [22] graded LH from 0 to 3 according to the inspection and palpation of the insulin injection site. Considering the limitations of LH severity assessment based only on the number of lesions, Ucieklak D [23] proposed a new LH severity scale considering both the number and size of LH lesions and categorized LH into four stages of advancement. Additionally, Hashem R [24] proposed a conceptual model of an LH grading system. However, the above grading methods did not refer to the metabolic outcomes of patients. In this study, it is relatively more objective to grade LH based on the abnormal ultrasonic echo of the subcutaneous fat layer of the patient and their blood glucose control indicators.

The pathophysiological mechanism of LH still remains unclear. Among various proposed mechanisms, it is widely accepted that LH is both a local effect caused by the reaction of adipocytes to the insulin injection and also the anabolic effect that insulin has on local adipocytes [25]. Many studies have found that LH is strongly associated with poor injection behavior [26,27], especially needle reuse and wrong injection site rotation. Additionally, standard injection technology training is essential in helping patients to reduce the occurrence of LH [28–30]. At the same time, what we all know is that insulin should be injected into undamaged skin and the subcutaneous fat layer to maintain its normal absorption [31]. So, for ethical reasons, when LHs were found, we informed the patient of correct injection methods and told them to avoid injection at the lesion site. Therefore, we could not observe the regression of LH in patients, and thus our hypothesis about LH progression is based on a reverse reasoning of the regression of existing LHs. This hypothesis still calls for further in-depth investigation. If possible, animal models may be recommended.

Our study further confirms the importance of timely LH screening for patients who need routine daily insulin injections, as early detection can help to avoid the deterioration of LH. China's technical guidelines for diabetes drug injection [32] state that patients with long-term insulin injections should be screened for skin complications at least once a year. It is also emphasized that the frequency of LH detection should be increased in patients who have already developed LH. Additionally, patients should be advised not to inject into the lesion site until the doctor confirms that LH has completely subsided so as not to interfere with insulin absorption.

5. Limitation

The data for TIR and CV in this study were only from 34 type 1 diabetes patients who wore an FGM system, and the results still need to be confirmed by further large-scale research participants.

Although HbA_{1C} is currently the "gold standard" for the evaluation of mean blood glucose control, we still need to pay additional attention to the hypoglycemia caused by injection insulin into LH, as severe hypoglycemia is a remarkable burden for patients with diabetes and increases the risk of adverse clinical outcomes [33], especially for patients with hypoechoic LH, as we mentioned previously. The relationship between various types of LH and patients' hypoglycemia or non-perceived hypoglycemia needs to be further strengthened in future studies.

6. Conclusions

This study once again confirmed the high prevalence of LH in patients with insulin injection and the effect of LH on blood glucose. The most important contribution of this study is to put forward a scientific hypothesis about the progress of LH according to the high-frequency ultrasound image characteristics of patients. Furthermore, the hypothesis was effectively verified when combined with blood glucose control indicators. We believe that the present study lays the groundwork for future research into the classification and grading of LH.

Author Contributions: Conceptualization, X.J., Y.S. and J.X.; Formal analysis, J.Y. and M.Z. (Meijing Zhou); Funding acquisition, X.J., J.X. and T.Y.; Investigation, H.W.; Methodology, J.Y., H.W., M.Z. (Min Zhu) and J.H.; Project administration, M.S. and J.X.; Supervision, J.H. and T.Y.; Writing—original draft, J.Y.; Writing—review and editing, M.Z. (Meijing Zhou) and Y.S. All authors have read and agreed to the published version of the manuscript.

Funding: Research reported in this paper is supported by Jiangsu Provincial Medical Key Discipline (ZDXK20220) and Hunan Sinocare Diabetes Foundation (2022SD01).

Institutional Review Board Statement: The study was conducted in accordance with the Declaration of Helsinki and approved by the Ethics Committee of the First Affiliated Hospital of Nanjing Medical University (2019-SR-268).

Informed Consent Statement: Informed consent was obtained from all subjects involved in the study.

Data Availability Statement: Data are available from the corresponding author upon reasonable request.

Conflicts of Interest: The authors declare no conflict of interest.

References

1. International Diabetes Federation. Diabetes Atlas 2021-10th Edition. Available online: www.diabetesatlas.org (accessed on 1 February 2022).
2. Gentile, S.; Strollo, F.; Satta, E.; Della Corte, T.; Romano, C.; Guarino, G. Insulin-Related Lipohypertrophy in Hemodialyzed Diabetic People: A Multicenter Observational Study and a Methodological Approach. *Diabetes Ther.* **2019**, *10*, 1423–1433. [CrossRef] [PubMed]
3. Ji, L.; Sun, Z.; Li, Q.; Qin, G.; Wei, Z.; Liu, J.; Chandran, A.B.A.B.; Hirsch, L.J.L.J. Lipohypertrophy in China: Prevalence, Risk Factors, Insulin Consumption, and Clinical Impact. *Diabetes Technol. Ther.* **2017**, *19*, 61–67. [CrossRef]
4. Volkova, N.I.; Davidenko, I.Y. Clinical significance of lipohypertrophy without visual and palpable changes detected by ultrasonography of subcutaneous fat. *Ter. arkhiv* **2019**, *91*, 62–66. [CrossRef]
5. Luo, D.; Shi, Y.; Zhu, M.; Wang, H.; Yan, D.; Yu, J.; Ji, J.; Liu, X.; Fan, B.; Xu, Y.; et al. Subclinical lipohypertrophy—Easily ignored complications of insulin therapy. *J. Diabetes Complicat.* **2020**, *35*, 107806. [CrossRef] [PubMed]
6. Kapeluto, J.E.; Paty, B.W.; Chang, S.D.; Meneilly, G.S. Ultrasound detection of insulin-induced lipohypertrophy in Type 1 and Type 2 diabetes. *Diabet. Med.* **2018**, *35*, 1383–1390. [CrossRef]
7. Bertuzzi, F.; Meneghini, E.; Bruschi, E.; Luzi, L.; Nichelatti, M.; Epis, O. Ultrasound characterization of insulin induced lipohypertrophy in type 1 diabetes mellitus. *J. Endocrinol. Investig.* **2017**, *40*, 1107–1113. [CrossRef] [PubMed]
8. Lin, Y.; Lin, L.; Wang, W.; Hong, J.; Zeng, H. Insulin-related lipohypertrophy: Ultrasound characteristics, risk factors, and impact of glucose fluctuations. *Endocrine* **2021**, *75*, 768–775. [CrossRef]

9. Yu, J.; Wang, H.; Zhu, M.; Yan, D.; Fan, B.; Shi, Y.; Shen, M.; Liu, X.; He, W.; Luo, D.; et al. Detection sensitivity of ultrasound scanning vs. clinical examination for insulin injection-related lipohypertrophy. *Chin. Med. J.* **2021**, *135*, 353–355. [CrossRef]
10. Tsadik, A.G.; Atey, T.M.; Nedi, T.; Fantahun, B.; Feyissa, M. Effect of Insulin-Induced Lipodystrophy on Glycemic Control among Children and Adolescents with Diabetes in Tikur Anbessa Specialized Hospital, Addis Ababa, Ethiopia. *J. Diabetes Res.* **2018**, *2018*, 4910962. [CrossRef]
11. Famulla, S.; Hövelmann, U.; Fischer, A.; Coester, H.-V.; Hermanski, L.; Kaltheuner, M.; Kaltheuner, L.; Heinemann, L.; Heise, T.; Hirsch, L. Insulin Injection Into Lipohypertrophic Tissue: Blunted and More Variable Insulin Absorption and Action and Impaired Postprandial Glucose Control. *Diabetes Care* **2016**, *39*, 1486–1492. [CrossRef]
12. Gupta, S.S.; Gupta, K.S.; Gathe, S.S.; Bamrah, P.; Gupta, S.S. Clinical Implications of Lipohypertrophy Among People with Type 1 Diabetes in India. *Diabetes Technol. Ther.* **2018**, *20*, 483–491. [CrossRef]
13. Rochester, D.; Bowie, J.D.; Kunzmann, A.; Lester, E. Ultrasound in the Staging of Lymphoma. *Radiology* **1977**, *124*, 483–487. [CrossRef] [PubMed]
14. Schüller, J.; Walther, V.; Schmiedt, E.; Staehler, G.; Bauer, H.; Schilling, A. Intravesical Ultrasound Tomography in Staging Bladder Carcinoma. *J. Urol.* **1982**, *128*, 264–266. [CrossRef]
15. Zhu, M.; Whang, H.; Shen, M.; Yu, J.; Yan, D.; Luo, D.; Shi, Y.; Hang, J.; Xu, J.; Yang, T. Clinical application of high-frequency ultrasound in the screening of lipohypertrophy in diabetic patients. *Chin. J. Diabetes Mellitus* **2021**, *13*, 848–853. [CrossRef]
16. Kapeluto, J.; Paty, B.W.; Chang, S.D.; Eddy, C.; Meneilly, G. Criteria for the Detection of Insulin-induced Lipohypertrophy Using Ultrasonography. *Can. J. Diabetes* **2015**, *39*, 534. [CrossRef]
17. Greenstein, Y.Y.; Guevarra, K. Point-of-Care Ultrasound in the Intensive Care Unit: Applications, Limitations, and the Evolution of Clinical Practice. *Clin. Chest Med.* **2022**, *43*, 373–384. [CrossRef]
18. Izzetti, R.; Nisi, M.; Aringhieri, G.; Vitali, S.; Oranges, T.; Romanelli, M.; Caramella, D.; Graziani, F.; Gabriele, M. Ultra-high frequency ultrasound in the differential diagnosis of oral pemphigus and pemphigoid: An explorative study. *Skin Res. Technol.* **2021**, *27*, 682–691. [CrossRef] [PubMed]
19. Abu Ghazaleh, H.; Hashem, R.; Forbes, A.; Dilwayo, T.R.; Duaso, M.; Sturt, J.; Halson-Brown, S.; Mulnier, H. A Systematic Review of Ultrasound-Detected Lipohypertrophy in Insulin-Exposed People with Diabetes. *Diabetes Ther.* **2018**, *9*, 1741–1756. [CrossRef] [PubMed]
20. American Diabetes Association. Standards of Medical Care in Diabetes—2010. *Diabetes Care* **2010**, *33* (Suppl. 1), S11–S61. [CrossRef]
21. Gentile, S.; Strollo, F.; Della Corte, T.; Marino, G.; Guarino, G. Skin complications of insulin injections: A case presentation and a possible explanation of hypoglycaemia. *Diabetes Res. Clin. Pract.* **2018**, *138*, 284–287. [CrossRef]
22. Demir, G.; Er, E.; Altınok, Y.A.; Özen, S.; Darcan, Ş.; Gökşen, D. Local complications of insulin administration sites and effect on diabetes management. *J. Clin. Nurs.* **2021**, *31*, 2530–2538. [CrossRef]
23. Ucieklak, D.; Mrozinska, S.; Wojnarska, A.; Malecki, M.T.; Klupa, T.; Matejko, B. Insulin-induced Lipohypertrophy in Patients with Type 1 Diabetes Mellitus Treated with an Insulin Pump. *Int. J. Endocrinol.* **2022**, *2022*, 9169296. [CrossRef] [PubMed]
24. Hashem, R.; Mulnier, H.; Abu Ghazaleh, H.; Halson-Brown, S.; Duaso, M.; Rogers, R.; Karalliedde, J.; Forbes, A. Characteristics and morphology of lipohypertrophic lesions in adults with type 1 diabetes with ultrasound screening: An exploratory observational study. *BMJ Open Diabetes Res. Care* **2021**, *9*, e002553. [CrossRef]
25. Xu, X.-H.; Carvalho, V.; Wang, X.-H.; Qiu, S.-H.; Sun, Z.-L. Lipohypertrophy: Prevalence, clinical consequence, and pathogenesis. *Chin. Med. J.* **2020**, *134*, 47–49. [CrossRef] [PubMed]
26. Gentile, S.; Guarino, G.; Della Corte, T.; Marino, G.; Fusco, A.; Corigliano, G.; Colarusso, S.; Piscopo, M.; Improta, M.R.; Corigliano, M.; et al. Insulin-Induced Skin Lipohypertrophy in Type 2 Diabetes: A Multicenter Regional Survey in Southern Italy. *Diabetes Ther.* **2020**, *11*, 2001–2017. [CrossRef] [PubMed]
27. Blanco, M.; Hernández, M.; Strauss, K.; Amaya, M. Prevalence and risk factors of lipohypertrophy in insulin-injecting patients with diabetes. *Diabetes Metab.* **2013**, *39*, 445–453. [CrossRef] [PubMed]
28. Smith, M.; Clapham, L.; Strauss, K. UK lipohypertrophy interventional study. *Diabetes Res. Clin. Pract.* **2017**, *126*, 248–253. [CrossRef] [PubMed]
29. Campinos, C.; Le Floch, J.-P.; Petit, C.; Penfornis, A.; Winiszewski, P.; Bordier, L.; Lepage, M.; Fermon, C.; Louis, J.; Almain, C.; et al. An Effective Intervention for Diabetic Lipohypertrophy: Results of a Randomized, Controlled, Prospective Multicenter Study in France. *Diabetes Technol. Ther.* **2017**, *19*, 623–632. [CrossRef]
30. Wang, W.; Huang, R.; Chen, Y.; Tu, M. Values of ultrasound for diagnosis and management of insulin-induced lipohypertrophy. *Medicine* **2021**, *100*, e26743. [CrossRef]
31. Perciun, R. Ultrasonographic aspect of subcutaneous tissue dystrophies as a result of insulin injections. *Med. Ultrason.* **2010**, *12*, 104–109.

32. Guidelines and Consensus Compilation Committee of Chinese Journal of Diabetes. Technical Guide for Diabetes Drug Injection in China (2016 edition). *Chin. J. Diabetes Mellit.* **2017**, *9*, 79–105.
33. Mantovani, A.; Grani, G.; Chioma, L.; Vancieri, G.; Giordani, I.; Rendina, R.; Rinaldi, M.E.; Andreadi, A.; Coccaro, C.; Boccardo, C.; et al. Severe hypoglycemia in patients with known diabetes requiring emergency department care: A report from an Italian multicenter study. *J. Clin. Transl. Endocrinol.* **2016**, *5*, 46–52. [CrossRef] [PubMed]

Disclaimer/Publisher's Note: The statements, opinions and data contained in all publications are solely those of the individual author(s) and contributor(s) and not of MDPI and/or the editor(s). MDPI and/or the editor(s) disclaim responsibility for any injury to people or property resulting from any ideas, methods, instructions or products referred to in the content.

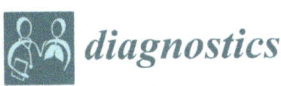

Brief Report

Multiparametric Skin Assessment in a Monocentric Cohort of Systemic Sclerosis Patients: Is There a Role for Ultra-High Frequency Ultrasound?

Marco Di Battista [1,2], Simone Barsotti [1], Saverio Vitali [3], Marco Palma [3], Giammarco Granieri [4], Teresa Oranges [4], Giacomo Aringhieri [3], Valentina Dini [4], Alessandra Della Rossa [1], Emanuele Neri [3], Marco Romanelli [4] and Marta Mosca [1,*]

1 Rheumatology Unit, University of Pisa, 56124 Pisa, Italy
2 Department of Medical Biotechnologies, University of Siena, 53100 Siena, Italy
3 Radiology Unit, University of Pisa, 56124 Pisa, Italy
4 Dermatology Unit, University of Pisa, 56124 Pisa, Italy
* Correspondence: marta.mosca@unipi.it

Abstract: *Background*: To assess skin involvement in a cohort of patients with systemic sclerosis (SSc) by comparing results obtained from modified Rodnan skin score (mRSS), durometry and ultra-high frequency ultrasound (UHFUS). *Methods*: SSc patients were enrolled along with healthy controls (HC), assessing disease-specific characteristics. Five regions of interest were investigated in the non-dominant upper limb. Each patient underwent a rheumatological evaluation of the mRSS, dermatological measurement with a durometer, and radiological UHFUS assessment with a 70 MHz probe calculating the mean grayscale value (MGV). *Results*: Forty-seven SSc patients (87.2% female, mean age 56.4 years) and 15 HC comparable for age and sex were enrolled. Durometry showed a positive correlation with mRSS in most regions of interest ($p = 0.025$, $\rho = 0.34$ in mean). When performing UHFUS, SSc patients had a significantly thicker epidermal layer ($p < 0.001$) and lower epidermal MGV ($p = 0.01$) than HC in almost all the different regions of interest. Lower values of dermal MGV were found at the distal and intermediate phalanx ($p < 0.01$). No relationships were found between UHFUS results either with mRSS or durometry. *Conclusions*: UHFUS is an emergent tool for skin assessment in SSc, showing significant alterations concerning skin thickness and echogenicity when compared with HC. The lack of correlations between UHFUS and both mRSS and durometry suggests that these are not equivalent techniques but may represent complementary methods for a full non-invasive skin evaluation in SSc.

Keywords: systemic sclerosis; ultra-high frequency ultrasound; durometry; skin score; skin imaging; skin fibrosis

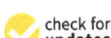

Citation: Di Battista, M.; Barsotti, S.; Vitali, S.; Palma, M.; Granieri, G.; Oranges, T.; Aringhieri, G.; Dini, V.; Della Rossa, A.; Neri, E.; et al. Multiparametric Skin Assessment in a Monocentric Cohort of Systemic Sclerosis Patients: Is There a Role for Ultra-High Frequency Ultrasound? *Diagnostics* **2023**, *13*, 1495. https://doi.org/10.3390/diagnostics13081495

Academic Editor: Po-Hsiang Tsui

Received: 30 March 2023
Revised: 16 April 2023
Accepted: 20 April 2023
Published: 21 April 2023

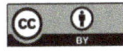

Copyright: © 2023 by the authors. Licensee MDPI, Basel, Switzerland. This article is an open access article distributed under the terms and conditions of the Creative Commons Attribution (CC BY) license (https://creativecommons.org/licenses/by/4.0/).

1. Introduction

Systemic sclerosis (SSc) is a rare connective tissue disorder characterized by diffuse microangiopathy and immune dysregulation, pathogenic elements that ultimately lead to the most known feature of this disease, namely tissue fibrosis of skin and internal organs [1,2]. Skin thickening is one of the most evident and studied aspects of SSc since it can be easily analyzed and mostly because it has been widely demonstrated that a more extensive skin involvement correlates with more severe internal organ damage, poor prognosis and increased disability [3,4]. Modified Rodnan Skin Score (mRSS) is a manual semi-quantitative score representing the most widespread clinometric tool to assess skin thickening in SSc. Despite the possible intra-reader and especially inter-reader variability, it is used as a primary or secondary outcome measure in clinical trials [5].

To improve the accuracy and sensitivity to change in the measurement of skin involvement, the use of semiquantitative/quantitative methods has been proposed. Among them, the durometer proved to be a non-invasive and easy-to-use instrument that can provide accurate and reliable measurements, gaining consideration as a complementary method to mRSS [6]. Recently, cutaneous ultrasonography emerged as a remarkable technique which allows for quantifying skin thickness, and studies regarding its use in SSc skin assessment have been published so far [7]. In the last few years, a growing interest has arisen in ultra-high frequency ultrasound (UHFUS), a method allowing a non-invasive detailed characterization of skin layers [8].

Our work aims to assess cutaneous involvement in a cohort of SSc patients, comparing results obtained from mRSS, durometry and UHFUS to obtain a complete and accurate multiparametric non-invasive evaluation of SSc skin.

2. Materials and Methods

2.1. Patients

We enrolled adult patients fulfilling 2013 EULAR/ACR criteria for SSc [9] attending a routine outpatient visit at the Rheumatology Unit of the University of Pisa between January and December 2019. We also enrolled 15 healthy controls (HC) with the same mean age and sex percentage of the SSc cohort. Full ethical approval was obtained from the local ethical committee (Comitato Etico Area Vasta Nord Ovest, approval number 13408). Each subject voluntarily agreed to participate and gave written informed consent to publish the material.

Each patient underwent a multidisciplinary (rheumatological, dermatological and radiological) evaluation at enrolment time. Initial data were collected through questions, medical records, and physical examination, including epidemiological data, disease duration and autoantibody profile (distinguishing between anti-centromere—ACA and anti-topoisomerase I—Scl70). All ongoing therapies were allowed. According to LeRoy classification [10], patients were classified into three skin subsets: sine scleroderma (ssSSc), limited (lcSSc) and diffuse cutaneous (dcSSc) groups. Moreover, the presence of hand contractures and the history of digital ulcers (DUs) were investigated. Ongoing DUs were an exclusion criterion. Afterwards, mRSS was performed either in the whole body (0–51 pts) or in some specific regions of interest (0–3 pts each) of the non-dominant upper limb:

- on the central dorsal side of the intermediate phalanx (IP) of the second finger.
- on the central dorsal side of the proximal phalanx (PP) of the second finger.
- on the dorsum of the hand (DH) (3 cm distally to the wrist joint).
- on the volar side of the forearm (VF) (5 cm proximally to the wrist joint).

2.2. Instrumental Assessment

Durometry assessment was performed by a single operator on five regions of interest of the non-dominant upper limb: distal phalanx (DP), IP and PP of the second finger, DH and VF. Skin hardness was measured with a portable durometer (Rex Model 1600, Rex Gauge Company, Buffalo Grove, IL, USA) in standard durometer units. The durometer was held in a vertical position keeping the foot of the gauge firmly against the skin. Each area was assessed three times, considering the mean value as the result.

UHFUS assessment was performed by a single operator with a 70 MHz probe (Vevo MD, VisualSonics, Toronto, ON, Canada). Images were acquired by placing a homogeneous layer of ultrasound gel between the transducer and the skin, keeping the various acquisition parameters constant. Five-second static clips of the skin were acquired at the five sites mentioned above DP, IP, PP, DH, and VF (Figure 1). A static image was extracted from each clip and was then analysed with Horos™ software v2.1.1 (Horos Project, Annapolis, MD, USA). Epidermal thickness, seen as a superficial hyperechoic band, was calculated as the mean value obtained from 5 measurements at different points of the image. Grayscale levels were then analyzed by positioning circular regions of interest (ROI) in the epidermal and dermal areas. Specifically, it was calculated the mean grayscale value (MGV) within the ROI, whose values range from 0 (totally black) to 255 (total white). The expert examiner was calibrated to improve intra-examiner repeatability on ten patients not included in the study until a k value > 0.8 was obtained.

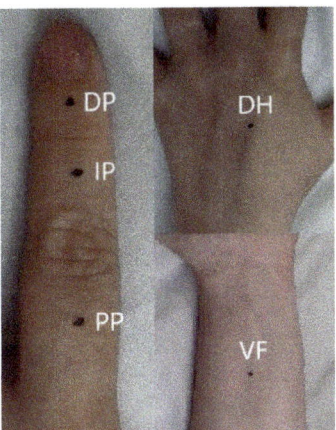

Figure 1. Skin regions of interest undergoing multiparametric non-invasive assessment. DP: distal phalanx; IP: intermediate phalanx; PP: proximal phalanx; DH: dorsum hand; VF: volar forearm.

2.3. Statistical Analysis

Categorical data were described by absolute and relative (%) frequency, whereas continuous data by mean and standard deviation. Comparisons between mean values were analyzed by Student's t test for independent samples (two-tailed) and one-way ANOVA. Comparisons between proportions were made with z-test for proportions. The correlation between variables was examined with Pearson's correlation coefficient (r). p values of less than 0.05 were considered significant, and all analyses were carried out with SPSS v.22 technology (IBM Corp., Armonk, NY, USA).

3. Results

3.1. Patients and mRSS

Forty-seven SSc patients were enrolled for this study, along with 15 HC comparable for age and sex. The baseline characteristics of the SSc cohort are reported in Table 1.

Table 1. Baseline characteristics of SSc cohort and HC.

	SSc (n = 47)	HC (n = 15)	p
Female	41 (87.2%)	11 (73.3%)	n.s.
Age (years)	56.4 ± 13.5	54.7 ± 14.3	n.s.
Disease duration (years)	10.8 ± 10.3		
ACA	27 (57.4%)		
Scl70	16 (34%)		
- ssSSc	9 (19.1%)		
- lcSSc	27 (57.4%)		
- dcSSc	11 (23.4%)		
DUs history	22 (46.8%)		
Hand contractures	5 (10.6%)		

Data are expressed in number (percentage) or mean ± standard deviation. SSc: systemic sclerosis; HC: healthy controls; ACA: anti-centromere autoantibodies; Scl70: anti-topoisomerase I autoantibodies; ssSSc: sine scleroderma SSc; lcSSc: limited cutaneous SSc; dcSSc: diffuse cutaneous SSc; DUs: digital ulcers; n.s.: not significant.

Among the possible correlations with disease characteristics, the mRSS performed in the whole body was found to be significantly higher in patients with Scl70 positivity

(p = 0.05) and hand contractures (p < 0.001). In contrast, lower values were associated with ACA positivity (p = 0.015). As expected, mRSS in dcSSc was significantly greater than lcSSc and ssSSc (p < 0.001 for both). Even when considering mRSS performed in the different regions of interest, dcSSc patients had significantly higher values than lcSSc and ssSSc (p < 0.001 for all).

3.2. Durometer

Durometer measurements performed in the different regions of interest highlighted that DH presented lower values in females (p = 0.025) and was inversely associated with disease duration (p = 0.012, ρ = −0.38). Among skin subsets, a statistical difference was found only at the level of IP, with dcSSc having higher values than lcSSc (p = 0.029) and ssSSc (p = 0.002). Durometer measurements were lower in ACA patients than Scl70 ones both in IP (p = 0.008) and PP (p = 0.001). Hand contractures were associated with higher values at DP (p = 0.009) and VF (p = 0.046). No other associations were found with other disease characteristics.

Evaluating possible relationships between the durometer and the total mRSS (whole body), it was found a direct correlation at the level of the IP (p = 0.025, ρ = 0.34), PP (p = 0.03, ρ = 0.33) and VF (p = 0.02, ρ = 0.35).

3.3. UHFUS

Table 2 summarizes the main UHFUS findings in our cohort. When performing UHFUS between SSc patients and HC, the former had a significantly thicker epidermal layer in all the different regions of interest (p < 0.001 for all)—Figure 2.

Table 2. UHFUS findings in SSc and HC.

	SSc (n = 47)	HC (n = 15)	p
Epidermal thickness (μm)			
- DP	258.6 ± 64.2	176.5 ± 21.1	<0.001
- IP	238.4 ± 77.7	173.3 ± 20.3	<0.001
- PP	206.9 ± 42.9	156.2 ± 18.1	<0.001
- DH	182.1 ± 33.3	146.7 ± 12.7	<0.001
- VF	180.1 ± 36.4	143.0 ± 18.0	<0.001
Epidermal MGV (0–255)			
- DP	168.6 ± 40.6	191.0 ± 23.7	0.01
- IP	168.2 ± 37.8	195.6 ± 20.9	0.01
- PP	174.2 ± 38.8	193.4 ± 18.8	0.01
- DH	184.5 ± 27.7	195.1 ± 19.2	n.s.
- VF	185.4 ± 24.6	190.1 ± 39.9	n.s.
Dermal MGV (0–255)			
- DP	62.9 ± 33.5	100.8 ± 27.2	<0.001
- IP	70.0 ± 35.6	98.3 ± 25.8	0.006
- PP	87.0 ± 37.9	107.4 ± 13.8	0.04
- DH	109.4 ± 32.7	118.1 ± 22.0	n.s.
- VF	124.7 ± 33.8	130.6 ± 31.5	n.s.

Data are expressed in mean ± standard deviation. SSc: systemic sclerosis; HC: healthy controls; MGV: mean grayscale value; DP: distal phalanx; IP: intermediate phalanx; PP: proximal phalanx; DH: dorsum hand; VF: volar forearm.; n.s.: not significant.

The SSc group also presented lower epidermal MGV at DP, IP and PP (p = 0.01 for all). Similarly, low values of dermal MGV reached statistical significance at DP (p < 0.001), IP (p = 0.006) and PP (p = 0.04)—Figure 3. When UHFUS results were diversified according to skin subset, both lcSSc and dcSSc reconfirmed a significantly thicker epidermal layer than HC for all the regions of interest. Noteworthy, when considering MGV differences between cutaneous subsets and HC, statistically significant lower values were detected for both skin subsets only at the dermal layer of DP ($p = 0.001$ for lcSSc; $p = 0.008$ for dcSSc) and IP ($p = 0.05$ for lcSSc; $p = 0.01$ for dcSSc).

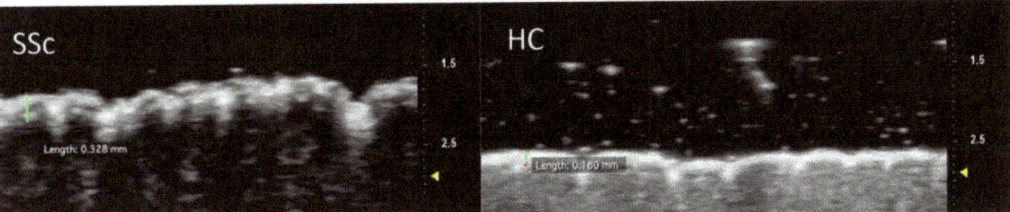

Figure 2. Measurement of epidermal thickness at the intermediate phalanx of the second finger. Note the increased thickness of the epidermal layer in the SSc patient compared to the control subject.

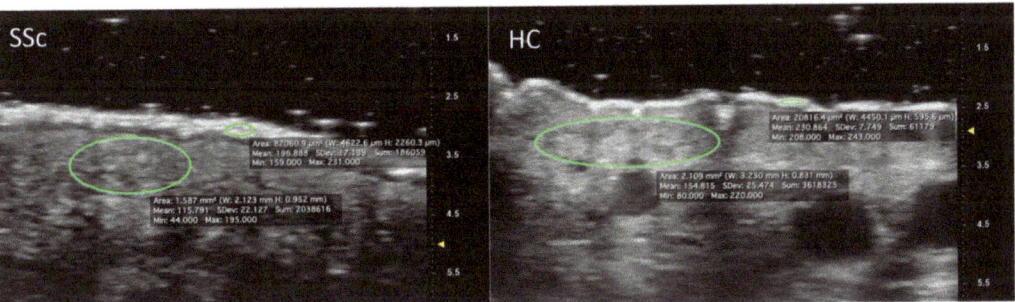

Figure 3. Measurement of epidermal and dermal grayscale values using ROIs positioned at the intermediate phalanx of the second finger. Note the reduction in the mean grayscale value in the SSc patient compared to the control subject in the epidermal and dermal areas.

Among SSc patients, epidermal thickness revealed an inverse correlation with disease duration at VF ($p = 0.017$, $\rho = -0.346$). No associations were found between UHFUS results and skin subsets, autoantibody profile, and disease characteristics.

No relationships were found between UHFUS results, and mRSS performed in the whole body or the different regions of interest. Furthermore, when comparing outcomes obtained from UHFUS with those from durometer, no relevant associations were found for any region of interest.

4. Discussion

Since skin thickness is the most evident feature of SSc, several techniques have been used over the years for its evaluation, always looking for the highest validity and reliability. In our work, we assessed skin involvement in a cohort of SSc patients through mRSS, durometry and UHFUS. Furthermore, the outcomes of these techniques were compared. In addition, UHFUS results from a group of HC were also analyzed, finding significant differences between the subgroups, interesting correlations with disease characteristics, and finally, obtaining a complete multiparametric non-invasive assessment of skin involvement in SSc.

Durometer measurements suggested that higher values are likely associated with the early phase of the disease and with some characteristics such as hand contractures and diffuse cutaneous subsets. Moreover, durometry showed a good correlation with mRSS performed in the whole body and a direct trend for the different regions of interest, reiterating the findings of previous studies [6,11].

The comparison of UHFUS outcomes between SSc patients and HC pointed out that the former had a diffusely thicker epidermal layer, even in limited cutaneous forms.

However, a significant dermal impairment (corresponding to a lower MGV) could be detected only in the distal part of the hand, likely reflecting the more impacting cutaneous and microvascular alterations that occur in the extremities. In this regard, an interesting negative correlation between UHFUS skin thickness and capillary density assessed by nailfold capillaroscopy was recently highlighted [12].

UHFUS showed that epidermal thickness was inversely correlated with disease duration. Hence, we confirm that skin is thicker in early phases and then becomes thinner, which was already demonstrated with HFUS by Hesselstrand et al., who found that patients with shorter disease duration had high skin thickness and low echogenicity [13]. They suggested that this ultrasonographic pattern could identify the edematous phase that precedes palpable skin involvement. This hint was somehow strengthened by an HFUS study that showed how skin thickness was more significant in SSc patients in the edematous phase and progressively decreased in those in the fibrotic and atrophic phases [14]. Moreover, a longitudinal evaluation revealed that a decrease in skin thickness and an increase in echogenicity were observed during a one-year follow-up [15].

The lack of correlations between UHFUS and both mRSS and durometry that emerged in our study is discordant with findings from other HFUS studies [13,14]. However, it could be explained by the fact that these are not equivalent techniques but complementary. The hypothesis that skin ultrasound can show something that other methods do not grasp was recently strengthened also by other studies. For example, HFUS revealed subclinical dermal involvement in areas with a normal mRSS in lcSSc patients [16], and there are other works besides ours that found no ultrasound differences between skin subsets [17]. Kissin et al., in 2006, tried to compare these three techniques for a skin assessment and found a good correlation between them all [18]. However, even leaving out the smaller number of patients analyzed, they used a 10 MHz probe, so it is reasonable to expect different and more accurate results with a 70 MHz probe. As pointed out by the Authors themselves, the durometer is designed to measure skin hardness, so it could not provide information about other pathological skin properties.

The results of this study indicate that, whereas mRSS and durometry are two techniques able to evaluate skin hardness reliably and unanimously, UHFUS appears as an autonomous method capable of showing different skin characteristics. The variation of the thickness and echogenicity of the various skin layers concerning the different phases of the disease represents an important reason for the larger use of this technique in SSc. Our data reconfirm the great potential of UHFUS in SSc skin assessment, as already highlighted by the previous work by Naredo et al. [8].

Recently, two systematic literature reviews on US assessment of skin involvement in SSc were published. They agree that the US, especially when applied with higher frequencies, is an effective and helpful tool for skin assessment in SSc, but some problems still limit its use. For example, image acquisition and analysis methods were heterogeneous and frequently under-reported, thus precluding data synthesis across studies. Moreover, there is limited or absent US evidence for sensitivity to change, test-retest reliability, clinical trial discrimination or thresholds of meaning. It was also underlined that US findings should be compared to skin histology. In this regard, although the US proved valid and reliable for skin thickness measurement, echogenicity seems to have a limited validity. Finally, developing a protocol for US skin assessment with image acquisition and analysis standardisation was deemed necessary for future research and to foster its clinical use [19,20].

Our work presents some limitations. The relatively small size of the cohort limits the generalizability of the findings to larger populations of SSc patients. Due to the intrinsic setting features of the device used for ultrasound assessment, it was impossible to measure the dermis's thickness as the boundaries of this layer were indistinguishable from the underlying hypodermis. As pointed out by a systematic literature review as part of a large international collaborative work on the assessment of skin involvement in SSc, it should also be considered that the disease progression rate of SSc before study entry may significantly impact the results [21]. The same applies to immunosuppressive therapies that may have affected skin involvement. The study's primary limitation is the lack of skin biopsy samples, which would have allowed us to directly validate the results obtained and the speculations formulated with the other techniques. This is even more true since a relationship between skin HFUS and dermal collagen content was found in SSc cutaneous biopsies [22]. Moreover, a good correlation between US-measured skin thickness and histological cutaneous thickness was demonstrated [23] as well as with circulating fibrocytes [24]. Skin US assessment, especially UHFUS, was performed in a few heterogeneous studies, so it still lacks validity criteria: further studies are then required. Finally, the design of the study does not provide information about the evolution of skin involvement. In this regard, a future study proposal could address UHFUS follow-up of SSc patients to assess the predictive value of UHFUS measurements in disease progression and outcomes.

In conclusion, skin evaluation in SSc patients could benefit from complementary methods to obtain a complete assessment, especially concerning UHFUS, a relatively new technique with great potential.

5. Conclusions

UHFUS is an emergent non-invasive diagnostic tool for skin assessment in SSc. It showed significant alterations concerning skin thickness and echogenicity when comparing SSc patients with HC. However, the lack of correlations between UHFUS and both mRSS and durometry suggests that these are not equivalent techniques but may represent complementary methods for a full skin evaluation in SSc. Therefore, future clinical use of UHFUS in the skin evaluation of SSc patients is conceivable.

Author Contributions: Conceptualization, S.B., S.V., V.D., A.D.R. and M.M.; methodology, M.D.B., S.B. and S.V.; validation, S.V. and V.D.; formal analysis, M.D.B. and S.B.; investigation, M.D.B., S.B., S.V., M.P., G.G., T.O., G.A. and V.D.; resources, A.D.R., E.N., M.R. and M.M.; data curation, M.D.B., S.B. and S.V.; writing—original draft preparation, M.D.B.; writing—review and editing, M.D.B., S.B., V.D., A.D.R. and M.M.; visualization, M.D.B., A.D.R. and M.M.; supervision, M.M. All authors have read and agreed to the published version of the manuscript.

Funding: This research received no external funding.

Institutional Review Board Statement: The study was conducted in accordance with the Declaration of Helsinki and approved by the Ethics Committee of Comitato Etico Area Vasta Nord Ovest (approval number 13408, 19 June 2018).

Informed Consent Statement: Informed consent was obtained from all subjects involved in the study. Written informed consent has been obtained from the patients to publish this paper.

Data Availability Statement: The datasets used and/or analysed during the current study are available from the corresponding author on reasonable request.

Acknowledgments: We wish to thank Bianca Benincasa and Rosa Maria Bruno for their precious help.

Conflicts of Interest: The authors declare no conflict of interest.

References

1. Di Battista, M.; Barsotti, S.; Orlandi, M.; Lepri, G.; Codullo, V.; Della Rossa, A.; Guiducci, S.; Del Galdo, F. One year in review 2021: Systemic sclerosis. *Clin. Exp. Rheumatol.* **2021**, *39*, 3–12. [CrossRef]
2. D'Oria, M.; Gandin, I.; Riccardo, P.; Hughes, M.; Lepidi, S.; Salton, F.; Confalonieri, P.; Confalonieri, M.; Tavano, S.; Ruaro, B. Correlation between Microvascular Damage and Internal Organ Involvement in Scleroderma: Focus on Lung Damage and Endothelial Dysfunction. *Diagnostics* **2023**, *13*, 55. [CrossRef]
3. Czirják, L.; Foeldvari, I.; Müller-Ladner, U. Skin involvement in systemic sclerosis. *Rheumatology* **2008**, *47*, v44–v45. [CrossRef]
4. Tieu, A.; Chaigne, B.; Dunogué, B.; Dion, J.; Régent, A.; Casadevall, M.; Cohen, P.; Legendre, P.; Terrier, B.; Costedoat-Chalumeau, N.; et al. Autoantibodies versus Skin Fibrosis Extent in Systemic Sclerosis: A Case-Control Study of Inverted Phenotypes. *Diagnostics* **2022**, *12*, 1067. [CrossRef]

5. Khanna, D.; Furst, D.E.; Clements, P.J.; Allanore, Y.; Baron, M.; Czirjak, L.; Distler, O.; Foeldvari, I.; Kuwana, M.; Matucci-Cerinic, M.; et al. Standardization of the modified Rodnan skin score for use in clinical trials of systemic sclerosis. *J. Scleroderma Relat. Disord.* **2017**, *2*, 11–18. [CrossRef]
6. Merkel, P.A.; Silliman, N.P.; Denton, C.P.; Furst, D.E.; Khanna, D.; Emery, P.; Hsu, V.M.; Streisand, J.B.; Polisson, R.P.; Åkesson, A.; et al. Validity, reliability, and feasibility of durometer measurements of scleroderma skin disease in a multicenter treatment trial. *Arthritis Rheumatol.* **2008**, *59*, 699–705. [CrossRef]
7. Santiago, T.; Santiago, M.; Ruaro, B.; Salvador, M.J.; Cutolo, M.; da Silva, J.A.P. Ultrasonography for the assessment of skin in systemic sclerosis: A systematic review. *Arthritis Care Res.* **2019**, *71*, 563–574. [CrossRef]
8. Naredo, E.; Pascau, J.; Damjanov, N.; Lepri, G.; Gordaliza, P.M.; Janta, I.; Ovalles-Bonilla, J.G.; López-Longo, F.J.; Matucci-Cerinic, M. Performance of ultra-high-frequency ultrasound in the evaluation of skin involvement in systemic sclerosis: A preliminary report. *Rheumatology* **2020**, *59*, 1671–1678. [CrossRef]
9. Van Den Hoogen, F.; Khanna, D.; Fransen, J.; Johnson, S.R.; Baron, M.; Tyndall, A.; Matucci-Cerinic, M.; Naden, R.P.; Medsger, T.A.; Carreira, P.E.; et al. 2013 classification criteria for systemic sclerosis: An American college of rheumatology/European league against rheumatism collaborative initiative. *Ann. Rheum. Dis.* **2013**, *72*, 1747–1755. [CrossRef]
10. LeRoy, E.; Black, C.; Fleischmajer, R.; Jablonska, S.; Krieg, T.; Medsger, T.A.; Wollheim, F. Scleroderma (systemic sclerosis): Classification, subsets and pathogenesis. *J. Rheumatol.* **1988**, *15*, 202–205.
11. Moon, K.W.; Song, R.; Kim, J.H.; Lee, E.Y.; Lee, E.B.; Song, Y.W. The correlation between durometer score and modified Rodnan skin score in systemic sclerosis. *Rheumatol. Int.* **2012**, *32*, 2465–2470. [CrossRef]
12. Dinsdale, G.; Wilkinson, S.; Wilkinson, J.; Moore, T.L.; Manning, J.B.; Berks, M.; Marjanovic, E.; Dickinson, M.; Herrick, A.L.; Murray, A.K. State-of-the-art technologies provide new insights linking skin and blood vessel abnormalities in SSc-related disorders. *Microvasc. Res.* **2020**, *130*, 104006. [CrossRef]
13. Hesselstrand, R.; Scheja, A.; Wildt, M.; Åkesson, A. High-frequency ultrasound of skin involvement in systemic sclerosis reflects oedema, extension and severity in early disease. *Rheumatology* **2008**, *47*, 84–87. [CrossRef]
14. Kaloudi, O.; Bandinelli, F.; Filippucci, E.; Conforti, M.L.; Miniati, I.; Guiducci, S.; Porta, F.; Candelieri, A.; Conforti, D.; Grassiri, G.; et al. High frequency ultrasound measurement of digital dermal thickness in systemic sclerosis. *Ann. Rheum. Dis.* **2010**, *69*, 1140–1143. [CrossRef]
15. Hesselstrand, R.; Carlestam, J.; Wildt, M.; Sandqvist, G.; Andréasson, K. High frequency ultrasound of skin involvement in systemic sclerosis—A follow-up study. *Arthritis Res. Ther.* **2015**, *17*, 329. [CrossRef]
16. Sulli, A.; Ruaro, B.; Smith, V.; Paolino, S.; Pizzorni, C.; Pesce, G.; Cutolo, M. Subclinical dermal involvement is detectable by high frequency ultrasound even in patients with limited cutaneous systemic sclerosis. *Arthritis Res. Ther.* **2017**, *19*, 61. [CrossRef]
17. Li, H.; Furst, D.E.; Jin, H.; Sun, C.; Wang, X.; Yang, L.; He, J.; Wang, Y.; Liu, A. High-frequency ultrasound of the skin in systemic sclerosis: An exploratory study to examine correlation with disease activity and to define the minimally detectable difference. *Arthritis Res. Ther.* **2018**, *20*, 181. [CrossRef]
18. Kissin, E.Y.; Schiller, A.M.; Gelbard, R.B.; Anderson, J.J.; Falanga, V.; Simms, R.W.; Korn, J.H.; Merkel, P.A. Durometry for the assessment of skin disease in systemic sclerosis. *Arthritis Rheumatol.* **2006**, *55*, 603–609. [CrossRef]
19. Santiago, T.; Santos, E.; Ruaro, B.; Lepri, G.; Green, L.; Wildt, M.; Watanabe, S.; Lescoat, A.; Hesselstrand, R.; Del Galdo, F.; et al. Ultrasound and elastography in the assessment of skin involvement in systemic sclerosis: A systematic literature review focusing on validation and standardization – WSF Skin Ultrasound Group. *Semin. Arthritis Rheum.* **2022**, *52*, 151954. [CrossRef]
20. Dźwigała, M.; Sobolewski, P.; Maślińska, M.; Yurtsever, I.; Szymańska, E.; Walecka, I. High-resolution ultrasound imaging of skin involvement in systemic sclerosis: A systematic review. *Rheumatol. Int.* **2021**, *41*, 285–295. [CrossRef]
21. Kumánovics, G.; Péntek, M.; Bae, S.; Opris, D.; Khanna, D.; Furst, D.E.; Czirják, L. Assessment of skin involvement in systemic sclerosis. *Rheumatology* **2017**, *56*, V53–V66. [CrossRef] [PubMed]
22. Flower, V.A.; Barratt, S.L.; Hart, D.J.; Mackenzie, A.B.; Shipley, J.A.; Ward, S.G.; Pauling, J.D. High-frequency ultrasound assessment of systemic sclerosis skin involvement: Intraobserver repeatability and relationship with clinician assessment and dermal collagen content. *J. Rheumatol.* **2021**, *48*, 867–876. [CrossRef] [PubMed]
23. Chen, C.; Cheng, Y.; Zhu, X.; Cai, Y.; Xue, Y.; Kong, N.; Yu, Y.; Xuan, D.; Zheng, S.; Yang, X.; et al. Ultrasound assessment of skin thickness and stiffness: The correlation with histology and clinical score in systemic sclerosis. *Arthritis Res. Ther.* **2020**, *22*, 197. [CrossRef]
24. Ruaro, B.; Soldano, S.; Smith, V.; Paolino, S.; Contini, P.; Montagna, P.; Pizzorni, C.; Casabella, A.; Tardito, S.; Sulli, A.; et al. Correlation between circulating fibrocytes and dermal thickness in limited cutaneous systemic sclerosis patients: A pilot study. *Rheumatol. Int.* **2019**, *39*, 1369–1376. [CrossRef] [PubMed]

Disclaimer/Publisher's Note: The statements, opinions and data contained in all publications are solely those of the individual author(s) and contributor(s) and not of MDPI and/or the editor(s). MDPI and/or the editor(s) disclaim responsibility for any injury to people or property resulting from any ideas, methods, instructions or products referred to in the content.

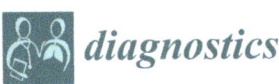

Article

Ultra-High Frequency Ultrasound Imaging of Bowel Wall in Hirschsprung's Disease—Correlation and Agreement Analyses of Histoanatomy

Tebin Hawez [1], Christina Graneli [1], Tobias Erlöv [2], Emilia Gottberg [3], Rodrigo Munoz Mitev [3], Kristine Hagelsteen [1], Maria Evertsson [4], Tomas Jansson [4], Magnus Cinthio [2] and Pernilla Stenström [1,*]

1. Department of Pediatric Surgery, Children's Hospital, Skåne University Hospital Lund, Lund University, 221 85 Lund, Sweden
2. Department of Biomedical Engineering, The Faculty of Engineering, Lund University, 223 63 Lund, Sweden
3. Department of Clinical Genetics and Pathology, Skåne University Hospital Lund, Lund University, 222 42 Lund, Sweden
4. Department of Biomedical Engineering, Skåne University Hospital Lund, The Faculty of Engineering, Lund University, 221 00 Lund, Sweden
* Correspondence: pernilla.stenstrom@med.lu.se

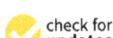

Citation: Hawez, T.; Graneli, C.; Erlöv, T.; Gottberg, E.; Munoz Mitev, R.; Hagelsteen, K.; Evertsson, M.; Jansson, T.; Cinthio, M.; Stenström, P. Ultra-High Frequency Ultrasound Imaging of Bowel Wall in Hirschsprung's Disease—Correlation and Agreement Analyses of Histoanatomy. *Diagnostics* **2023**, *13*, 1388. https://doi.org/10.3390/diagnostics13081388

Academic Editor: Takuji Tanaka

Received: 9 February 2023
Revised: 2 April 2023
Accepted: 4 April 2023
Published: 11 April 2023

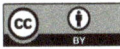

Copyright: © 2023 by the authors. Licensee MDPI, Basel, Switzerland. This article is an open access article distributed under the terms and conditions of the Creative Commons Attribution (CC BY) license (https://creativecommons.org/licenses/by/4.0/).

Abstract: Hirschsprung's disease (HD) is characterized by aganglionosis in the bowel wall, requiring resection. Ultra-high frequency ultrasound (UHFUS) imaging of the bowel wall has been suggested to be an instantaneous method of deciding resection length. The aim of this study was to validate UHFUS imaging of the bowel wall in children with HD by exploring the correlation and systematic differences between UHFUS and histopathology. Resected fresh bowel specimens of children 0–1 years old, operated on for rectosigmoid aganglionosis at a national HD center 2018–2021, were examined ex vivo with UHFUS center frequency 50 MHz. Aganglionosis and ganglionosis were confirmed by histopathological staining and immunohistochemistry. Histoanatomical layers of bowel wall in histopathological and UHFUS images, respectively, were outlined using MATLAB programs. Both histopathological and UHFUS images were available for 19 aganglionic and 18 ganglionic specimens. The thickness of muscularis interna correlated positively between histopathology and UHFUS in both aganglionosis ($R = 0.651$, $p = 0.003$) and ganglionosis ($R = 0.534$, $p = 0.023$). The muscularis interna was systematically thicker in histopathology than in UHFUS images in both aganglionosis (0.499 vs. 0.309 mm; $p < 0.001$) and ganglionosis (0.644 versus 0.556 mm; $p = 0.003$). Significant correlations and systematic differences between histopathological and UHFUS images support the hypothesis that UHFUS reproduces the histoanatomy of the bowel wall in HD accurately.

Keywords: Hirschsprung's disease; bowel wall; ultra-high frequency ultrasound; histopathology; children

1. Introduction

Hirschsprung's disease is a congenital bowel motility disorder characterized by aganglionosis in the bowel wall. Inhibiting relaxation, aganglionosis leads to a life-threatening functional obstruction [1–3]. Treatment of Hirschsprung's disease is by surgery, including resection of the aganglionic and transition zone segments, followed by the establishment of bowel continuity [4,5]. Aganglionosis always stretches in an oral direction from the anus. In the majority of patients, only the rectosigmoid colon is affected, but aganglionosis can also extend over a longer distance [6]. When deciding upon the length of bowel to be resected, intraoperative fresh frozen biopsies are required to confirm the level of ganglionosis. Acknowledged clinical problems are that the frozen biopsy method is a rather blunt technique, and that resection of a too short or a too long bowel segment can cause severe postoperative problems [7,8]. Additionally, waiting times for frozen biopsy analyses during surgery can be considerable, up to several hours, especially if multiple biopsies are needed as a result of an unexpected aganglionic extension, thus burdening the child with having to endure prolonged anesthesia. A more precise and instant intraoperative diagnostic method is warranted to make Hirschsprung's disease surgery quicker and safer. Ultra-high frequency ultrasonography (UHFUS) has been suggested to be such an instant method that could potentially replace frozen biopsy [9]. UHFUS with frequencies of <70 MHz captures superficial depths of a few millimeters with a resolution down to 30 µm [10]. This is compared to conventional ultrasound with 2–15 MHz frequencies used in clinical settings and imaging depths of 2–20 cm. UHFUS imaging has been reported to have diagnostic potential within the fields of dermatology, vascular medicine, musculoskeletal evaluation, and gastrointestinal surgery with regard to Hirschsprung's disease [9,11]. In diagnostics of Hirschsprung's disease, a pilot study showed that UHFUS can potentially be useful in differentiating between the aganglionic and ganglionic bowel wall [9]. This could be because histoanatomical landmarks have been shown to differ between ganglionosis and aganglionosis [9,12]. However, there remains a gap in knowledge regarding the accuracy of UHFUS in reproducing the histoanatomical layers of the bowel wall.

Therefore, the overall aim of this study was to explore whether the histoanatomical layers of the bowel wall could be imaged accurately by UHFUS. The first research question was to establish whether the thicknesses of the histoanatomical layers of the muscularis interna and muscularis externa, as seen on UHFUS images of fresh bowel wall ex vivo, correlate to those of the histopathologically-prepared specimen. The second question was to ascertain whether any systematic differences and low agreement of histoanatomical thicknesses were evident when comparing the bowel wall thicknesses as measured on histopathology and UHFUS images.

The first hypothesis was that morphometrics, i.e., thicknesses of histoanatomical layers as measured by UHFUS imaging and histopathological specimens, respectively, would correlate well. The second hypothesis was that systematic differences and a low agreement between morphometrics of bowel walls on histoanatomy and UHFUS would be evident as a result of histopathology preparation effects of specimens [13–15].

2. Materials and Methods

2.1. Patients

This study was a translational observational study performed at a national referral center for Hirschsprung's disease covering a geographical uptake area of 5 million residents. Morphometrics of formalin-prepared hematoxylin–eosin-stained bowel wall specimens were compared with those of the same patient's fresh bowel wall imaged on UHFUS ex vivo.

All children with Hirschsprung's disease who were to undergo surgery with resection of the aganglionic bowel segment at the Department of Pediatric Surgery (a national center for Hirschsprung's disease) from April 2018 to December 2021 were eligible for inclusion. Information about the patient's age, weight, and length of resected bowel segments were retrieved from the local Hirschsprung's disease register with data collected prospectively. The inclusion criterion for correlation analyses was rectosigmoid aganglionosis stretching 5–30 cm, according to the pathology report, in children weighing under 10 kg and being younger than 1 year of age. The surgical resection length of aganglionosis was decided based upon the pathologist's analysis of intraoperative fresh frozen biopsies taken by the pediatric surgeon, confirming the presence of ganglionic bowel wall. The accuracy of the frozen biopsy results was confirmed by full histopathological analyses by histopathological staining with hematoxylin–eosin and immunohistochemistry (calretinin and S-100) [16–18] in a final pathology report of the whole resected specimen.

2.2. Specimen Treatments—Fresh and Histopathological

For UHFUS imaging, the Vevo MD ultrasound scanner (FUJIFILM VisualSonics Inc., Toronto, ON, Canada) equipped with a UHF70 transducer, delivering a center frequency of 50 MHz, was used. After surgical resection of the bowel, the retrieved fresh bowel specimen was pinned to a cork mat and examined ex vivo using UHFUS from the serosal (outer) surface (Figure 1). A gel layer was used as a conductor between the transducer and the bowel wall. Minimal pressure was applied to the bowel during the examination in order to avoid manipulation of the examined specimen. UHFUS images were taken longitudinally and saved as B-mode images. For each patient, UHFUS images of both aganglionic and ganglionic bowel walls were saved prospectively in a database. We used a predefined ultrasound acquisition protocol that included center frequency (50 MHz), power (100%), gain (48 dB), depth (7 mm), width (9.73 mm), persistence (off), and dynamic range (65 dB). The settings, including the depth-depending gain, could be optimized during scanning. Two pediatric surgeons (CG, PS) performed all the UHFUS examinations together. They established the working procedure together and assisted each other in imaging and sampling. The bowel specimen was thereafter treated with formalin and sent to the Department of Clinical Genetics and Pathology, where aganglionic and ganglionic segments were confirmed by microscopy after paraffin embedding and standard histopathological staining with hematoxylin–eosin and immunohistochemistry (calretinin and S-100). Histoanatomical images were saved cross-sectioned in the data system Laboratory Information Management System (LIMS) RS Pathology®. Images with hematoxylin–eosin staining were assessed. UHFUS and histopathological images of poor quality, as a result of damaged tissue, broken specimens, or air interfaces causing shadows in the UHFUS imaging, were excluded from the study.

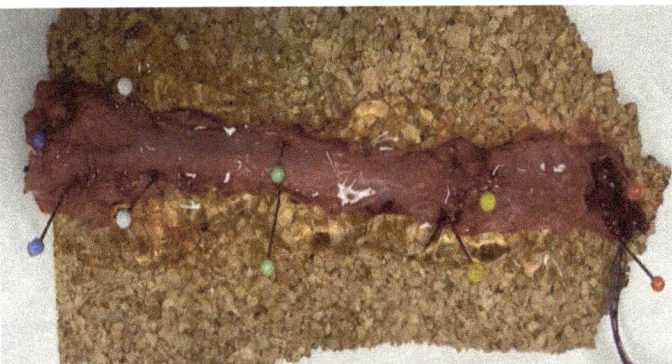

Figure 1. Resected bowel of a child with Hirschsprung's disease. Pinpointed aganglionic bowel (blue pins) and ganglionic bowel (yellow pins) represent the sites where the histoanatomical thicknesses on ultra-high frequency ultrasound (UHFUS) (ex vivo) and histopathology were correlated and compared.

2.3. Assessment and Measurements

Histopathological and UHFUS images were assessed using two in-house software programs based on MATLAB (MathWorks Inc., Natick, MA, USA). One program for histopathology and one for UHFUS, respectively, were developed within the research project. In the histopathological MATLAB program, the external and internal borders of the muscular layers were delineated manually for the muscularis externa and muscularis interna, respectively (Figure 2). The histopathology images could be assessed either whole or in parts. White areas within the tissue were automatically erased before calculations, as programmed. This was decided upon by the assessor in order to avoid sections with image or specimen artifacts. In the UHFUS images, a 5 mm long region of interest (ROI) in the MATLAB program was selected by the assessor and decided upon with respect to image quality and well-represented histoanatomy in the B-mode. The ROI was selected by the same pediatric surgeons who performed the UHFUS examinations. Within this ROI, the presumed muscularis externa and interna were delineated manually, in a similar manner to the procedure when taking the histopathology images. Muscular layer thicknesses were generated automatically from measurement intervals of every 14 μm in the histopathology images and 32 μm in the UHFUS images, respectively (Figure 2).

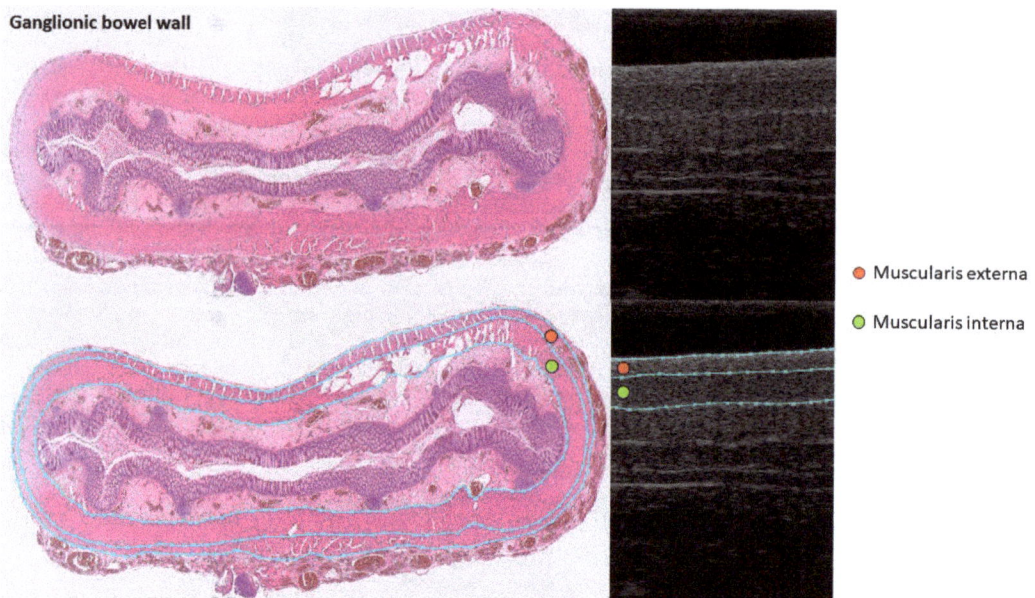

Figure 2. Histoanatomical and ultra-high frequency ultrasound (UHFUS) images of the ganglionic bowel wall of the same patient. The histopathological specimens (**left**) were stained with hematoxylin–eosin. UHFUS imaging (**right**) was performed on bowel ex vivo with center frequency 50 MHz. The method of how to delineate muscularis externa's and interna's outermost limits using MATLAB software is shown in the lower images.

2.4. Statistics

Measurements of the muscularis externa and interna, generated from delineation in MATLAB, were given as mean thickness with standard deviation (SD), and median thickness with range (minimum to maximum). These calculations were performed for both aganglionosis and ganglionosis in histopathological and UHFUS images, respectively. Data management and statistical analyses were performed using Microsoft® Excel and IBM® SPSS® statistics version 27. Ratios of the muscularis interna and externa thicknesses were calculated and used in systematic difference analyses (paired testing). Correlation between histopathological and UHFUS images, and their strength and direction, was assessed by the Spearman correlation test on a group level. For exploring systematic differences between the modalities, the Wilcoxon Signed Rank Test was used, in which the patient served as their own control. A *p*-value of <0.05 was considered to be statistically significant.

Agreement referred to whether histoanatomical thicknesses were close or differed between the histopathological specimen and UHFUS images. Agreement between thicknesses was visualized and interpreted by Bland–Altman plots: a method that has proven to be useful in comparing diagnostic modalities [19,20].

2.5. Ethical Considerations

Ethical approval was obtained from the local ethics review board (DNR 2017/769). Oral and written information was given, and the guardians' written consents were obtained.

3. Results

3.1. Patient and Specimen Characteristics

During the study period, 36 children underwent surgery for Hirschsprung's disease. According to the study criteria, 16 children were excluded (Figure 3). Two histopathological specimen images (one aganglionic and one ganglionic) and one UHFUS image (ganglionic) were excluded as a result of artifacts in the specimen and/or images. Thus, in total, 19 aganglionic and 18 ganglionic bowel specimens from 20 patients were included. The median age of the included patients was 29 days (range: 11–174 days) and their median weight was 4012 g (range: 2600–7700 g) at the time of surgery. The median length of the formalin-fixed resected bowel specimen was 17 cm (range 7–26 cm).

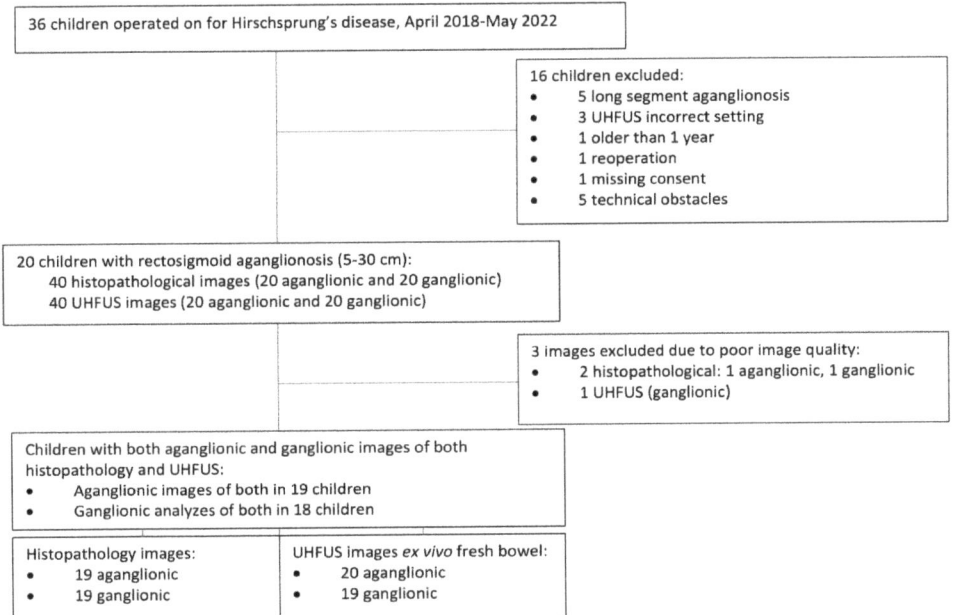

Figure 3. Flow chart of patients and images included in the study. UHFUS: ultra-high frequency ultrasound.

3.2. Aganglionic Bowel Wall

In aganglionosis, the thickness of the muscularis interna correlated positively between histopathology results and UHFUS in aganglionosis, i.e., the thicker the muscularis interna was in the histopathological specimen, the thicker it was on UHFUS imaging ($R = 0.651$, $p = 0.003$, Spearman correlation analyses) (Figure 4a and Appendix A). This correlation housed a systematic difference in the thickness of the muscularis interna, which was, on average, 0.168 mm thicker in histopathological images than on UHFUS ($p < 0.001$) (Table 1).

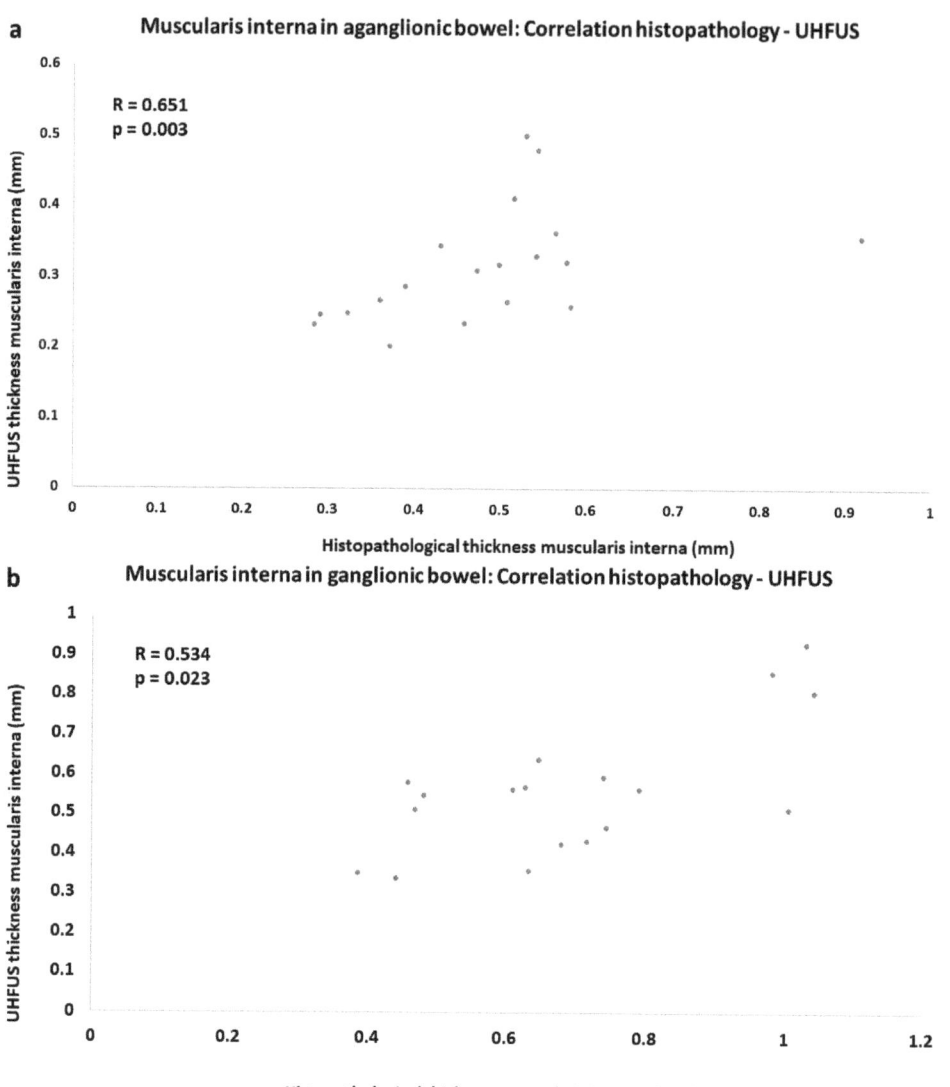

Figure 4. Correlation between muscularis interna thickness in histologically prepared specimens and ultra-high frequency ultrasound (UHFUS) images of (**a**) aganglionic bowel wall, $n = 19$, and (**b**) ganglionic bowel wall, $n = 18$. Spearman rank correlation coefficient (R).

Table 1. Systematic differences of histoanatomical dimensions in bowel wall comparing histopathologically-prepared bowel specimens and ultra-high frequency ultrasound (UHFUS) of ex vivo examined bowel samples. Thicknesses were assessed using MATLAB programs. Median was calculated as the 50th percentile of individual mean measurements of histoanatomical thicknesses.

Histoanatomical Layer	Thickness in Aganglionosis n = 19			Thickness in Ganglionosis n = 18		
	Histopathology (mm) Median (Range)	UHFUS Image (mm) Median (Range)	Systematic Difference p-Value [1]	Histopathological Bowel Wall Specimen (mm) Median (Range)	UHFUS Image (mm) Median (Range)	Systematic Difference p-Value [1]
Muscularis interna (mm)	0.499 (0.284–0.918)	0.309 (0.202–0.500)	<0.001	0.664 (0.386–1.042)	0.556 (0.338–0.931)	0.003
Muscularis externa (mm)	0.291 (0.165–1.285)	0.322 (0.175–0.830)	0.872	0.297 (0.186–0.556)	0.433 (0.169–0.668)	0.006
Ratio: muscularis interna/ muscularis externa	1.253 (0.492–2.257)	0.888 (0.382–2.074)	0.064	2.101 (1.290–3.247)	1.333 (0.723–2.059)	<0.001

[1] Related-Samples Wilcoxon Signed Rank Test.

3.3. Ganglionic Bowel Wall

In ganglionic bowel wall specimens, the thickness of the muscularis interna also correlated positively between histopathology results and UHFUS (R = 0.534, p = 0.023) (Figure 4b and Appendix A). The correlation housed a systematic difference, being, on average, 0.136 mm thicker in histopathology images compared to images achieved using UHFUS (p = 0.003) (Table 1). In ganglionosis, the muscularis externa differed systematically, being thinner in histopathological specimens than on UHFUS images (p = 0.006) (Table 1). The ratio of the thickness of the muscularis interna/muscularis externa in ganglionosis was systematically greater in histopathological specimens than on UHFUS (p < 0.001) (Table 1).

3.4. Agreements

In line with the result of systematic differences, agreements between histoanatomical thicknesses of muscularis interna and externa in histopathological and UHFUS images were low (Figure 5).

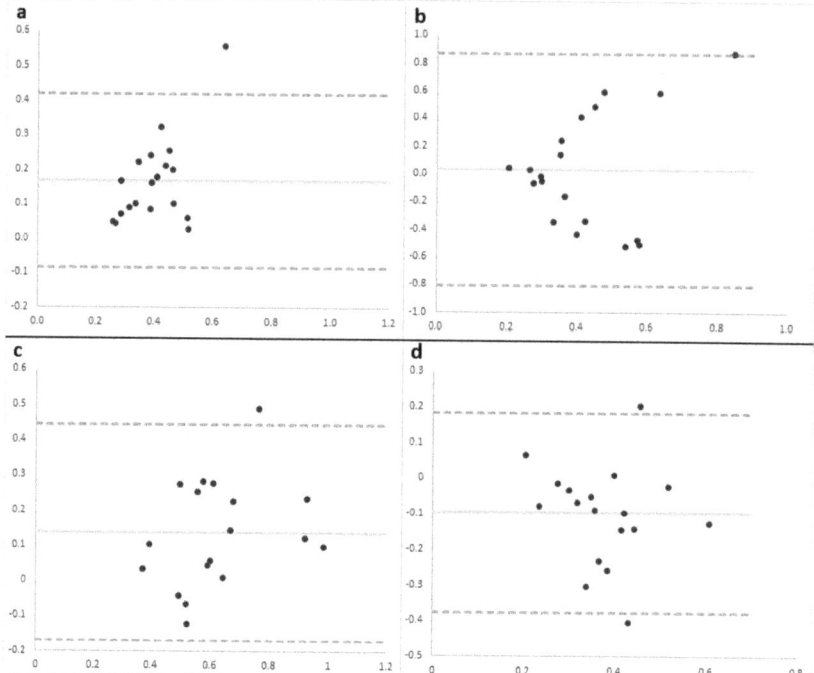

Figure 5. Agreement scatterplots (Bland–Altman) showing low agreement (uneven distribution) of thicknesses (mm) of histoanatomical layers as measured in histopathological and UHFUS images. The X-axis shows the mean thickness of the histoanatomical layer of histopathology and UHFUS in the same patient. The Y-axis shows the mean difference of thickness between the histoanatomical and UHFUS layer thickness in the same patient. The yellow horizontal lines represent degrees of agreement. The blue dashed horizontal lines represent ± 2 SD of histoanatomical thickness difference. Aganglionosis: Agreement of thicknesses of (**a**) muscularis interna and (**b**) muscularis externa, $n = 19$. Ganglionosis: Agreement of thicknesses of (**c**) muscularis interna and (**d**) muscularis externa. $n = 18$.

4. Discussion

According to the study results, UHFUS visualized histoanatomical muscular layers of bowel walls in children with Hirschsprung's disease accurately. The histoanatomical muscular layer thicknesses, and especially those of the muscularis interna, correlated well between UHFUS imaging and histopathology. As expected, as a result of speculated histopathological preparation effects, systematic differences and low agreement were evident between the UHFUS images and histopathology results. The study's confirmation of a reliable reproduction by UHFUS of the thicknesses of the bowel wall's histoanatomical muscular layers supports our previous report on the potential of UHFUS in imaging the bowel wall [9].

Studies aiming to correlate the histoanatomy of the bowel wall to findings on ultrasound have been carried out previously, but only by exploring the use of lower frequency ultrasound and never UHFUS. In these previous reports, the use of ultrasound of 8.5 and 25 MHz on human bowel did not visualize histological layer thicknesses convincingly [21,22]. The lack of correlation was attributed to the small histoanatomical sizes and the physical principles of ultrasound, i.e., how the soundwaves interacted differently with various tissues. These studies were limited by the use of low- and normo-resolution ultrasound, leading to less detailed images compared to those that can be visualized by UHFUS on small tissues over short distances [11]. Advantages of ultra-high resolution imaging over short distances, such as when visualizing bowel wall, and our here-reported UHFUS results, are supported by one animal study suggesting strong and positive correlations between histological and ultrasound morphometrics of both the muscularis interna and muscularis externa in bowel wall [23].

One factor to be taken into consideration is that ultrasound accuracy might depend upon the examiner's handling and positioning of the transducer. This is also of concern in the validation of UHFUS. In the animal study referred to above [23], the transducer was positioned in water at 1 cm from the sample, in order to avoid any modifying pressure on the tissue. This meticulous methodology was not repeated in our study because we aimed for a clinically feasible setting, implying an almost direct contact between the transducer and bowel. Therefore, we cannot exclude the possibility that pressing the transducer on the bowel wall might have influenced the muscular thicknesses in the UHFUS images. This could have affected the muscularis externa in particular, which is the layer closest to the transducer and could, therefore, be most influenced by external pressure. However, the external pressure imposed by the transducer will also be the case in the clinic, requiring consideration in our forthcoming further methodological validation and refining work. The individual learning curve can influence the accuracy and reliability of the detailed UHFUS, and this needs to be taken into consideration and addressed before diagnostics can be implemented in clinical work.

Another factor to be considered, both in the validation process and in the clinic, is the user-dependent quality of imaging and subjective interpretation of images. In the present study, two surgeons performed the UHFUS assessments, and interpretations were confirmed using MATLAB programming. Nevertheless, before clinical implementation of the UHFUS technique can occur, interpersonal variability testing of the UHFUS on the bowel will be required as part of the validation process.

As expected, significant systematic differences were observed. These were hypothesized to be a result of the expected effects of histopathological preparation. Our finding that the muscularis interna was systematically thicker on histopathological imaging than on UHFUS was in line with the results of a preclinical animal model study suggesting a swelling of muscular tissue post-formalin fixation [24]. Notably, there are also studies suggesting a shrinkage of the bowel due to formalin fixation [13–15]. However, in contrast to our study, those bowel specimens were analyzed regarding total specimen length, while analyses in our study were cross-sectional, focusing on separate muscularis layers. Speculating, one explanation for the shrinking versus swelling of the tissue could be the direction of the assessment. This is because a whole bowel specimen comprises a mix of several histoanatomical layers, and their various fiber directions might lead to a total shrinking effect in length. Still, within the whole specimen, separate histoanatomical layers might swell, which could possibly be identified when the specimen is studied cross-sectionally.

A strength of our study was the fairly homogenous cohort, including only children with recto-sigmoid aganglionosis who were of similar ages and weights. The majority of specimens and UHFUS images were generally of high quality, containing well-preserved histoanatomical bowel wall layers. Although limited, a need for the exclusion of samples as a result of low image quality was evident in three of 40 cases. Image quality requires full consideration in the clinic because safe diagnostics must be secured for all patients. Greater experience, methodological refinements, and technical improvements are expected to contribute to an improved image quality. Specific strategies for improving image quality could be to repeat imaging in every patient, in order to secure the highest quality of results.

Another strength of the study was that both aganglionic and ganglionic areas were pinpointed specifically on both fresh and fixated bowel samples and, therefore, allowed correlation of exactly the same areas. This also enabled the patient to serve as their own control in paired statistical tests, minimizing effects by confounding factors, such as increased bowel wall thickness with age [12,25]. Furthermore, the two MATLAB programs, developed specifically for analyses of UHFUS and histopathological imaging, enabled precise delineations of the histoanatomical muscle layers and the programs supported the generation of outcomes objectively. These MATLAB programs enable the unique, novel, and exact technique to assess the histoanatomy of the bowel wall, which will be useful in future studies.

One obvious limitation of the study was the sparse number of specimens which diminished the probability of revealing the absence of differences. In addition to pressure effects, there were only a few patients who might have contributed inconsistent findings of aganglionic muscularis externa. Additionally, as a result of the great diversity in thicknesses of the muscularis externa, particularly in aganglionosis, the statistical power was low. Moreover, the UHFUS examinations were not standardized with regard to the transducer angle or gel amount, which might have impacted the measured layer thicknesses of the bowel wall. Additionally, histopathological images were cross-sectioned while UHFUS images were sectioned longitudinally. Since thicknesses might appear differently if cross- or longitudinally sectioned, the direction of the transducer might have influenced the outcome. For statistical limitations, assessments using MATLAB programming of both histopathology and UHFUS were performed by only one person, which might have skewed data. Similarly, the Bland–Altman agreement analyses were, by their nature, linked to a subjective interpretation; however, this potential bias was minimized by having a statistician assist in the interpretation of the results. For an intervariability control, analyses between UHFUS users will be analyzed separately (cohen kappa) in a next step. Then, for transparency, objectivity, and to collect more data, a multicenter study for validation of the use of UHFUS in the diagnostics of bowel wall pathology is warranted. This is now planned, in the form of a long-term outcome report.

This study is part of a larger project aiming to develop and validate the use of UHFUS in Hirschsprung's disease, as a novel and immediate method to delineate between aganglionic and ganglionic bowel. Adding knowledge about the validity of UHFUS in the histoanatomical preciseness of the bowel wall, this study serves as an important and essential start for more studies on UHFUS in the diagnostics of Hirschsprung's disease.

5. Conclusions

This study reveals that UHFUS imaging replicates the histoanatomy of the bowel wall adequately. The thicknesses of the histoanatomical muscular layers, and especially the muscularis interna, correlated well between histopathological and UHFUS images, and the expected systematic differences as a result of histopathological preparations were confirmed. This study serves as a profound base for the use of UHFUS as a novel method in the diagnostics of Hirschsprung's disease.

Author Contributions: Conceptualization: C.G. and P.S.; Methodology: T.H., T.E., R.M.M., T.J., M.C. and P.S.; Software: T.E., T.H. and E.G.; Validation: T.H., M.E. and P.S.; Formal analysis: T.H. and P.S.; Investigation: C.G., K.H., E.G., M.C. and P.S.; Resources: P.S. and C.G.; Data Curation: T.H., K.H. and R.M.M.; Writing—Original Draft Preparation: T.H. and P.S., Writing—Review and editing: C.G., T.E., K.H., M.E., R.M.M., E.G. and P.S.; Visualization: T.H., P.S., K.H., R.M.M. and M.C.; Project administration, P.S., Supervision, P.S. All authors have read and agreed to the published version of the manuscript.

Funding: Open access funding was provided by Lund University, Sweden. Swedish Regional Research funding (ALF 2022-0215) Region Skåne, Skåne University Hospital's Funding (SUS Fonder och Stiftelser), Swedish Research Council Starting grants 2021–01569.

Institutional Review Board Statement: The study was conducted in accordance with the Declaration of Helsinki, and ethical approval was obtained from the local ethics review board: Lund University (DNR 2017/769).

Informed Consent Statement: Oral and written information was given, and the guardians' written consents were obtained.

Data Availability Statement: The data presented in this study are available on reasonable request from the corresponding author.

Acknowledgments: Ros Kenn, Medical Editor/Writer who performed the language editing; http://roskenn.co.uk (accessed on 3 April 2023).

Conflicts of Interest: The authors declare no conflict of interest.

Appendix A

Table A1. Correlation of histoanatomical dimensions in bowel wall in histologically prepared bowel specimen and ex vivo ultra-high frequency ultrasound (UHFUS) examined bowel, in aganglionic and ganglionic bowel wall, respectively. Median was calculated as the 50th percentile of all individual mean measurements of histoanatomical thicknesses assessed in an in-house programmed MATLAB program. A p-value of <0.05 was considered to be statistically significant.

Histoanatomical Layer	Thickness in Aganglionosis				Thickness in Ganglionosis			
	Histopathological Bowel Wall Specimen (mm) Median (Range)	UHFUS Image (mm) Median (Range)	R [1]	Correlation p-Value	Histopathological Bowel Wall Specimen (mm) Median (Range)	UHFUS Image (mm) Median (Range)	R [1]	Correlation p-Value
Muscularis interna (mm)	0.499 (0.284–0.918)	0.309 (0.202–0.500)	0.651	0.003	0.664 (0.386–1.042)	0.556 (0.338–0.931)	0.534	0.023
Muscularis externa (mm)	0.291 (0.165–1.285)	0.322 (0.175–0.830)	−0.309	0.198	0.297 (0.186–0.556)	0.433 (0.169–0.668)	0.240	0.338

[1] R = Spearman rank correlation coefficient.

References

1. Langer, J.C. Hirschsprung disease. *Curr. Opin. Pediatr.* **2013**, *25*, 368–374. [CrossRef]
2. Butler Tjaden, N.E.; Trainor, P.A. The developmental etiology and pathogenesis of Hirschsprung disease. *Transl. Res.* **2013**, *162*, 1–15. [CrossRef] [PubMed]
3. Gosain, A.; Brinkman, A.S. Hirschsprung's associated enterocolitis. *Curr. Opin. Pediatr.* **2015**, *27*, 364–369. [CrossRef] [PubMed]
4. Kyrklund, K.; Sloots, C.E.J.; De Blaauw, I.; Bjørnland, K.; Rolle, U.; Cavalieri, D.; Francalanci, P.; Fusaro, F.; Lemli, A.; Schwarzer, N.; et al. Ernica guidelines for the management of rectosigmoid Hirschsprung's disease. *Orphanet J. Rare Dis.* **2020**, *15*, 164. [CrossRef]
5. Langer, J.C. Surgical approach to Hirschsprung disease. *Semin. Pediatr. Surg.* **2022**, *31*, 151156. [CrossRef] [PubMed]
6. Ramachandran, V.; Nguyen, J.; Caruso, C.; Rao, D. Hirschsprung's disease: Two cases of total intestinal aganglionosis. *Am. J. Clin. Pathol.* **2020**, *154*, S73. [CrossRef]
7. Ghose, S.; Squire, B.; Stringer, M.; Batcup, G.; Crabbe, D. Hirschsprung's disease: Problems with transition-zone pull-through. *J. Pediatr. Surg.* **2000**, *35*, 1805–1809. [CrossRef]
8. Lawal, T.A.; Chatoorgoon, K.; Collins, M.H.; Coe, A.; Peña, A.; Levitt, M.A. Redo pull-through in Hirschsprung's [corrected] disease for obstructive symptoms due to residual aganglionosis and transition zone bowel. *J. Pediatr. Surg.* **2011**, *46*, 342–347. [CrossRef]
9. Granéli, C.; Erlöv, T.; Mitev, R.M.; Kasselaki, I.; Hagelsteen, K.; Gisselsson, D.; Jansson, T.; Cinthio, M.; Stenström, P. Ultra-high frequency ultrasonography to distinguish ganglionic from aganglionic bowel wall in Hirschsprung disease: A first report. *J. Pediatr. Surg.* **2021**, *56*, 2281–2285. [CrossRef]
10. Boczar, D.; Forte, A.J.; Serrano, L.P.; Trigg, S.D.; Clendenen, S.R. Use of ultra-high-frequency ultrasound on diagnosis and management of lipofibromatous hamartoma: A technical report. *Cureus* **2019**, *11*, e5808. [CrossRef]
11. Izzetti, R.; Vitali, S.; Aringhieri, G.; Nisi, M.; Oranges, T.; Dini, V.; Ferro, F.; Baldini, C.; Romanelli, M.; Caramella, D.; et al. Ultra-high frequency ultrasound, a promising diagnostic technique: Review of the literature and single-center experience. *Can. Assoc. Radiol. J.* **2021**, *72*, 418–431. [CrossRef]
12. Graneli, C.; Patarroyo, S.; Mitev, R.M.; Gisselsson, D.; Gottberg, E.; Erlöv, T.; Jansson, T.; Hagelsteen, K.; Cinthio, M.; Stenström, P. Histopathological dimensions differ between aganglionic and ganglionic bowel wall in children with Hirschsprung's disease. *BMC Pediatr.* **2022**, *22*, 723. [CrossRef]
13. Eid, I.; El-Muhtaseb, M.S.; Mukherjee, R.; Renwick, R.; Gardiner, D.S.; Macdonald, A. Histological processing variability in the determination of lateral resection margins in rectal cancer. *J. Clin. Pathol.* **2007**, *60*, 593–595. [CrossRef]
14. Goldstein, N.S.; Soman, A.; Sacksner, J. Disparate surgical margin lengths of colorectal resection specimens between in vivo and in vitro measurements. The effects of surgical resection and formalin fixation on organ shrinkage. *Am. J. Clin. Pathol.* **1999**, *111*, 349–351. [CrossRef]
15. Lam, D.; Kaneko, Y.; Scarlett, A.; D'Souza, B.; Norris, R.; Woods, R. The effect of formalin fixation on resection margins in colorectal cancer. *Int. J. Surg. Pathol.* **2019**, *27*, 700–705. [CrossRef]

16. Chan, J.K. The wonderful colors of the hematoxylin-eosin stain in diagnostic surgical pathology. *Int. J. Surg. Pathol.* **2014**, *22*, 12–32. [CrossRef]
17. Bachmann, L.; Besendörfer, M.; Carbon, R.; Lux, P.; Agaimy, A.; Hartmann, A.; Rau, T.T. Immunohistochemical panel for the diagnosis of Hirschsprung's disease using antibodies to MAP2, calretinin, GLUT1 and S100. *Histopathology* **2015**, *66*, 824–835. [CrossRef]
18. Galazka, P.; Szylberg, L.; Bodnar, M.; Styczynski, J.; Marszalek, A. Diagnostic algorithm in Hirschsprung's disease: Focus on immunohistochemistry markers. *In Vivo* **2020**, *34*, 1355–1359. [CrossRef]
19. Bland, J.M.; Altman, D.G. Statistical methods for assessing agreement between two methods of clinical measurement. *Lancet* **1986**, *1*, 307–310. [CrossRef]
20. Joekel, J.; Eggemann, H.; Costa, S.D.; Ignatov, A. Should the hyperechogenic halo around malignant breast lesions be included in the measurement of tumor size? *Breast Cancer Res. Treat.* **2016**, *156*, 311–317. [CrossRef]
21. Kimmey, M.; Martin, R.; Haggitt, R.; Wang, K.; Franklin, D.; Silverstein, F. Histologic correlates of gastrointestinal ultrasound images. *Gastroenterology* **1989**, *96*, 433–441. [CrossRef] [PubMed]
22. Wiersema, M.J.; Wiersema, L.M. High-resolution 25-megahertz ultrasonography of the gastrointestinal wall: Histologic correlates. *Gastrointest. Endosc.* **1993**, *39*, 499–504. [CrossRef]
23. Le Roux, A.B.; Granger, L.A.; Wakamatsu, N.; Kearney, M.T.; Gaschen, L. Ex vivo correlation of ultrasonographic small intestinal wall layering with histology in dogs. *Vet. Radiol. Ultrasound* **2016**, *57*, 534–545. [CrossRef] [PubMed]
24. Docquier, P.-L.; Paul, L.; Cartiaux, O.; Lecouvet, F.; Dufrane, D.; Delloye, C.; Galant, C. Formalin fixation could interfere with the clinical assessment of the tumor-free margin in tumor surgery: Magnetic resonance imaging-based study. *Oncology* **2010**, *78*, 115–124. [CrossRef] [PubMed]
25. Haber, H.P.; Stern, M. Intestinal ultrasonography in children and young adults: Bowel wall thickness is age dependent. *J. Ultrasound Med.* **2000**, *19*, 315–321. [CrossRef]

Disclaimer/Publisher's Note: The statements, opinions and data contained in all publications are solely those of the individual author(s) and contributor(s) and not of MDPI and/or the editor(s). MDPI and/or the editor(s) disclaim responsibility for any injury to people or property resulting from any ideas, methods, instructions or products referred to in the content.

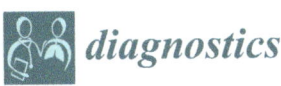

Review

Quantitative Ultrasound Techniques Used for Peripheral Nerve Assessment

Saeed Jerban [1,2,3,*], Victor Barrère [2,3], Michael Andre [1,2], Eric Y. Chang [1,2] and Sameer B. Shah [2,3,4,*]

1. Department of Radiology, University of California, San Diego, CA 92093, USA
2. Research Service, Veterans Affairs San Diego Healthcare System, San Diego, CA 92161, USA
3. Department of Orthopaedic Surgery, University of California, San Diego, CA 92093, USA
4. Department of Bioengineering, University of California, San Diego, CA 92093, USA
* Correspondence: sjerban@health.ucsd.edu (S.J.); sbshah@health.ucsd.edu (S.B.S.); Tel.: +1-858-246-2229 (S.J.); +1-858-822-0720 (S.B.S.); Fax: +1-888-960-5922 (S.J.); +1-858-822-3807 (S.B.S.)

Abstract: Aim: This review article describes quantitative ultrasound (QUS) techniques and summarizes their strengths and limitations when applied to peripheral nerves. Methods: A systematic review was conducted on publications after 1990 in Google Scholar, Scopus, and PubMed databases. The search terms "peripheral nerve", "quantitative ultrasound", and "elastography ultrasound" were used to identify studies related to this investigation. Results: Based on this literature review, QUS investigations performed on peripheral nerves can be categorized into three main groups: (1) B-mode echogenicity measurements, which are affected by a variety of post-processing algorithms applied during image formation and in subsequent B-mode images; (2) ultrasound (US) elastography, which examines tissue stiffness or elasticity through modalities such as strain ultrasonography or shear wave elastography (SWE). With strain ultrasonography, induced tissue strain, caused by internal or external compression stimuli that distort the tissue, is measured by tracking detectable speckles in the B-mode images. In SWE, the propagation speed of shear waves, generated by externally applied mechanical vibrations or internal US "push pulse" stimuli, is measured to estimate tissue elasticity; (3) the characterization of raw backscattered ultrasound radiofrequency (RF) signals, which provide fundamental ultrasonic tissue parameters, such as the acoustic attenuation and backscattered coefficients, that reflect tissue composition and microstructural properties. Conclusions: QUS techniques allow the objective evaluation of peripheral nerves and reduce operator- or system-associated biases that can influence qualitative B-mode imaging. The application of QUS techniques to peripheral nerves, including their strengths and limitations, were described and discussed in this review to enhance clinical translation.

Keywords: peripheral nerve; quantitative ultrasound; B-mode; elastography; shear wave; ultrasound echogenicity

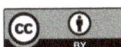

Citation: Jerban, S.; Barrère, V.; Andre, M.; Chang, E.Y.; Shah, S.B. Quantitative Ultrasound Techniques Used for Peripheral Nerve Assessment. *Diagnostics* 2023, *13*, 956. https://doi.org/10.3390/diagnostics13050956

Academic Editors: Rossana Izzetti and Marco Nisi

Received: 20 January 2023
Revised: 14 February 2023
Accepted: 17 February 2023
Published: 2 March 2023

Copyright: © 2023 by the authors. Licensee MDPI, Basel, Switzerland. This article is an open access article distributed under the terms and conditions of the Creative Commons Attribution (CC BY) license (https://creativecommons.org/licenses/by/4.0/).

1. Introduction

Ultrasound (US) is an increasingly popular modality for imaging peripheral nerves in the clinic, providing important information about nerve microstructure [1,2]. Many peripheral nerves are located superficially and, hence, are easily accessible for US examination. Although neurophysiological assessments are often considered the gold standard for peripheral nerve assessment [3], US-based techniques can be used as a complementary tool, providing anatomical information and localizing lesions more specifically [4], and providing additional data to guide clinical interventions [4–7]. Using US for peripheral nerve evaluation is advantageous compared to other imaging modalities, particularly in pediatric [4,8] and geriatric [9,10] populations, due to its rapid scanning capability and wide in-clinic availability.

The dominant US imaging technique in medical studies is reflection or pulse-echo technology (echo-ultrasonography), which analyzes the signals returned to the transducer from the macro- and microstructures within and between studied tissues [11,12]. This technique is based on the principle of sonar (i.e., sound navigation and ranging), where the pulse transmitter and pulse receiver are located on the same side of the studied tissues. Sound waves are typically produced by piezoelectric transducers within the US probe that are stimulated by electrical pulses to vibrate or ring at a desired frequency (e.g., 2 to 18 MHz in common clinical probes). The generated sound waves can be focused at a desired depth by using the phased-array technique, which rings individual or subgroups of elements of the transducer array with a specific delayed calculated sequence [11,12].

Four main operational states (modes) of US have been used in medical imaging, including A-, B-, M-, and Doppler mode [11,12]. A-mode, or amplitude modulation mode, is the simplest type of US. A single transducer transmits a sound pressure wave along a line through the skin into the tissue of interest and receives echoes back from interfaces that are encountered. The echoes are plotted on screen as spikes of different amplitude depending on the echo intensity along the line of propagation. The location along the line corresponds to the depth from the probe and is determined by the round-trip time for the echo assuming a value for the speed of sound, commonly 1540 m/s [11,12]. B-mode, or brightness modulation, is the most common form of US imaging; in this mode, a transducer array simultaneously scans a plane through the tissue and displays a two-dimensional (2D) image reconstructed from A-mode data from each transducer [11–13]. Echo-ultrasonography's concept and A-mode data as well as B-mode image generation are presented in Figure 1 in schematics. The brightness of pixels in B-mode images depends on the amplitude of the echoes arising from the depth captured in the corresponding A-mode data. Tissue contrast in B-mode images is obtained based on the differences in the soft tissues' acoustic properties, including density, sound speed, scattering, and absorption encountered by the propagating sound waves [12]. M-mode, or motion modulation, displays a one-dimensional A-mode line that is displaced horizontally with time. This mode is typically used for measuring the rate and the range of motion in moving body parts, such as imaging the dynamic cardiac chamber walls and valves [14]. The time-displacement graph is generated by continuously measuring the distance of the object in a selected region of interest from its nearest transducer, using the A-mode data of that transducer. Finally, the Doppler mode utilizes the Doppler effect to assess the velocity (direction and speed) of moving structures in the body, most typically blood [14,15]. Using a known transmitted US frequency, echoes received from blood moving toward the transducer are shifted to a higher frequency, while echoes received from blood moving away from the transducer are shifted to a lower frequency. By calculating the frequency shift of a particular sample volume, for example, a jet of blood flow within arteries, its speed and direction can be determined, mapped onto the B-mode image, and thus visualized. This is particularly useful in cardiovascular studies and can be helpful in identifying peripheral nerves and blood vessels. Doppler speed information is quantitative and is often displayed graphically using an overlaid color scheme (directional Doppler) on a co-registered B-mode image.

US devices and transducers are often categorized based on their nominal operating frequencies into the following three ranges: 1–15 MHz is typical for current clinical scanners; 15–30 MHz is typically designated as high-frequency ultrasound (HFUS); and 30–100 MHz is typically designated as ultra-high-frequency ultrasound (UHFUS) [16–18]. HFUS and UHFUS developments have resulted in improved image resolution and quality when evaluating superficial tissues in the human body [13,19,20] such as peripheral nerves [21,22], eye [19,23], and skin [13,17,18,20]. Commonly utilized clinical HFUS transducers for nerve imaging operate with peak frequencies of >20 MHz, which produce very high-resolution US images at shallow depths < 5 cm. In current clinical practice, peripheral nerves are evaluated qualitatively using grey-scale B-mode images, which provide information about nerve structure, and using color Doppler images to show vascularity [1,5–7].

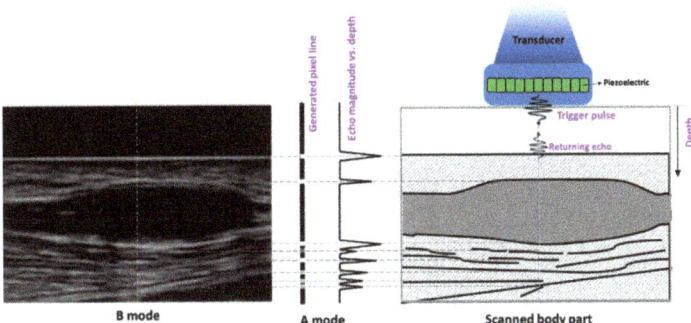

Figure 1. Schematic description of echo-ultrasonography technique as well as A- and B-mode data generation concepts. The returning pulse from the scatterers (schematically shown on the **right**) encountered by the trigger pulse, generated by an exemplary piezoelectric transducer within the US probe, is used to generate A-mode data as well as a pixel line (shown in the **middle**) of the final B-mode image (shown on the **left**).

US is a promising modality for assessing the peripheral nerve status, but it is limited by its qualitative basis as well as system- and operator-dependency [12]. Thus, the qualitative interpretation of US images is often variable or inconclusive. For example, neuropathy often leads to altered nerve echogenicity and even the disappearance of fascicular architecture in B-mode images. Increased vascularity, abnormal anatomical structures, and reduced nerve mobility, indicative of tethering, can also be considered in a neuropathy diagnosis with US [5–7]. However, such qualitative nerve characterizations may vary for different operators and imaging setups. Morphometric assessments of B-mode images may provide more objective metrics for evaluating nerve structure. For example, the increased cross-sectional area (CSA) of median nerves has often been correlated with the diagnosis of carpal tunnel syndrome (CTS) [5,24]. To account for differences in patient anthropometric characteristics, dimensionless CSA ratios of nerves (e.g., carpal tunnel inlet-to-outlet) have also been used to assess neuropathy [25]. Nevertheless, even these indices may be confounded by operator-induced and platform-specific sources of variability. Moreover, such morphometric measures lack information about the nerves' microstructure. Figure 2 shows B-mode images on the transverse plane (short axis plane) of the median nerve in an exemplary healthy participant compared with a CTS patient. Remarkably, the fascicles detected in the healthy median nerve cannot be seen in the CTS patient [5].

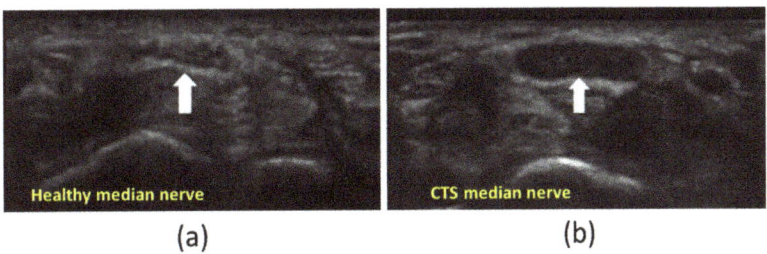

Figure 2. US B-mode images in the transverse plane (short axis plane) of the median nerve (white arrow) in (**a**) a healthy participant and (**b**) a patient with carpal tunnel syndrome (CTS). The fascicles detected in the healthy median nerve cannot be seen in the CTS patient. This figure was previously presented by Vlassakov and Sala-Blanch [5]. Reprinting permission is granted through Rightslink system. Minor modifications were performed for presentation purposes.

Quantitative ultrasound (QUS) techniques offer the potential for a more objective evaluation of peripheral nerves, promising the improved diagnosis of neuropathy and nerve injury. QUS approaches have the potential to more reliably reflect differences in the multi-scale composite structure of the nerves (e.g., fascicles, organized bundles of nerve fibers within a fascicle, and axons), which cannot be directly observed by qualitative methods. QUS investigations performed on peripheral nerves can be categorized into three main groups: (1) B-mode echogenicity-based outcomes, (2) elastography, and (3) backscattered RF signal characterization. B-mode echogenicity measures employ post-processing algorithms in B-mode images to determine the visualized microstructure of the tissue. The underlying physical principle of elastography is that tissue stiffness and other tissue mechanical properties can be quantitatively estimated by analyzing the response of the tissue to an applied force. Strain ultrasonography and shear wave elastography (SWE) are the two major classes of US elastography techniques [26]. In strain ultrasonography, tissue strain, as a response to internal or external compression stimuli, is measured by tracking the motion of speckles detectable in B-mode images [26,27]. In SWE, the speed of shear waves generated by external vibrations or tissue compression is measured and correlated to tissue elasticity or stiffness [26,27]. Finally, backscattered RF signal characterization permits the measurement and modeling of fundamental tissue acoustic parameters that relate to composition and microstructure [12,28]. The signals needed to measure these fundamental tissue parameters are often discarded during machine-dependent B-mode image formation.

In this review, we describe the three main categories of QUS techniques and summarize QUS-based investigations performed on peripheral nerves. The focus of this review will be the employed techniques rather than the results of each application case. In addition to summarizing the strengths and the use cases for each approach, this review also describes the potential limitations associated with each QUS technique.

2. Materials and Methods

This review conducted between 2020 and 2022 aimed to provide a thorough description of the current QUS techniques including the advantages and limitations. The literature search was performed in PubMed, Scopus, and Google Scholar databases using the following keywords: "peripheral nerve" and "quantitative ultrasound" or "elastography ultrasound" published after the year 1990. The results were first screened automatically and then through title and abstract reading for excluding duplicated records, non-English written reports, non-ultrasound or non-quantitative studies, and review articles. Study selection was performed following the PRISMA 2020 guidelines as summarized in Figure 3. All reviewed QUS-based investigations performed on peripheral nerves are summarized in Table 1.

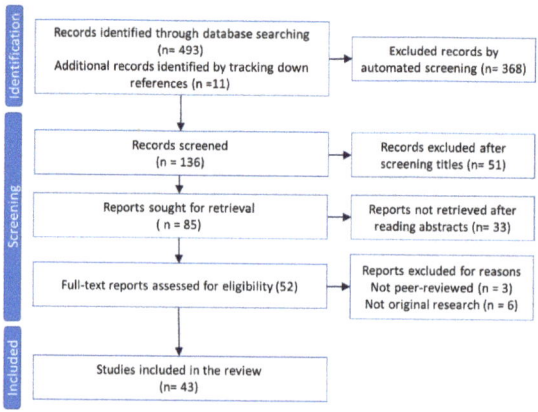

Figure 3. Study selection flowchart based on PRISMA 2020 guidelines.

Table 1. QUS-based investigations performed on peripheral nerves.

Type of QUS	Study	Goal	Anatomy	Scanner	Probe Frequency	Findings
B-mode echogenicity measurement	Tagliafico et al., 2010 [29]	To investigate the feasibility of using US-based measure of the peripheral nerve density (hypoechoic fraction) in detecting CTS and neurofibromas.	• Median nerve 35 CTS and 30 neurofibroma patients vs. 65 controls • Transverse plane	iU-22, Philips (Eindhoven, The Netherlands)	• Linear array transducer 5 to 17 MHz frequency range	• Nerve density in the median nerve was significantly higher in CTS patients and significantly lower in neurofibroma patients compared with the healthy normal subjects.
	Boom and Visser, 2012 [30]	To investigate the feasibility of using hypoechoic fraction obtained with various thresholding methods in detecting neuropathy.	• Ulnar nerve 56 patients with neuropathy vs. 37 controls • Transverse plane	Xario XG, Toshiba (Tokyo, Japan)	• Linear array transducer (PLT-1204BT) 7 to 18 MHz frequency range	• Significantly lower average hypoechoic fraction was found in the patient group compared with the controls using several different thresholding methods.
	Bignotti et al., 2015 [22]	To investigate the feasibility of using US nerve density index in evaluating patients with limited cutaneous systemic sclerosis (lcSSc).	• Median nerve 40 lcSSc patients vs. 40 controls • Transverse plane	iU-22, Philips (Eindhoven, The Netherlands)	• Linear array transducer 5 to 17 MHz frequency range	• US nerve density index was found significantly lower in lcSSc patients than in healthy controls. • Symptomatic patients demonstrated lower nerve density compared to non-symptomatic patients.
	Simon et al., 2015 [31]	To study the relationship between US B-mode hypoechoic fraction and electrophysiologic measures of the peripheral nerve.	• Ulnar nerve in vivo 16 neuropathy patients vs. 52 controls • Transverse plane	A Mindray M7 (Shenzen, China)	• Linear array transducer (L14-6) 6 to 14 MHz frequency range	• Nerve hypoechoic fraction and CSA were significantly increased in patients. • Hypoechoic fraction was similar in the asymptomatic and symptomatic limbs of patients. • Motor nerve conduction velocity correlated with the maximum hypoechoic fraction and CSA.
	Byra et al., 2020 [21]	To investigate correlations between collagen/myelin content (histology) of nerves with a US-based texture feature, gray level co-occurrence matrix (GLCM).	• Ulnar nerve 6 control cadavers, 85 fascicles • Transverse plane	Vevo MD, FUJIFILM (Toronto, Canada)	• Linear array transducer (UHF48) Center frequency at 30 MHz	• GLCM showed a significant correlation with the combined collagen and myelin content of fascicles.
	Byra et al., 2020 [24]	To investigate the feasibility of using the nerve–tissue contrast index (NTI) method in detecting CTS, by considering echogenicity differences in the surrounding tissue.	• Median nerve in vivo 10 CTS patients vs. 21 controls • Transverse plane	Vevo MD, FUJIFILM (Toronto, Canada)	• Linear array transducer (UHF48) Center frequency at 30 MHz	• NTI and CSA were significantly higher in patients.

Table 1. *Cont.*

Type of QUS	Study	Goal	Anatomy	Scanner	Probe Frequency	Findings
Strain ultrasonography	Palmeri et al., 2009 [32]	To investigate nerves' contrast improvement of strain US vs. B-mode US.	• Distal sciatic, brachial plexus, femoral nerves • 2 healthy subjects • Longitudinal and transverse planes	SONOLINE Antares, Siemens (Erlangen Germany)	• Linear array transducer (VF 7-3 and VF I0-5 • 3 to 7 and 5 to 10 frequency ranges	• The strain sonography with ARFI significantly increased the contrast with muscle helping localize nerves for anesthetic injection.
	Orman et al., 2013 [33]	To investigate the potential of strain US (pure strain) free-hand compression in detecting CTS.	• Median nerve • 41 CTS patients vs. 24 controls • Transverse plane	Aplio XG, SSA 790A, Toshiba(Nasushiobara, Japan)	• Linear array transducer 12 to 17 MHz frequency ranges	• Strain was significantly lower in the patients with CTS. • Nerve perimeter and CSA of patients with CTS were significantly higher.
	Miyamoto et al., 2014 [34]	To investigate the capability of free-hand compression strain US technique (strain ratio (SR) with respect to acoustic coupler rubber, ACR) in detecting CTS.	• Median nerve • 31 CTS patients vs. 22 controls • Longitudinal and transverse planes	HI VISION Preirus Hitachi-Aloka Medical (Tokyo, Japan)	• Linear array transducer • 5 to 18 MHz frequency range • AC (Hitachi-Aloka Medical)	• Both the strain ratio (AC/nerve) and the CSA in the patients with CTS were significantly higher (stiffer nerves). • The presence of CTS was predicted by means of AC/nerve SR and CSA cutoff values of 4.3% and 11 mm^2, respectively.
	Yoshii et al., 2015 [35]	To investigate the capability of strain US technique with a cyclic compression apparatus (strain and SR with respect to ACR) in detecting CTS.	• Median nerve • 8 CTS patients vs. 30 controls • Transverse plane	HI VISION Avius, Hitachi Aloka Medical (Tokyo, Japan)	• Linear array transducer • 5 to 18 MHz frequency range • AC (Hitachi-Aloka Medical)	• Nerve strains of the patients were significantly lower. • Strain ratios, CSA, and perimeters were significantly higher in the patients.
	Ghajarzadeh et al., 2015 [36]	To investigate the capability of free-hand compression strain US technique (blue and red pixel counts in strain image) in detecting CTS severity.	• Median nerve • 31 CTS patients vs. 22 controls • Transverse plane	MYLAB 70 XVG, Esaote (Genoa, Italy)	• Linear array transducer • 5 to 13 MHz frequency range	• Blue indexes in strain images and nerve CSA were significantly different between controls and CTS patients with different levels of disease severity.
	Tatar et al., 2016 [37]	To investigate the capability of free-hand compression strain ultrasonography (SR and strain difference between two nerve sections) in detecting CTS and its severity.	• Median nerve • 15 mild CTS, 20 moderate CTS patients vs. 18 controls • Transverse plane	MYLAB 60, Esaote (Genoa, Italy)	• Linear array transducer • 4 to 13 MHz frequency range	• CTS groups showed significantly stiffer nerves compared with control group. • Despite SR-related indexes, CSA-based measures were significantly different between mild and moderate CTS.

Table 1. Cont.

Type of QUS	Study	Goal	Anatomy	Scanner	Probe Frequency	Findings
Strain ultrasonography—Continued	Ishibashi et al., 2016 [38]	To investigate the capability of free-hand compression strain US (SR ratio nerve/ACR) in detecting neuropathy in type 2 diabetes patients.	• Tibial nerve • 198 type II diabetic patients vs. 29 controls • Transverse plane	HI VISION Ascendus, Hitachi Medical (Tokyo, Japan)	• Linear array transducer • Center frequency at 18 MHz • AC (Hitachi-Aloka Medical)	• SR in patients without neuropathy was lower compared with controls, further decreasing after developing neuropathy. • The tibial nerve CSA in diabetic patients was larger, and increased significantly relative to neuropathy severity. • Greater performance was shown for SR versus CSA in detecting nerve neuropathy.
	Kesikburun et al., 2016 [39]	To investigate the capability of free-hand strain US technique (using SR) in detecting CTS.	• Median nerve • 1 CTS patient (case study) • Longitudinal plane	GE LOGIQ S7, GE Healthcare (Yizhuang, China)	• Linear array transducer • 5 to 12 MHz frequency range	• Four-fold increase in nerve elasticity was reported in the symptomatic nerve compared with the healthy wrist.
	Yoshii et al., 2017 [40]	To investigate the capability of strain US technique with a cyclic compression apparatus (strain, AC/nerve SR, strain/applied pressure ratio) in detecting CTS	• Median nerve • 35 CTS patients vs. 15 controls. • Transverse plane	HI VISION Avius, Hitachi Aloka Medical (Tokyo, Japan)	• Linear array transducer • 5 to 18 MHz frequency range • AC (Hitachi-Aloka Medical)	• Nerve strain was significantly lower in patients. • Pressure and pressure/strain ratio were significantly higher in patients. • The ROC curve analyses showed that pressure/strain ratio slightly improved the CTS detection compared with using strain alone
	Nogueira-Barbosa et al., 2017 [41]	To investigate the feasibility of employing the free-hand strain US technique (using SR) in detecting leprosy.	• Median nerve • 18 leprosy patients vs. 26 controls • Transverse and longitudinal planes	SonixRP, Ultrasonix (Richmond, Canada)	• Linear array transducer (L14-5) • 5 to 14 MHz frequency range	• Significantly lower SR was observed for the leprosy patients compared with controls. • Leprosy patients with reactions showed lower SR compared with patients without reactions.
	Martin and Cartwright, 2017 [42]	To investigate the feasibility of employing the ambient strain US technique (SR was used) in detecting CTS.	• Median nerve • 17 CTS patients vs. 26 controls • Transverse and longitudinal planes	iU-22, Philips (Eindhoven, The Netherlands)	• Linear array transducer • 5 to 12 MHz frequency range	• Despite the previous literature, no significant differences were found in SR between CTS patients and controls.
	Tezcan et al., 2019 [43]	To investigate the feasibility of employing the strain US technique (SR) in evaluating low-level laser therapy on CTS patients.	• Median nerve • 34 CTS patients with therapy vs. 17 patients without therapy • Transverse plane	ACUSON S3000, Siemens (Erlangen, Germany)	• Linear array transducer • 4 to 9 MHz frequency range	• Mean SR, CSA, and clinical severity scores (SSS, and FSS) decreased significantly after laser therapy.

Table 1. Cont.

Type of QUS	Study	Goal	Anatomy	Scanner	Probe Frequency	Findings
Shear wave elastography (SWE)	Kantarci et al., 2014 [44]	To investigate the potential of SWE (stiffness) with ARFI push pulses in detecting CTS.	• Median nerve • 37 CTS patients vs. 18 controls • Longitudinal plane	Aixplorer; SuperSonic Imagine (Les Jardins de la Duranne, France)	• Linear array transducer 4 to 15 MHz frequency range	• Nerve stiffness was significantly higher in the CTS group compared with controls. • Stiffness was significantly higher in the severe CTS group compared with the mild or moderate severity group.
	Andrade et al., 2016 [45]	To employ SWE (shear wave velocity, SWV) to detect the changes in sciatic nerve stiffness during human ankle motion.	• Sciatic nerve • 9 healthy volunteers • Longitudinal plane	Aixplorer; SuperSonic Imagine (Les Jardins de la Duranne, France)	• Linear array transducer (SL 10–2) 2 to 10 MHz frequency range	• SWV in the sciatic nerve significantly increased during dorsiflexion when the knee was extended (knee 180°), but no changes were observed for the knee at 90°. • SWV in the nerve decreased non-significantly after five ankle dorsiflexions.
	Inal et al., 2017 [46]	To investigate the feasibility of optic nerve evaluations with free-hand compression strain US and SWE in Behcet's patients.	• Optic nerve • 46 Behcet's patients vs. 54 controls • Longitudinal plane	LOGIQ E9, GE Healthcare (Wauwatosa, USA)	• Linear array transducer 6 to 9 MHz frequency range	• Significantly higher stiffness and lower strain were observed in the optic nerve of Behcet's patients compared with healthy volunteers.
	Inal et al., 2017 [47]	To investigate the feasibility of optic nerve evaluations with free-hand compression strain US and SWE (stiffness) in patients with MS.	• Optic nerve in vivo • 54 MS patients vs. 59 controls • Longitudinal plane	LOGIQ E9, GE Healthcare (Wauwatosa, USA)	• Linear array transducer 6 to 9 MHz frequency range	• Significantly higher stiffness and lower strain were observed in the optic nerve in MS patients compared with healthy volunteers.
	Dikici et al., 2017 [48]	To investigate the feasibility of using SWE (stiffness) for the diagnosis of diabetic peripheral neuropathy.	• Tibial nerve • 20 diabetic patients with neuropathy, 20 without neuropathy, and 20 controls • Longitudinal plane	Aixplorer; SuperSonic Imagine (Les Jardins de la Duranne, France)	• Linear array transducer 4 to 15 MHz frequency range	• Diabetic patients without neuropathy had significantly higher stiffness and CSA values compared with control subjects. • Patients with neuropathy had much higher stiffness and CSA compared with patients without neuropathy and controls.
	Bortolotto et al., 2017 [49]	To investigate the "bone-proximity" hardening artifacts affecting SWE.	• Median nerve • 36 healthy volunteers • Transverse plane	Aplio 500, Toshiba (Tokyo, Japan)	• Linear array transducer 14 MHz frequency	• Higher stiffness was reported in nerve sections near bone, and carpel tunnel, compared with the mid-arm.

Table 1. Cont.

Type of QUS	Study	Goal	Anatomy	Scanner	Probe Frequency	Findings
Shear wave elastography (SWE)	Arslan et al., 2018 [50]	To examine the efficiency of SWE (stiffness) in CTS detection and determining CTS severity level.	• Median nerve 19 severe, 38 moderate, and 39 mild CTS patient vs. 21 controls • Longitudinal plane	ACUSON S2000, Siemens (Mountain View, USA)	• Linear array transducer 4 to 9 MHz frequency range	• Severe CTS groups showed significantly higher stiffness than mild or moderate severity group. • The CSA also showed significant increasing pattern by the severity of CTS.
	Zhu et al., 2018 [51]	To examine the nerve tension impacts on the SWE results (SWS) at different nerve sections.	• Median nerve 40 healthy volunteers • Longitudinal plane	Aixplorer; SuperSonic Imagine (Les Jardins de la Duranne, France)	• Linear array transducer 4 to 15 MHz frequency range	• Stretching nerves resulted in a significant increase in SWS. The SWS at wrist was significantly higher than the SWS at the midarm.
	Cingoz et al., 2018 [52]	To compare the SWE evaluation of nerves with MRI diffusion.	• Median nerve 35 mild, 9 moderate, 15 severe CTS wrists vs. 18 controls • Longitudinal plane	Aplio 500, Toshiba (Tokyo, Japan)	• Linear array transducer 14 MHz frequency	• CTS patients showed higher stiffness than healthy subjects. Patients with moderate–severe CTS had higher stiffness than patients with mild CTS.
	Bedewi et al., 2018 [53]	To investigate the feasibility of SWE (stiffness) in evaluating the brachial plexus nerves.	• Brachial plexus root nerves 40 healthy volunteers • Transverse plane	Aixplorer; SuperSonic Imagine (Les Jardins de la Duranne, France)	• Linear array transducer 4 to 15 MHz frequency range	• Significant differences were found in C6 and C7 nerves between male and female participants. • Significant inverse correlation with height was noted at the C6 nerve root.
	Aslan and Analan, 2018 [54]	To study the effects of chronic flexed wrist posture among chronic stroke patients using SWE (SWS).	• Median nerve of 24 chronic stroke patients • Longitudinal plane	ACUSON S2000, Siemens (Erlangen, Germany)	• Linear array transducer 4 to 9 MHz frequency range	• SWS on the affected side was significantly higher than on the unaffected side. • CSA on the affected side was significantly lower than that of the unaffected side. • The time elapsed since the stroke showed a significant correlation with CSA.
	Kültür et al., 2018 [55]	To evaluate the brachial plexus after radiotherapy for breast cancer using SWE (stiffness).	• Brachial plexus 23 patients underwent radiotherapy. • Transverse plane	LOGIQ E9, GE (Waukesha, USA)	• Linear array transducer 6 to 9 MHz frequency range	• Significantly higher stiffness was estimated for brachial plexuses receiving radiotherapy compared with the contralateral side.

Table 1. Cont.

Type of QUS	Study	Goal	Anatomy	Scanner	Probe Frequency	Findings
Shear wave elastography (SWE)—Continued	Paluch et al., 2018 [56]	To investigate the feasibility of the ulnar neuropathy diagnosis using SWE (stiffness).	• Ulnar nerve • 34 patients with neuropathy vs. 38 healthy controls • Longitudinal axis	iAplio 900, Canon (Tokyo, Japan)	• Linear array transducer • 5 to 18 MHz frequency range	• Patients with ulnar neuropathy presented significantly greater ulnar nerve stiffness in the cubital tunnel and the cubital tunnel to distal and mid-arm stiffness ratio compared with controls. • Mean CSA of the ulnar nerve in the cubital tunnel was significantly larger in patients with neuropathy than in controls.
	Burulday et al., 2018 [57]	To evaluate the median nerve of patients with acromegaly using SWE.	• Median nerves • 15 CTS patients vs. 20 controls • Transverse and longitudinal planes	LOGIQ E9, GE (Waukesha, USA)	• Linear array transducer • 6 to 15 MHz frequency range	• Median nerve stiffness and CSA were significantly higher in the patients with acromegaly compared with the control group for both axial and longitudinal nerve planes
	Neto et al., 2019 [58]	To investigate the immediate impact of slump neurodynamics technique on sciatic nerve stiffness using SWE.	• Sciatic nerve • 14 healthy controls • Longitudinal plane	Aixplorer; SuperSonic Imagine (Les Jardins de la Duranne, France)	• Linear array transducer (SL 10-2) • 2 to 10 MHz frequency range	• The sciatic nerve stiffness of healthy participants did not change immediately after a slump neurodynamic technique
	Tiago Neto et al., 2019 [59].	To investigate the impact of chronic lower-back-related pain in legs on sciatic nerve stiffness using SWE.	• Sciatic nerve • 8 patients with lower-back related pain in legs vs. 8 healthy controls • Longitudinal plane	Aixplorer; SuperSonic Imagine (Les Jardins de la Duranne, France)	• Linear array transducer (SL 10-2) • 2 to 10 MHz frequency range	• The affected limb showed higher sciatic nerve stiffness compared to the unaffected limb of the patients. • No differences were observed between the unaffected limb of patients and the healthy controls.
	Jiang et al., 2019 [60]	To investigate the feasibility of using SWE (stiffness) for the diagnosis of diabetic peripheral neuropathy (DPN).	• Tibial nerve • 70 diabetic patients with DPN and without DPN vs. 20 healthy controls • Longitudinal plane	Aixplorer; SuperSonic Imagine (Les Jardins de la Duranne, France)	• Linear array transducer • 4 to 15 MHz frequency range	• The tibial nerve stiffness was found to be significantly higher in patients with DPN than that in patients without DPN and control subjects.
	He et al., 2019 [61]	To evaluate patients with diabetic peripheral neuropathy using SWE (stiffness).	• Tibial/median nerves • 40 diabetic patients with and 40 without peripheral neuropathy vs. 40 controls • Longitudinal plane	Aixplorer; SuperSonic Imagine (Les Jardins de la Duranne, France).	• Linear array transducer • 4 to 15 MHz frequency range	• The diabetic patients with neuropathy showed significantly higher nerve stiffness and CSA • No significant difference in nerve stiffness was found between the nerves in the left and right limbs in patients.

Table 1. Cont.

Type of QUS	Study	Goal	Anatomy	Scanner	Probe Frequency	Findings
Shear wave elastography (SWE)—Continued	Aslan et al., 2019 [62]	To evaluate adolescent patients with type-I diabetic without peripheral neuropathy using SWE (stiffness).	• Tibial and median nerves • 25 diabetic patients vs. 32 healthy controls • Transverse and Longitudinal planes	Resona 7, Mindray (Shenzhen, China)	• Linear array transducer (ComboWave) • 4 to 15 MHz frequency range	• Both the median nerve and posterior tibial nerve were smaller, and stiffer in the patient group.
	Şahan et al., 2019 [63]	To investigate the feasibility of optic nerve evaluations with free-hand compression strain US and SWE (stiffness) in patients with migraine.	• Optic nerve in vivo • 30 patients with migraine (16 with and 14 without visual auras) vs. 30 controls. • Longitudinal plane	LOGIQ E9, GE Healthcare (Wauwatosa, USA)	• Linear array transducer • 6 to 15-MHz frequency range	• Stiffness from SWE was significantly higher in the optic nerve in patients with migraine compared with controls. • A positive correlation was reported between the duration of the disease and the shear modulus.
	Moran et al., 2020 [64]	To examine the efficiency of SWE (stiffness) compared with CSA changes in CTS detection and determining CTS severity level.	• Median nerve in vivo • 8 severe, 35 moderate, and 36 mild CTS patients vs. and negative EDT controls • Longitudinal plane	Aplio 500, Toshiba (Tokyo, Japan)	• Linear array transducer • 5 to 14 MHz frequency	• Stiffness and CSA increased according to the CTS severity level. • Stiffness was not different between patients with negative and mild CTS findings.
	Wei and Ye, 2020 [65]	To evaluate patients with diabetic peripheral neuropathy using SWE (stiffness).	• Tibial nerve • 14 diabetic patients with peripheral neuropathy, 13 diabetic patients without peripheral neuropathy vs. 20 healthy controls • Longitudinal plane	ACUSON S2000, Siemens (Erlangen, Germany)	• Linear array transducer • 4 to 9 MHz frequency range	• Tibial nerve stiffness in patients with neuropathy and without neuropathy were significantly higher than controls. • CSA did not show any significant differences. • No significant difference in nerve stiffness was found between the patient with neuropathy and those without neuropathy.

Table 1. Cont.

Type of QUS	Study	Goal	Anatomy	Scanner	Probe Frequency	Findings
Shear wave elastography (SWE)—Continued	Bedewi et al., 2020 [66]	To investigate the feasibility of SWE (stiffness) to evaluate the saphenous nerves.	• Saphenous nerves of 36 healthy subjects • Transverse and Longitudinal plane	Aixplorer, SuperSonic Imagine (Les Jardins de la Duranne, France)	• Linear array transducer • 5 to 18 MHz frequency range	• Stiffness of the saphenous nerve was found to be very similar in the short and long axes. • No correlations of SEW results were found with age, height, weight, and BMI.
	Schrier et al., 2020 [67]	To examine the SWE sensitivity to increasing tensile loading on cadaver nerves at different nerve sections.	• Median nerves 10 normal cadaveric wrists • Transverse and Longitudinal plane	LOGIQ E9, GE (Waukesha, USA)	• Linear array transducer (9LD) • 2 to 8 MHz frequency range	• SWE- and indentation-based nerve stiffness increased significantly with tensile loading. • Acquisition in a transverse plane showed lower values compared with the longitudinal plane. • Stiffness did not change when measured proximal to the carpal tunnel.
	Rugel et al., 2020 [68]	To study the limb position impact on the SWE (SWS).	• Median and ulnar nerves 16 healthy controls • Longitudinal plane	Aixplorer, SuperSonic Imagine (Les Jardins de la Duranne, France)	• Linear array transducer • 4 to 15 MHz frequency range	• SWS increased for limb positions that induced greater tension on the nerves. • SWS in median nerve increased by elbow extension. • SWS in ulnar nerve increased by elbow flexion.
Backscattered radiofrequency (RF) signal characterization	Byra et al., 2019 [21]	To investigate correlations between collagen/myelin content (histology) of nerves with back backscatter coefficient (BSC), attenuation coefficient (AC), Nakagami parameter, and entropy.	• Ulnar nerve 6 control cadavers, 85 fascicles • Transverse plane	Vevo MD, FUJIFILM (Toronto, Canada)	• Linear array transducer (UHF48) • Center frequency at 30 MHz	• BSC and entropy showed significant correlations with the combined collagen and myelin.

3. B-Mode Echogenicity Measurement

In B-mode images, sonographers typically identify peripheral nerves based on fascicular boundaries; in the transverse plane, nerves appear honeycomb-like, while in the longitudinal plane, nerves display parallel hyperechoic fascicular borders. Figure 4 shows B-mode images in the transverse and longitudinal planes of the median nerve in a healthy volunteer generated with UFH22 (7–10 MHz) and UFH48 (10–22 MHz) US probes on a Vevo MD, FUJIFILM machine. The honeycomb-like structure of the nerves in the transverse plane becomes more obvious in images generated with higher-frequency probes. Nerves differ from tendons, which display a dense fibrillar structure in B-mode [7,69,70], and are additionally distinguished from blood vessels by using Doppler US [5–7,68]. B-mode echogenicity carries information about the nerve structure. Specifically, B-mode images comprise both the information of specular reflections at the tissue interfaces (large structures compared to the wavelength), displayed as hyperechoic areas, and the information of the backscattered signal from the microstructure of the tissue (equal to or smaller than the wavelength), displayed as speckle texture in the image.

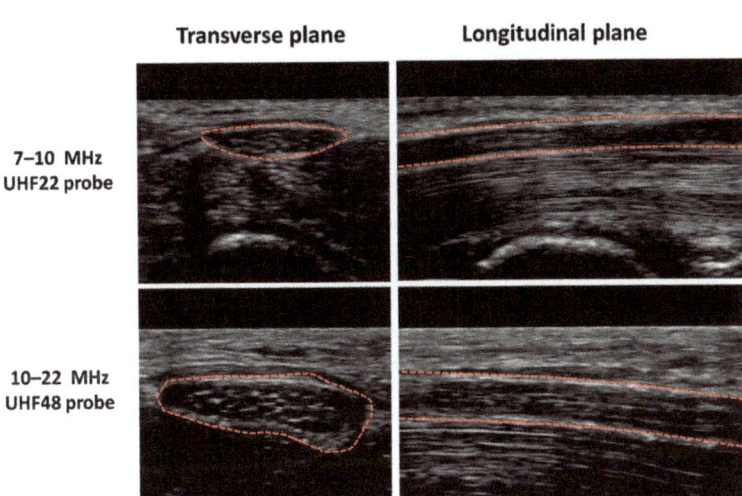

Figure 4. US B-mode images in transverse and longitudinal planes of the median nerve (indicated in red dashed lines) in a healthy volunteer generated with UFH22 (7–10 MHz) and UFH48 (10–22 MHz) US probes on a Vevo MD, FUJIFILM machine. The honeycomb-like structure of the nerves in the transverse plane becomes more obvious in images generated with higher-frequency probes.

The measurement of the hypoechoic fractional area of the nerves in US B-mode images, or so-called nerve density index, has been suggested as an objective measurement of overall nerve echogenicity, capable of distinguishing between normal and abnormal nerves. Tagliafico et al. investigated the feasibility of using the peripheral nerve density index for distinguishing between CTS and neurofibromas in the median nerve [29]. Nerve density was found to be significantly higher in patients with CTS and significantly lower in patients with neurofibromas compared with healthy normal subjects. Using an analogous approach, Bignotti et al. concluded that the median nerve density index was significantly lower in patients with limited cutaneous systemic sclerosis compared to healthy controls [22]. Moreover, symptomatic patients demonstrated lower nerve density compared to non-symptomatic patients. Such approaches have been further refined by normalizing nerve echogenicity to its surrounding tissue environment, thus potentially offsetting machine effects and absolute patient-to-patient differences in echogenicity. For example, Byra et al. investigated the nerve–tissue contrast index (NTI), the ratio between the average brightness of the surrounding tissue to the median nerve, in the context of a CTS diagnosis [24]. NTI was found to be significantly higher in CTS patients compared with healthy volunteers. Boom and Visser employed a variety of thresholding methods to measure the hypoechoic fraction (similar to US nerve density) of the ulnar nerve to detect ulnar neuropathy, with a significantly lower average hypoechoic fraction found in a patient group compared with controls [30]. In an attempt to correlate echogenicity measures with more conventional diagnostic approaches, Simon et al. [31] studied the relation between the ulnar nerve hypoechoic fraction and the electrophysiologic "inching" measures [31]. Hypoechoic fraction and CSA were significantly increased in patients with neuropathy immediately distal and proximal to the medial epicondyle. The above-elbow ulnar motor conduction velocity was inversely correlated with both CSA and hypoechoic fraction in limbs with neuropathy. As an example of the potential ambiguity of such approaches, though, asymptomatic and symptomatic limbs of patients demonstrated similar hypoechoic fractions. In addition to these more common echogenicity measures, the texture of US B-mode images may also be evaluated in peripheral nerves, offering a more nuanced assessment of structural heterogeneity within nerves. For example, in cadaveric ulnar nerves, a texture feature index obtained using the gray level co-occurrence matrix algorithm correlated to combined collagen and myelin concentrations obtained from histology [21].

4. US Elastography

The concept of US elastography was introduced by Ophir et al. [71], as a generalization of Eisenscher's echosonography method [72]. Elastography in general can be explained as analogous to a palpation exam performed on the entire tissue volume. During a palpation exam, the physician taps (shears) the tissue with his or her fingers, and qualitatively senses the deformability or stiffness of the examined tissues. Similarly, US elastography estimates tissue elasticity by analyzing the response of the tissue to an applied force monitored with US [26,27]. Strain ultrasonography and SWE are the two major classes of US elastography techniques [26]. In strain ultrasonography, the tissue strain, as a response to internal or external compression stimuli, is measured by tracking the motion of speckles detectable in B-mode images [26,27]. In SWE, the speed of shear waves induced by external vibrations or tissue compression is measured, which is correlated to tissue elasticity or stiffness [26,27]. These basic mechanical parameters are defined and presented schematically in Table 2.

Table 2. Definition of the basic mechanical parameters described in this study.

Mechanical Parameters	Definition	Formula	Schematics
Normal stress	The magnitude of the force applied to the unit area perpendicular to the force direction	$\sigma = \frac{F}{A}$	
Normal strain	The change in length of the tissue per its unit length parallel to the force direction	$\varepsilon = \frac{\Delta L}{L_0}$	
Young's modulus (i.e., normal modulus)	Elasticity defined in applied force direction but perpendicular to the unit volume surface	$E = \frac{\sigma}{\varepsilon}$	
Shear stress	The magnitude of the force applied to the unit area parallel to the force direction	$\tau = \frac{F}{A}$	
Shear strain	The angular change in originally right angles of the unit volume after shear stress application	$\gamma = \frac{\Delta X}{L_0}$	
Shear modulus	Elasticity defined in applied force direction and parallel to the unit volume surface	$G = \frac{\tau}{\gamma}$ $G = \frac{E}{2(1+v)}$	
Bulk modulus	Elasticity defined over the unit of volume when a uniform volumetric stress is applied, and a uniform strain is induced	$K = \frac{E}{3(1-2v)}$	

Elasticity and strain are two important concepts in strain elastography and SWE. The elasticity of a material describes its tendency to retain its original size and shape after being subjected to a deforming force or stress. Solids possess shear and volume elasticity such that they resist changes in shape and volume. Liquids, however, possess only volume elasticity such that they resist changes in their volume, but not in their shapes. Soft tissues are comprised of both liquids and solids; therefore, they possess shear and volume elasticities, yet their shear elasticity is significantly lower than their volume elasticity. Strain can be described as the change in the length of the tissue per its unit length (Table 2). The magnitude of the force applied to the unit area, which induces the strain, is known as stress. The modulus of elasticity can be quantified as the ratio of stress to strain (units of N/m^2, or Pa). It can be quantified depending on the stress and strain direction, such that Young's modulus (i.e., normal modulus), E, quantifies elasticity in the direction normal to the unit volume surface while the shear modulus, G, quantifies elasticity in the tangential direction to the unit volume surface. However, when uniform volumetric stress and strain can be assumed (e.g., liquids under pressure), the bulk or volume elastic modulus, K, can be described over the unit of volume.

4.1. Strain Ultrasonography

In strain ultrasonography, US is employed to measure the induced tissue displacement in the same direction as the applied stress. As shown in Figure 5, the required cyclic mechanical compression can be applied by (a) free-hand cyclic compression (palpation), (b) cardiovascular pulsation or respiratory motion, (c) acoustic radiation force impulse (ARFI), or (d) external mechanical vibration [2]. The induced strain, regardless of the stress application method, can be measured using different approaches depending on the manufacturer: RF echo correlation-based tracking, Doppler processing, or a combination of the two methods [2]. For example, in RF echo correlation-based tracking, RF A-lines are acquired along the axis of displacement; then, their changes in time between different acquisitions allow the measurement of the tissue displacement and the estimation of the normal strain.

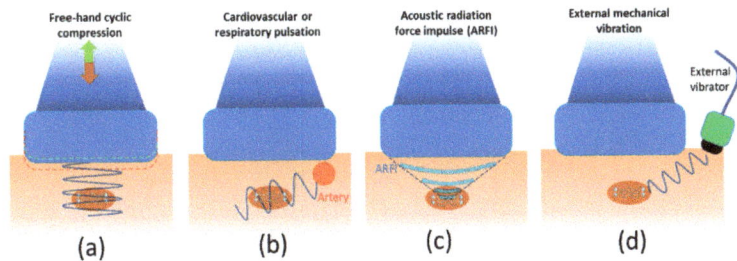

Figure 5. Strain ultrasonography techniques categorized by their excitation methods (generating pressure wave sources) to induce strain in the tissue of interest. (**a**) Free-hand cyclic compression (palpation), (**b**) cardiovascular or respiratory pulsation, (**c**) acoustic radiation force impulse (ARFI), and (**d**) external mechanical vibration have been used as excitation sources in strain ultrasonography.

In the free-hand compression technique, compression–decompression cycles are performed using the US transducer itself, with force and frequency adjusted by the sonographer to an appropriate range according to a strain indicator on the US screen [34]. It is very important that the compression occurs vertically, without over-compression, and that the tissue does not slip out of the compression plane [33]. Strain ratios (SRs) are often calculated to provide more reproducible indices from strain-ultrasonography-generated images, as the applied stresses cannot be well-controlled [2].

In ARFI-based compression, a long-duration (e.g., 0.1–0.5 ms vs. 0.02 ms pulses in B-mode imaging), high-intensity (e.g., spatial peak pulse average = 1400 W/cm^2, spatial peak temporal average = 0.7 W/cm^2) acoustic "pushing pulse" (i.e., ARFI) is used to displace tissue (displacement of ~10–20 µm) perpendicular to the surface. The magnitude of the applied acoustic radiation force, F, can be estimated by the acoustic absorption rate in the tissue, α, the speed of sound in the tissue, c, and the temporal average intensity of the acoustic beam, I, according to Equation (1) [2,26,27].

$$F = \frac{2\alpha I}{c} \qquad (1)$$

Strain Ultrasonography Applied to Peripheral Nerves

Orman et al. [33] investigated the application of free-hand compression in strain ultrasonography to evaluate median nerve mechanical properties. The mean tissue strain was significantly lower in patients with CTS compared to controls, implying higher tissue stiffness. Given that the mean median nerve perimeter and its CSA in patients were also significantly higher than those of controls, the authors concluded that the enlarged nerves were entrapped by the surrounding tissue structures in carpal tunnel. This entrapment created a pre-stressed condition, resulting in increased apparent stiffness; it was hypothesized that freeing the nerve would reduce the apparent stiffness. The reproducibility of the free-hand compression strain ultrasonography technique in detecting CTS was improved by calculating SR against an acoustic coupler rubber (ACR, made of elastic resin) as an external reference (Figure 6, [34]). The higher SR (ACR/nerve) in CTS patients compared with healthy volunteers implied lower nerve strain, similar to earlier studies [33]. Kesikburun et al. [39] later attempted using bone as an internal reference for SR calculation in median nerve evaluation in CTS patients, reporting a four-fold increase in nerve elasticity for the symptomatic wrist versus the asymptomatic wrist. However, considering bone as the reference for SR measurements is challenging, given the differences in sound speed within soft tissues versus bone. Moreover, near-zero values are expected for strains in bone using free-hand compression. In contrast, Nogueira-Barbosa et al. [41] used the flexor digitorum superficialis muscle (i.e., a soft tissue) as an internal reference for SR calculation in the median nerve in patients with chronic leprosy. A significantly lower SR was observed in the leprosy patients compared with the control group. Later, Tezcan et al. [43] used fat as the reference for SR measurement in the median nerve in patients with CTS undergoing low-level laser therapy and reported a significant drop in nerve stiffness (increased strain) after the therapy. Despite the promise of using muscle or fat as internal references, one caveat is that muscle, fat, and nerves may also be affected by a given pathological condition.

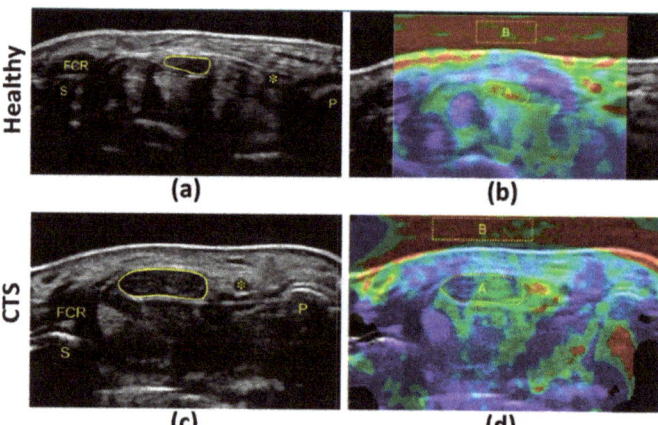

Figure 6. (a) B-mode and (b) strain images in the transverse plane of the median nerve in a healthy subject (57-year-old female). (c) B-mode and (d) strain images in the transverse plane of the median nerve in a CTS patient (64-year-old female). Strain ratio (SR) was measured by comparing the strain values in the median nerve (indicated with A in (b,d)) with an acoustic coupler rubber (ACR) as an external reference (indicated with B in (b,d)). The median nerve in the CTS patient showed a higher SR (ACR/Median nerve) and CSA. These figures were previously presented by Miyamoto et al. [34]. Reprinting permission is granted by the Radiological Society of North America, which is the copyright holder. Minor modifications were performed for presentation purposes. * = Ulnar artery, FCR = flexor carpi radialis, P = pisiform bone, S = scaphoid bone.

Free-hand compression strain ultrasonography was also used to probe neuropathic severity in several studies, including a comparatively subjective colorimetric assessment of strain levels [36] and a more repeatable SR-based approach [37], to distinguish between individuals with and without CTS. For the latter, the outcomes could not distinguish between mild and moderate CTS [37]. However, a comparable SR-based approach (reciprocal of SR) was successfully used to identify individuals with diabetic neuropathy in tibial nerves; here, the outcomes differentiated between neuropathic severity and correlated with morphometric changes [38].

Ambient or passive strain ultrasonography was also deployed to probe neuropathy; however, the measured SR between the median nerve and nearby tendons was insufficient to identify significant differences between CTS and control groups [42]. It is likely that cardiorespiratory pulsations induced inconsistent deformations in the nerve and reference tendons, which resulted in higher variability compared to free-hand compression strain ultrasonography. In contrast, strain ultrasonography with a cyclic compression apparatus improved repeatability by means of a pre-determined cyclic displacement of the transducer (4 mm displacement at 1.5 Hz) [35]. Using this approach, consistent with freehand compression studies, strains were significantly lower while SR and CSA were significantly higher in CTS patients versus controls. In a later study, the same research group [40] added a strain gauge to the cyclic compression apparatus, to measure pressure. The pressure and pressure/strain ratio (a more realistic index to determine elasticity) were both significantly higher in the CTS patients than in controls.

The feasibility of strain ultrasonography using ARFI push pulses was first investigated by Palmeri et al. [32] to visualize peripheral nerves with adequate contrast versus their surrounding tissues (e.g., muscle, fat, and fascia). The purpose was to improve US guidance in monitoring the distribution of injected anesthetic around the targeted nerves. ARFI strain ultrasonography images yielded significant contrast improvements for the distal sciatic nerve structures and brachial plexus peripheral nerves compared with B-mode imaging. B-mode and ARFI image acquisitions were ECG-triggered for in vivo imaging at locations adjacent to arteries. Several ARFI-based strain ultrasonography investigations have also been reported in the literature as parts of SWE-focused studies, which are summarized in the next section. A limitation of ARFI-based approaches is that the intensity of the radiation force is limited by the potential tissue damage by a push at high acoustic power. As a consequence, the magnitude of the displacements as well as the imaging depth are restricted. In the next section, the assessment of shear elastic modulus (G) will be discussed, as it has more recently been preferred for its fast and reliable assessment, and its wider range of measurable values.

4.2. Shear Wave Elastography (SWE)

In contrast to strain ultrasonography, which measures physical tissue displacement parallel to the applied normal stress, SWE employs dynamic stress to generate shear waves in perpendicular directions. The measurement of the shear wave speed (SWS) results in an estimation of the tissue's shear and normal elastic moduli (G and E) [27]. SWE was developed based on the fact that the shear elastic modulus, G ($G \approx E/3$ for semi-incompressible tissues), determines the propagation speed of mechanical waves, SWS, at a magnitude of the square root of G divided by tissue density, ρ, as presented in Equation (2).

$$SWS = \sqrt{\frac{G}{\rho}} \approx \sqrt{\frac{E}{3\rho}} \qquad (2)$$

Thus, by evaluating SWS, the elastic modulus of a medium can be estimated. SWS remains below 10 m/s on average in soft tissues and can be adequately tracked by B-mode US images [27]. Shear waves propagate faster through stiffer and denser tissues, as well as along the tissue axis aligned with organized fibers (e.g., the long axis in tendons) [73]. As shown in Figure 7, the shear wave generation methods in nerve SWE studies can be categorized mainly as (a) external mechanical vibration, (b) single-point-focused ARFI, and (c) multiple-point-focused ARFI [2].

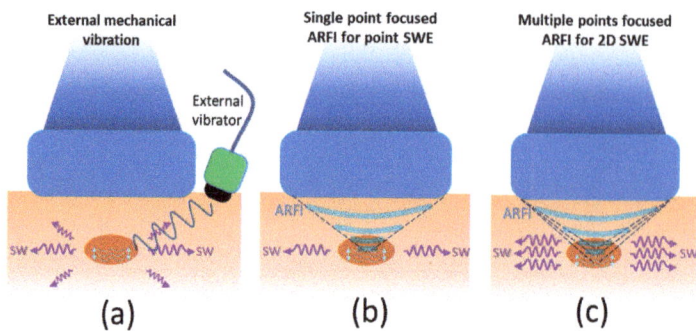

Figure 7. Shear wave elastography (SWE) techniques categorized by their excitation methods to generate shear waves in the tissue of interest: (**a**) external mechanical vibration, (**b**) single-point-focused ARFI for point SWE, and (**c**) multiple-point-focused ARFI for 2D SWE.

Although an external vibration device can induce shear waves, as initially proposed by Krouskop et al. [74], most clinical SWE studies utilize ARFI pulses to induce shear waves, as first proposed by Sugimoto et al. in 1990 [75]. ARFI pushing pulses perpendicular to the tissue surface, as noted in Section 3, result in tissue vibration at an ultrasonic frequency and consequent tissue deformation (displacement) within the region of US excitation (ROE), due to sound wave absorption and scattering. The induced deformation generates shear waves that laterally propagate away from the ROE at a much slower velocity (<10 m/s) compared with US pressure pulses (1500 m/s). Although shear wave mode conversion also occurs with conventional B-mode imaging, the force magnitudes are too small to generate tissue motion detectable with conventional US. ARFI pulses can be applied at a single focal location (point shear wave elastography, pSWE) (Figure 7b) or a multi-focal configuration such that each focal zone is interrogated in rapid succession, leading to a cylindrically shaped shear wave extending over a larger depth, enabling real-time shear wave images to be formed (Figure 7c) [2,26,27]. SWE with multi-focal ARFI configuration is called 2D shear wave elastography (2D-SWE) and allows the real-time monitoring of shear waves in 2D for an SWS measurement. Notably, for 2D SWE, shorter propagation distances are utilized due to the limitations in the number of US tracking pulses.

Considering shear wave generation as the first step in SWE, during the second step, US rapid plane wave excitations are used to track tissue displacement while shear waves propagate. In the third step, changes in tissue displacement maps over time are used to calculate SWS. Frame rates for tracking shear waves are typically between 2 kHz and 10 kHz [73]. Scanners may display different versions of a quality index as a measure of confidence in the estimated SWS, which is calculated from the correlation coefficients between frames of the speckle-tracking images. If the frame rate is too low, there is motion of the patient or probe, or there is no well-developed speckle in the region, then the quality index is low.

SWE Applied to Peripheral Nerves

ARFI-SWE has been investigated in several studies to detect CTS. The median nerve stiffness and SWS were reported to be significantly higher in CTS patients compared with controls, and often accompanied by an increase in nerve CSA [44,50,52,64]. Stiffness also accurately differentiated between patients with severe CTS and those with mild or moderate [44,50,52,64]. Figure 8 shows the B-mode image, estimated stiffness in kPa, and the shear wave propagation map in the median nerves of a healthy participant (a, b) and a CTS patient (c, d) [52], who demonstrated a higher stiffness and larger CSA. Notably, the shear wave propagation map displays the arrival time of a shear wave using a series of wave contour lines. ARFI-based SWE also revealed similar changes in the median nerve (higher nerve stiffness and CSA) for patients with acromegaly [57].

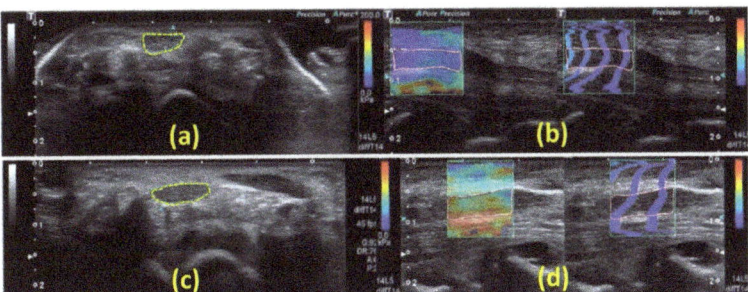

Figure 8. (**a**,**c**) B-mode images of the transverse plane of median nerves of a healthy subject and a CTS patient, respectively. The median nerve cross-section is identified by the dashed line. CSAs of the median nerve were 16 and 27 mm^2 for the healthy subject and CTS patient, respectively. (**b**,**d**) SWE-based stiffness and propagation maps from SWE on the longitudinal planes of the median nerves of the same healthy subject (**b**) and CTS patient (**d**), respectively. The average stiffnesses measured along the longitudinal plane of the median nerve were 35 and 113 kPa for the healthy subject and CTS patient, respectively. These figures were previously presented by Cingoz et al. [52]. Reprinting permission is granted through Rightslink system. Minor modifications were performed for presentation purposes.

Several studies have focused on the SWE-based assessment of peripheral nerve neuropathy. Aslan and Analan [54] used SWE to study the effects of chronic flexed wrist posture among chronic stroke patients on median nerve elasticity and CSA. SWS was significantly higher, but CSA was significantly lower (unlike CTS) for the affected side than the unaffected side; however, SWS did not correlate with the elapsed time since stroke. Similarly, SWE revealed significantly greater ulnar nerve stiffness within the cubital tunnel in patients with ulnar neuropathy (i.e., cubital tunnel syndrome) compared to healthy controls [56]; tibial nerve stiffness in patients with diabetic neuropathy compared to non-neuropathic diabetics and healthy controls [48,60,62,65]; and median nerve stiffness in patients with diabetic neuropathy compared to controls [61,62]. Neuropathic changes were often accompanied by increased CSA [60–62]; however, some studies have reported a reversed trend in the tibial nerve [65]. Interestingly, though, both the median and tibial nerves were often found to be thinner in diabetic patients who did not display neuropathy, suggestive of nerve atrophy before neuropathy onset [62]. Conversely, other studies have reported higher CSAs in the tibial nerves of patients with diabetic neuropathy [65]. Such controversial findings in CSA changes emphasize the utility of combining QUS and morphometric imaging.

A number of other nerves have also been studied using SWE. SWE and free-hand compression strain ultrasonography in optic nerves of patients with Behcet's syndrome (a chronic autoimmune disease) [46] and multiple sclerosis [47] showed significantly higher stiffness and lower strains compared with the control group. Optic nerve stiffness was also examined in patients with migraine using SWE and free-hand compression strain ultrasonography; patients displayed an insignificant decrease in calculated strain (stiffness increase), but a significant increase in SWS [63]. In another study, SWE revealed higher elastic moduli in the brachial plexus nerves of patients receiving radiotherapy compared to their contralateral nerves [55]. SWE has also been used to evaluate healthy nerves; for example, sex-dependent differences between elastic moduli in cervical nerve roots have been noted in healthy volunteers [53].

Considerations for Evaluating Peripheral Nerves with SWE

Despite its broad utility, the scale of a targeted nerve should be carefully considered when interpreting SWE outcomes. In one study, the mean stiffness of the saphenous nerve was found to be very similar in the short and long axes [66], a finding inconsistent with multiple other investigations showing a higher shear wave speed in the longitudinal plane [1,67]. It is likely that reliable elasticity data could not be acquired in the transverse plane of the nerves [51], potentially due to the similar scale of nerve diameter and the wavelength of the shear waves and a higher signal from wave reflections at the fiber bundles, apparent in the nerve's transverse plane [1,67]. SWE measures in thinner nerves may also be less accurate as they are spanned by a smaller number of shear wavelengths to be tracked by US. In addition, the speckle tracking is confounded by the fact that the US beam is larger than the nerve, which introduces a partial volume effect that creates additional influences of the surrounding tissues on reported SWS.

Nerve anatomy and tension should also be considered in evaluating SWE outcomes. Median nerves stretched via wrist extension showed a significant increase in SWS (i.e., nerve stiffness) at the wrist compared to mid-forearm [51], possibly due to the (carpal) bone proximity artifact [49], which occurs when the studied structure is near a rigid plane such as the bone cortex that prevents homogeneous shear wave propagation. Alternatively, increased SWS may reflect nerve tension due to nerve deformation over the extended wrist [76] or increased pressure within the carpal tunnel [77]. Similar phenomena were observed in sciatic nerves, where increased SWS was noted after tensioning through ankle dorsiflexion in combination with knee extension [45], in median nerves with elbow extension [68], and in ulnar nerves with elbow flexion [68].

The correlation between increased tensile loading and increased SWS has also been validated through the ex vivo application of tensile loads [51]. Nerve viability may also influence SWE outcomes; unlike the above study [51], Schrier et al. [67] reported no differences in median nerve elasticity between the median nerve at the wrist and forearm, as measured in cadaveric nerves using SWE and lateral mechanical compression tests. Such differences might be due to the loss of in vivo loading and intra-nerve pressure or post-mortem tissue changes. More recently, Neto et al. [58] investigated the immediate impact of the slump neurodynamics technique, an exercise for the purpose of improving neural mechanosensitivity, on sciatic nerve stiffness using SWE. SWS was measured during passive foot dorsiflexion in a healthy group before and immediately after slump neurodynamics training. Despite significant differences in the sciatic nerve SWS caused by dorsiflexion, SWS did not change after slump neurodynamic loading, suggesting that nerves likely returned to their natural biomechanical state immediately after releasing the tensile load imposed by the slump. The impact of chronic lower-back-related leg pain on sciatic nerve stiffness was investigated during passive foot dorsiflexion by the same research group [59]. The affected limb showed higher sciatic nerve stiffness compared to the unaffected limb of patients; however, no differences were observed between the unaffected limb of patients versus the healthy controls.

5. Backscattered Radiofrequency (RF) Signal Characterization

US scanners increasingly permit access to the beam-formed backscattered RF signals through a research interface. Quantifying such raw RF US data allows an assessment of fundamental acoustic tissue parameters, which can be scanner-independent [12,28]. Commonly used RF signal quantifications, such as backscatter coefficient (BSC), attenuation coefficient (AC), structure–function, and stochastic modeling of envelope statistics of backscattered echoes, are highly likely to be related to the tissue composition and microstructure [12,28].

BSC indicates the tissue's ability to scatter US waves back to the transducer analogous to echogenicity, providing information about tissue structure and composition. Indeed, the backscattered coefficient represents the energy backscattered by the biological tissue as a fraction of the emitted signal. A reliable assessment requires accounting for all the causes of the loss of energy of the emitted wave in addition to the backscatter, such as the quantitative assessment of the tissue AC, but also the diffraction of the transducer and settings on the gain and processing in the scanner. AC indicates the magnitude of the loss of energy (absorption and scattering) during the US wave propagation into and back from tissues. The entropy of the backscattered echo amplitude can also be used as a model-free approach to analyze the backscattered echo statistics [78]. Such model-free approaches in general do not directly provide an estimation of the tissue microstructure, even though statistical correlations can be found between such coefficients and the tissue microstructural parameters.

In addition to model-free approaches to analyze backscattered echo statistics, some model-based methods have been proposed to estimate the microstructural properties of the tissues [12,79]. Such techniques often require solving an inverse equation problem by fitting the accurately measured BSC and AC parameters (functions of the RF spectrum) in a predefined model of the scatterers in the tissue of interest. For example, stochastic models of the backscattered echo statistics provide an indirect estimate of the spatial and size distributions of scattering microstructures within the studied tissue. Envelope statistics can be also modeled using various distribution functions such as Nakagami distribution, which models random distributions of scatterers in the resolution cells (pre-Rayleigh to Rician distributions) [80].

Raw backscattered RF signal characteristics have been used for several soft tissue assessments [12] including liver [81], breast [82], muscle [83], annular pulleys (tendons) of the fingers [84], and skin [85]. Recently, Byra et al. [21] investigated cadaveric ulnar nerves using raw RF signal measures including BSC, AC, Nakagami parameter, and entropy. These specimens were also assessed with histology; the combined collagen/myelin content demonstrated significant correlations with the BSC and entropy.

6. QUS Limitations in Nerve Evaluation

Employing any US technique for peripheral nerve assessment is affected by well-described sonography artifacts such as shadowing, insonation angle, reverberation, and clutter artifacts. Moreover, US techniques are affected by variations in the system settings and parameters such as RF frequency, sampling rate, and gains, which occasionally lead to biased results. Since the structures of interest in peripheral nerves are small, higher US frequencies are often preferred for qualitative and quantitative nerve imaging. The higher US frequencies result in a sharp decrease in the signal-to-noise ratio (SNR) as a function of the depth, due to the higher capacity of biological tissues to attenuate high-frequency RF waves. Therefore, the effective imaging depth for quantitative US techniques is often limited to a few centimeters for nerve imaging, which is more challenging for in vivo investigations when considering the variability in the dimensions of the intermediate tissue layers (e.g., skin, muscle, and fat) between the transducer and the nerves.

B-mode echogenicity measures performed on post-processed images (e.g., nerve density) are limited due to their dependence on the scanner settings and manual identification of tissue boundaries [1,2,73].

US elastography-based measures of tissues are limited by assumptions about the tissue's material behavior (e.g., linear, elastic, isotropic, homogenous, and incompressible material) to simplify the analysis and interpretation of the strain ultrasonography and SWE measurements [2,73]. However, soft tissues are known to be inherently nonlinear, viscoelastic, and heterogeneous [2]. Specifically, including viscosity in the tissue model means that the tissue stiffness and SWS both depend on the excitation ARFI pulse frequency (or frequency of the external mechanical vibrations), which may vary for different US systems and transducers [2]. Moreover, the mechanical nonlinearity in soft tissue's behavior means that the induced level of strain in response to an ARFI pulse or other external loads depends on the initial strain state of the material; in other words, operator-dependent transducer orientation and initial compression [1,2]. SWE and strain ultrasonography studies of peripheral nerves have recommended single cutoff values for strain, strain ratio, stiffness, and stiffness ratio between different nerve sections, which, in general, showed better sensitivity and specificity levels in neuropathy diagnosis compared with CSA values and their ratio, despite the codependence of CSA and SWS [1]. However, such single cutoff values show large variations depending on the US system and transducer [1].

Backscattered RF signal characterizations often require analyzing the tissue scans relative to a tissue-mimicking calibration phantom, with a known BSC and AC profile in a range of targeting frequencies. These extra calibration scans may be considered highly resource- or time-consuming, and require specialized training. Therefore, backscattered RF signal characterization methods may be especially challenging for patient-oriented in vivo experimental acquisitions. Notably, methods without extra calibration scans have been reported in other tissues (liver and breast) and may serve to guide future peripheral nerve assessments. In such methods, a smaller reference phantom can be scanned concurrently with the tissue and utilized for further BSC corrections. On the other hand, clinical US systems have been shown to have very stable acoustic output and gain, suggesting calibration scans can be stored once and then applied to the subsequent data analysis for extended periods, reducing the impact on clinical throughput. Moreover, the backscattered RF signal characterizations involve more sophisticated data processing, perhaps offline, compared with other QUS categories. As described in Section 5, the model-based backscattered-signal-related measures often require solving an inverse equation problem by fitting the accurately measured BSC and AC parameters in a predefined model of the scatterers in the medium of interest. More sophisticated models may be required for a more accurate assessment of the backscattered RF signal from peripheral nerves by considering their specific microstructure, surrounding tissue, and microenvironment as quantified using immunohistochemical approaches [86]. As is the case for other QUS techniques, raw RF signal characterization can be influenced by the transducer orientation and compression applied by the operator.

7. Conclusions

Three main classes of QUS techniques were described and their reported applications on peripheral nerves in the literature were summarized in this study. Neuropathy and nerve injury may affect the composite structure of the nerves at different scales (i.e., fascicles, organized bundles of nerve fibers within a fascicle, and axons), which can be potentially assessed by QUS techniques. Among the discussed QUS techniques, SWE is more appropriate for the mechanical assessment of peripheral nerves while backscattered RF signal characterization is recommended for the microstructural assessment of the nerves. These approaches are important topics for further investigation.

Author Contributions: Conceptualization, S.J., M.A., E.Y.C. and S.B.S.; methodology, S.J., V.B., M.A., E.Y.C. and S.B.S.; investigation, S.J., V.B., M.A., E.Y.C. and S.B.S.; resources, E.Y.C. and S.B.S.; writing—original draft preparation, S.J., V.B., M.A., E.Y.C. and S.B.S.; writing—review and editing, S.J., V.B., M.A., E.Y.C. and S.B.S.; visualization, S.J. and V.B.; supervision, M.A., E.Y.C. and S.B.S. All authors have read and agreed to the published version of the manuscript.

Funding: This research was funded by the Department of Defense (W81XWH-20-1-0927), Department of Veterans Affairs (I01CX002118-01 and I01CX001388), and National Institutes of Health (K01AR080257).

Institutional Review Board Statement: Not applicable.

Informed Consent Statement: Not applicable.

Data Availability Statement: All data used for this review study are publicly available.

Acknowledgments: We gratefully acknowledge funding from the Department of Defense (W81XWH-20-1-0927), Department of Veterans Affairs (I01CX002118-01 and I01CX001388), and National Institutes of Health (K01AR080257).

Conflicts of Interest: The authors declare no conflict of interest.

Abbreviations

AC: attenuation coefficient; ACR: acoustic coupler rubber; ARFI: acoustic radiation force impulse; BSC: backscatter coefficient; CSA: cross-sectional area; CTS: carpel tunnel syndrome; E: normal elastic moduli; G: shear elastic modulus; HF: high-frequency; NTI: nerve–tissue contrast index; pSWE: point shear wave elastography; QUS: quantitative ultrasound; RF: radiofrequency; ROE: region of US excitation; SNR: signal-to-noise ratio; SR: strain ratio; SWE: shear wave elastography; SWS: shear wave speed; 2D: two-dimensional; US: ultrasound; W: Watt.

References

1. Wee, T.C.; Simon, N.G. Ultrasound Elastography for the Evaluation of Peripheral Nerves: A Systematic Review. *Muscle Nerve* **2019**, *60*, 501–512. [CrossRef]
2. Shiina, T.; Nightingale, K.R.; Palmeri, M.L.; Hall, T.J.; Bamber, J.C.; Barr, R.G.; Castera, L.; Choi, B.I.; Chou, Y.H.; Cosgrove, D.; et al. WFUMB Guidelines and Recommendations for Clinical Use of Ultrasound Elastography: Part 1: Basic Principles and Terminology. *Ultrasound Med. Biol.* **2015**, *41*, 1126–1147. [CrossRef]
3. Pelosi, L.; Arányi, Z.; Beekman, R.; Bland, J.; Coraci, D.; Hobson-Webb, L.D.; Padua, L.; Podnar, S.; Simon, N.; van Alfen, N.; et al. Expert Consensus on the Combined Investigation of Ulnar Neuropathy at the Elbow Using Electrodiagnostic Tests and Nerve Ultrasound. *Clin. Neurophysiol.* **2021**, *132*, 2274–2281. [CrossRef]
4. Allen, K.W.; Moake, M.M. Ultrasound-Guided Paravenous Saphenous Nerve Block for Lower Extremity Abscess Incision and Drainage in a Male Adolescent. *Pediatr. Emerg. Care* **2022**, *1*, 1–10. [CrossRef]
5. Vlassakov, K.V.; Sala-Blanch, X. Ultrasound of the Peripheral Nerves. *Nerves Nerve Inj.* **2015**, *1*, 227–250. [CrossRef]
6. Jacobson, J.A.; Wilson, T.J.; Yang, L.J.S. Sonography of Common Peripheral Nerve Disorders with Clinical Correlation. *J. Ultrasound Med.* **2016**, *35*, 683–693. [CrossRef]
7. Suk, J.I.; Walker, F.O.; Cartwright, M.S. Ultrasonography of Peripheral Nerves. *Curr. Neurol. Neurosci. Rep.* **2013**, *13*, 328. [CrossRef] [PubMed]
8. VanHorn, T.A.; Cartwright, M.S. Neuromuscular Ultrasound in the Pediatric Population. *Diagnostics* **2020**, *10*, 1012. [CrossRef]
9. Tsai, T.-Y.; Cheong, K.M.; Su, Y.-C.; Shih, M.-C.; Chau, S.W.; Chen, M.-W.; Chen, C.-T.; Lee, Y.-K.; Sun, J.-T.; Chen, K.-F.; et al. Ultrasound-Guided Femoral Nerve Block in Geriatric Patients with Hip Fracture in the Emergency Department. *J. Clin. Med.* **2022**, *11*, 2778. [CrossRef]
10. Can, B.; Kara, M.; Kara, Ö.; Ülger, Z.; Frontera, W.R.; Özçakar, L. The Value of Musculoskeletal Ultrasound in Geriatric Care and Rehabilitation. *Int. J. Rehabil. Res.* **2017**, *40*, 285–296. [CrossRef]
11. Carovac, A.; Smajlovic, F.; Junuzovic, D. Application of Ultrasound in Medicine. *Acta Inform. Med.* **2011**, *19*, 168. [CrossRef] [PubMed]
12. Mamou, J.; Oelze, M.L. *Quantitative Ultrasound in Soft Tissues*; Springer: Berlin/Heidelberg, Germany, 2013; ISBN 9789400769519.
13. Levy, J.; Barrett, D.L.; Harris, N.; Jeong, J.J.; Yang, X.; Chen, S.C. High-Frequency Ultrasound in Clinical Dermatology: A Review. *Ultrasound J.* **2021**, *13*, 24. [CrossRef] [PubMed]
14. Moran, C.M.; Thomson, A.J.W. Preclinical Ultrasound Imaging—A Review of Techniques and Imaging Applications. *Front. Phys.* **2020**, *8*. [CrossRef]
15. Oglat, A.; Matjafri, M.; Suardi, N.; Oqlat, M.; Abdelrahman, M.; Oqlat, A. A Review of Medical Doppler Ultrasonography of Blood Flow in General and Especially in Common Carotid Artery. *J. Med. Ultrasound* **2018**, *26*, 3. [CrossRef]
16. Chen, H.-C.; Kadono, T.; Mimura, Y.; Saeki, H.; Tamaki, K. High-Frequency Ultrasound as a Useful Device in the Preliminary Differentiation of Lichen Sclerosus et Atrophicus from Morphea. *J. Dermatol.* **2004**, *31*, 556–559. [CrossRef]
17. Izzetti, R.; Oranges, T.; Janowska, A.; Gabriele, M.; Graziani, F.; Romanelli, M. The Application of Ultra-High-Frequency Ultrasound in Dermatology and Wound Management. *Int. J. Low. Extrem. Wounds* **2020**, *19*, 334–340. [CrossRef]
18. Izzetti, R.; Vitali, S.; Aringhieri, G.; Nisi, M.; Oranges, T.; Dini, V.; Ferro, F.; Baldini, C.; Romanelli, M.; Caramella, D.; et al. Ultra-High Frequency Ultrasound, A Promising Diagnostic Technique: Review of the Literature and Single-Center Experience. *Can. Assoc. Radiol. J.* **2021**, *72*, 418–431. [CrossRef]
19. Shung, K.K. High Frequency Ultrasonic Imaging. *J. Med. Ultrasound* **2009**, *17*, 25–30. [CrossRef]
20. Wortsman, X. Ultrasound in dermatology: Why, how, and when? *Semin. Ultrasound CT MRI* **2013**, *34*, 177–195. [CrossRef]
21. Byra, M.; Wan, L.; Wong, J.H.; Du, J.; Shah, S.B.; Andre, M.P.; Chang, E.Y. Quantitative Ultrasound and B-Mode Image Texture Features Correlate with Collagen and Myelin Content in Human Ulnar Nerve Fascicles. *Ultrasound Med. Biol.* **2019**, *45*, 1830–1840. [CrossRef]
22. Bignotti, B.; Ghio, M.; Panico, N.; Tagliafico, G.; Martinoli, C.; Tagliafico, A. High-Resolution Ultrasound of Peripheral Nerves in Systemic Sclerosis: A Pilot Study of Computer-Aided Quantitative Assessment of Nerve Density. *Skelet. Radiol.* **2015**, *44*, 1761–1767. [CrossRef]
23. Coleman, D.J.; Silverman, R.H.; Rondeau, M.J.; Lloyd, H.O.; Daly, S. Explaining the Current Role of High Frequency Ultrasound in Ophthalmic Diagnosis (Ophthalmic Ultrasound). *Expert Rev. Ophthalmol.* **2006**, *1*, 63–76. [CrossRef] [PubMed]

24. Byra, M.; Hentzen, E.; Du, J.; Andre, M.; Chang, E.Y.; Shah, S. Assessing the Performance of Morphologic and Echogenic Features in Median Nerve Ultrasound for Carpal Tunnel Syndrome Diagnosis. *J. Ultrasound Med.* **2020**, *39*, 1165–1174. [CrossRef] [PubMed]
25. Fu, T.; Cao, M.; Liu, F.; Zhu, J.; Ye, D.; Feng, X.; Xu, Y.; Wang, G.; Bai, Y. Carpal Tunnel Syndrome Assessment with Ultrasonography: Value of Inlet-to-Outlet Median Nerve Area Ratio in Patients versus Healthy Volunteers. *PLoS ONE* **2015**, *10*, e0116777. [CrossRef] [PubMed]
26. Li, G.Y.; Cao, Y. Mechanics of Ultrasound Elastography. *Proc. R. Soc. A Math. Phys. Eng. Sci.* **2017**, *473*, 20160841. [CrossRef]
27. Sigrist, R.M.S.; Liau, J.; Kaffas, A.E.; Chammas, M.C.; Willmann, J.K. Ultrasound Elastography: Review of Techniques and Clinical Applications. *Therasonics* **2017**, *7*, 1303–1328. [CrossRef] [PubMed]
28. Oelze, M.L.; Mamou, J. Review of Quantitative Ultrasound: Envelope Statistics and Backscatter Coefficient Imaging and Contributions to Diagnostic Ultrasound. *IEEE Trans. Ultrason. Ferroelectr. Freq. Control.* **2016**, *63*, 336–351. [CrossRef]
29. Tagliafico, A.; Tagliafico, G.; Martinoli, C. Nerve Density: A New Parameter to Evaluate Peripheral Nerve Pathology on Ultrasound. Preliminary Study. *Ultrasound Med. Biol.* **2010**, *36*, 1588–1593. [CrossRef]
30. Boom, J.; Visser, L.H. Quantitative Assessment of Nerve Echogenicity: Comparison of Methods for Evaluating Nerve Echogenicity in Ulnar Neuropathy at the Elbow. *Clin. Neurophysiol.* **2012**, *123*, 1446–1453. [CrossRef]
31. Simon, N.G.; Ralph, J.W.; Poncelet, A.N.; Engstrom, J.W.; Chin, C.; Kliot, M. A Comparison of Ultrasonographic and Electrophysiologic "inching" in Ulnar Neuropathy at the Elbow. *Clin. Neurophysiol.* **2015**, *126*, 391–398. [CrossRef]
32. Palmeri, M.L.; Dahl, J.J.; Macleod, D.B.; Grant, S.A.; Nightingale, K.R. On the Feasibility of Imaging Peripheral Nerves Using Acoustic Radiation Force Impulse Imaging. *Ultrason. Imaging* **2009**, *31*, 172–182. [CrossRef]
33. Orman, G.; Ozben, S.; Huseyinoglu, N.; Duymus, M.; Orman, K.G. Ultrasound Elastographic Evaluation in the Diagnosis of Carpal Tunnel Syndrome: Initial Findings. *Ultrasound Med. Biol.* **2013**, *39*, 1184–1189. [CrossRef] [PubMed]
34. Miyamoto, H.; Halpern, E.J.; Kastlunger, M.; Gabl, M.; Arora, R.; Bellmann-Weiler, R.; Feuchtner, G.M.; Jaschke, W.R.; Klauser, A.S. Carpal Tunnel Syndrome Diagnosis by Means of Median Nerve Elasticity—Improved Diagnostic Accuracy of US with Sonoelastography. *Radiology* **2014**, *270*, 481–486. [CrossRef]
35. Yoshii, Y.; Ishii, T.; Tanaka, T.; Tung, W.L.; Sakai, S. Detecting Median Nerve Strain Changes with Cyclic Compression Apparatus: A Comparison of Carpal Tunnel Syndrome Patients and Healthy Controls. *Ultrasound Med. Biol.* **2015**, *41*, 669–674. [CrossRef] [PubMed]
36. Ghajarzadeh, M.; Dadgostar, M.; Sarraf, P.; Emami-Razavi, S.Z.; Miri, S.; Malek, M. Application of Ultrasound Elastography for Determining Carpal Tunnel Syndrome Severity. *Jpn. J. Radiol.* **2015**, *33*, 273–278. [CrossRef]
37. Tatar, I.G.; Kurt, A.; Yavasoglu, N.G.; Hekimoglu, B. Carpal Tunnel Syndrome: Elastosonographic Strain Ratio and Crosssectional Area Evaluation for the Diagnosis and Disease Severity. *Med. Ultrason.* **2016**, *18*, 305–311. [CrossRef]
38. Ishibashi, F.; Taniguchi, M.; Kojima, R.; Kawasaki, A.; Kosaka, A.; Uetake, H. Elasticity of the Tibial Nerve Assessed by Sonoelastography Was Reduced before the Development of Neuropathy and Further Deterioration Associated with the Severity of Neuropathy in Patients with Type 2 Diabetes. *J. Diabetes Investig.* **2016**, *7*, 404–412. [CrossRef] [PubMed]
39. Kesikburun, S.; Adigüzel, E.; Kesikburun, B.; Yaşar, E. Sonoelastographic Assessment of the Median Nerve in the Longitudinal Plane for Carpal Tunnel Syndrome. *PMR* **2016**, *8*, 183–185. [CrossRef]
40. Yoshii, Y.; Tung, W.L.; Ishii, T. Measurement of Median Nerve Strain and Applied Pressure for the Diagnosis of Carpal Tunnel Syndrome. *Ultrasound Med. Biol.* **2017**, *43*, 1205–1209. [CrossRef]
41. Nogueira-Barbosa, M.H.; Lugão, H.B.; Gregio-Júnior, E.; Crema, M.D.; Kobayashi, M.T.T.; Frade, M.A.C.; Pavan, T.Z.; Carneiro, A.A.O. Ultrasound Elastography Assessment of the Median Nerve in Leprosy Patients. *Muscle Nerve* **2017**, *56*, 393–398. [CrossRef]
42. Martin, M.J.; Cartwright, M.S. A Pilot Study of Strain Elastography in the Diagnosis of Carpal Tunnel Syndrome. *J. Clin. Neurophysiol.* **2017**, *34*, 114–118. [CrossRef]
43. Tezcan, S.; Ozturk, F.U.; Uslu, N.; Nalbant, M.; Yemisci, O.U. Carpal Tunnel Syndrome Evaluation of the Effects of Low-Level Laser Therapy with Ultrasound Strain Imaging. *J. Ultrasound Med.* **2019**, *38*, 113–122. [CrossRef] [PubMed]
44. Kantarci, F.; Ustabasioglu, F.E.; Delil, S.; Olgun, D.C.; Korkmazer, B.; Dikici, A.S.; Tutar, O.; Nalbantoglu, M.; Uzun, N.; Mihmanli, I. Median Nerve Stiffness Measurement by Shear Wave Elastography: A Potential Sonographic Method in the Diagnosis of Carpal Tunnel Syndrome. *Eur. Radiol.* **2014**, *24*, 434–440. [CrossRef] [PubMed]
45. Andrade, R.J.; Nordez, A.; Hug, F.; Ates, F.; Coppieters, M.W.; Pezarat-Correia, P.; Freitas, S.R. Non-Invasive Assessment of Sciatic Nerve Stiffness during Human Ankle Motion Using Ultrasound Shear Wave Elastography. *J. Biomech.* **2016**, *49*, 326–331. [CrossRef] [PubMed]
46. Inal, M.; Tan, S.; Demirkan, S.; Burulday, V.; Gündüz, Ö.; Örnek, K. Evaluation of Optic Nerve with Strain and Shear Wave Elastography in Patients with Behçet's Disease and Healthy Subjects. *Ultrasound Med. Biol.* **2017**, *43*, 1348–1354. [CrossRef] [PubMed]
47. Inal, M.; Tan, S.; Yumusak, M.E.; Sahan, M.H.; Alpua, M.; Örnek, K. Evaluation of the Optic Nerve Using Strain and Shear Wave Elastography in Patients with Multiple Sclerosis and Healthy Subjects. *Med. Ultrason.* **2017**, *19*, 39–44. [CrossRef] [PubMed]
48. Dikici, A.S.; Ustabasioglu, F.E.; Delil, S.; Nalbantoglu, M.; Korkmaz, B.; Bakan, S.; Kula, O.; Uzun, N.; Mihmanli, I.; Kantarci, F. Evaluation of the Tibial Nerve with Shear-Wave Elastography: A Potential Sonographic Method for the Diagnosis of Diabetic Peripheral Neuropathy. *Radiology* **2017**, *282*, 494–501. [CrossRef]

49. Bortolotto, C.; Turpini, E.; Felisaz, P.; Fresilli, D.; Fiorina, I.; Raciti, M.V.; Belloni, E.; Bottinelli, O.; Cantisani, V.; Calliada, F. Median Nerve Evaluation by Shear Wave Elastosonography: Impact of "Bone-Proximity" Hardening Artifacts and Inter-Observer Agreement. *J. Ultrasound* **2017**, *20*, 293–299. [CrossRef]
50. Arslan, H.; Yavuz, A.; Ilgen, F.; Aycan, A.; Ozgokce, M.; Akdeniz, H.; Batur, A. The Efficiency of Acoustic Radiation Force Impulse (ARFI) Elastography in the Diagnosis and Staging of Carpal Tunnel Syndrome. *J. Med. Ultrason.* **2018**, *45*, 453–459. [CrossRef]
51. Zhu, B.; Yan, F.; He, Y.; Wang, L.; Xiang, X.; Tang, Y.; Yang, Y.; Qiu, L. Evaluation of the Healthy Median Nerve Elasticity. *Medicine* **2018**, *97*, e12956. [CrossRef]
52. Cingoz, M.; Kandemirli, S.G.; Alis, D.C.; Samanci, C.; Kandemirli, G.C.; Adatepe, N.U. Evaluation of Median Nerve by Shear Wave Elastography and Diffusion Tensor Imaging in Carpal Tunnel Syndrome. *Eur. J. Radiol.* **2018**, *101*, 59–64. [CrossRef]
53. Bedewi, M.A.; Nissman, D.; Aldossary, N.M.; Maetani, T.H.; El Sharkawy, M.S.; Koura, H. Shear Wave Elastography of the Brachial Plexus Roots at the Interscalene Groove. *Neurol. Res.* **2018**, *40*, 805–810. [CrossRef]
54. Aslan, H.; Analan, P.D. Effects of Chronic Flexed Wrist Posture on the Elasticity and Crosssectional Area of the Median Nerve at the Carpal Tunnel among Chronic Stroke Patients. *Med. Ultrason.* **2018**, *20*, 71–75. [CrossRef] [PubMed]
55. Kültür, T.; Okumuş, M.; Inal, M.; Yalçın, S. Evaluation of the Brachial Plexus with Shear Wave Elastography after Radiotherapy for Breast Cancer. *J. Ultrasound Med.* **2018**, *37*, 2029–2035. [CrossRef] [PubMed]
56. Paluch, Ł.; Noszczyk, B.; Nitek, Ż.; Walecki, J.; Osiak, K.; Pietruski, P. Shear-Wave Elastography: A New Potential Method to Diagnose Ulnar Neuropathy at the Elbow. *Eur. Radiol.* **2018**, *28*, 4932–4939. [CrossRef] [PubMed]
57. Burulday, V.; Doğan, A.; Şahan, M.H.; Arıkan, Ş.; Güngüneş, A. Ultrasound Elastography of the Median Nerve in Patients with Acromegaly: A Case-Control Study. *J. Ultrasound Med.* **2018**, *37*, 2371–2377. [CrossRef] [PubMed]
58. Neto, T.; Freitas, S.R.; Andrade, R.J.; Gomes, J.; Mendes, B.; Mendes, T.; Nordez, A.; Oliveira, R. Sciatic Nerve Stiffness Is Not Changed Immediately after a Slump Neurodynamics Technique. *Muscle Ligaments Tendons J.* **2019**, *07*, 583. [CrossRef]
59. Neto, T.; Freitas, S.R.; Andrade, R.J.; Vaz, J.R.; Mendes, B.; Firmino, T.; Bruno, P.M.; Nordez, A.; Oliveira, R. Noninvasive Measurement of Sciatic Nerve Stiffness in Patients with Chronic Low Back Related Leg Pain Using Shear Wave Elastography. *J. Ultrasound Med.* **2019**, *38*, 157–164. [CrossRef] [PubMed]
60. Jiang, W.; Huang, S.; Teng, H.; Wang, P.; Wu, M.; Zhou, X.; Xu, W.; Zhang, Q.; Ran, H. Diagnostic Performance of Two-Dimensional Shear Wave Elastography for Evaluating Tibial Nerve Stiffness in Patients with Diabetic Peripheral Neuropathy. *Eur. Radiol.* **2019**, *29*, 2167–2174. [CrossRef]
61. He, Y.; Xiang, X.; Zhu, B.H.; Qiu, L. Shear Wave Elastography Evaluation of the Median and Tibial Nerve in Diabetic Peripheral Neuropathy. *Quant. Imaging Med. Surg.* **2019**, *9*, 273–282. [CrossRef]
62. Aslan, M.; Aslan, A.; Emeksiz, H.C.; Candan, F.; Erdemli, S.; Tombul, T.; Gunaydın, G.D.; Kabaalioğlu, A. Assessment of Peripheral Nerves with Shear Wave Elastography in Type 1 Diabetic Adolescents Without Diabetic Peripheral Neuropathy. *J. Ultrasound Med.* **2019**, *38*, 1583–1596. [CrossRef]
63. Şahan, M.H.; Doğan, A.; İnal, M.; Alpua, M.; Asal, N. Evaluation of the Optic Nerve by Strain and Shear Wave Elastography in Patients with Migraine. *J. Ultrasound Med.* **2019**, *38*, 1153–1161. [CrossRef]
64. Moran, L.; Royuela, A.; de Vargas, A.P.; Lopez, A.; Cepeda, Y.; Martinelli, G. Carpal Tunnel Syndrome: Diagnostic Usefulness of Ultrasound Measurement of the Median Nerve Area and Quantitative Elastographic Measurement of the Median Nerve Stiffness. *J. Ultrasound Med.* **2020**, *39*, 331–339. [CrossRef]
65. Wei, M.; Ye, X. Feasibility of Point Shear Wave Elastography for Evaluating Diabetic Peripheral Neuropathy. *J. Ultrasound Med.* **2020**, *39*, 1135–1141. [CrossRef]
66. Bedewi, M.A.; Elsifey, A.A.; Kotb, M.A.; Bediwy, A.M.; Ahmed, Y.M.; Swify, S.M.; Abodonya, A.M. Shear Wave Elastography of the Saphenous Nerve. *Medicine* **2020**, *99*, e22120. [CrossRef]
67. Schrier, V.J.M.M.; Lin, J.; Gregory, A.; Thoreson, A.R.; Alizad, A.; Amadio, P.C.; Fatemi, M. Shear Wave Elastography of the Median Nerve: A Mechanical Study. *Muscle Nerve* **2020**, *61*, 826–833. [CrossRef]
68. Rugel, C.L.; Franz, C.K.; Lee, S.S.M. Influence of Limb Position on Assessment of Nerve Mechanical Properties by Using Shear Wave Ultrasound Elastography. *Muscle Nerve* **2020**, *61*, 616–622. [CrossRef]
69. Bruno, F.; Palumbo, P.; Arrigoni, F.; Mariani, S.; Aringhieri, G.; Carotti, M.; Natella, R.; Zappia, M.; Cipriani, P.; Giacomelli, R.; et al. Advanced Diagnostic Imaging and Intervention in Tendon Diseases. *Acta Biomed.* **2020**, *91*, 98–106. [CrossRef]
70. Chianca, V.; Di Pietto, F.; Zappia, M.; Albano, D.; Messina, C.; Sconfienza, L.M. Musculoskeletal Ultrasound in the Emergency Department. *Semin. Musculoskelet. Radiol.* **2020**, *24*, 167–174. [CrossRef]
71. Ophir, J.; Céspedes, I.; Ponnekanti, H.; Yazdi, Y.; Li, X. Elastography: A Quantitative Method for Imaging the Elasticity of Biological Tissues. *Ultrason. Imaging* **1991**, *13*, 111–134. [CrossRef]
72. Eisenscher, A.; Schweg-Toffler, E.; Pelletier, G.; Jacquemard, P. Rhythmic Echographic Palpation. Echosismography. A New Technic of Differentiating Benign and Malignant Tumors by Ultrasonic Study of Tissue Elasticity. *J. Radiol.* **1983**, *64 4*, 255–261.
73. Taljanovic, M.S.; Gimber, L.H.; Giles, W.B.; Latt, L.D.; Melville, D.M.; Gao, L.; Witte, R.S. Shear-Wave Elastography: Basic Physics and Musculoskeletal Applications. *Imaging Phys.* **2017**, *37*, 855–870. [CrossRef]
74. Krouskop, T.A.; Dougherty, D.R.; Vinson, F.S. A Pulsed Doppler Ultrasonic System for Making Noninvasive Measurements of the Mechanical Properties of Soft Tissue. *J. Rehabil. Res. Dev.* **1987**, *24*, 1–8.
75. Sugimoto, T.; Ueha, S.; Itoh, K. Tissue Hardness Measurement Using the Radiation Force of Focused Ultrasound. In Proceedings of the IEEE Symposium on Ultrasonics, Honolulu, HI, USA, 4–7 December 1990; Volume 3, pp. 1377–1380.

76. Wright, T.W.; Glowczewskie, F.; Wheeler, D.; Miller, G.; Cowin, D. Excursion and Strain of the Median Nerve. *J. Bone Jt. Surg.* **1996**, *78*, 1897–1903. [CrossRef]
77. Kubo, K.; Zhou, B.; Cheng, Y.S.; Yang, T.H.; Qiang, B.; An, K.N.; Moran, S.L.; Amadio, P.C.; Zhang, X.; Zhao, C. Ultrasound Elastography for Carpal Tunnel Pressure Measurement: A Cadaveric Validation Study. *J. Orthop. Res.* **2018**, *36*, 477–483. [CrossRef]
78. Tsui, P.H.; Wan, Y.L. Effects of Fatty Infiltration of the Liver on the Shannon Entropy of Ultrasound Backscattered Signals. *Entropy* **2016**, *18*, 341. [CrossRef]
79. Han, A.; O'Brien, W.D. Structure Function Estimated from Histological Tissue Sections. *IEEE Trans. Ultrason. Ferroelectr. Freq. Control.* **2016**, *63*, 1296–1305. [CrossRef]
80. Shankar, P.M. A General Statistical Model for Ultrasonic Backscattering from Tissues. *IEEE Trans. Ultrason. Ferroelectr. Freq. Control.* **2000**, *47*, 727–736. [CrossRef]
81. Lin, S.C.; Heba, E.; Wolfson, T.; Ang, B.; Gamst, A.; Han, A.; Erdman, J.W.; O'Brien, W.D.; Andre, M.P.; Sirlin, C.B.; et al. Noninvasive Diagnosis of Nonalcoholic Fatty Liver Disease Andquantification of Liver Fat Using a New Quantitative Ultrasound Technique. *Clin. Gastroenterol. Hepatol.* **2015**, *13*, 1337–1345.e6. [CrossRef]
82. Byra, M.; Nowicki, A.; Wróblewska-Piotrzkowska, H.; Dobruch-Sobczak, K. Classification of Breast Lesions Using Segmented Quantitative Ultrasound Maps of Homodyned K Distribution Parameters. *Med. Phys.* **2016**, *43*, 5561. [CrossRef]
83. Weng, W.C.; Tsui, P.H.; Lin, C.Y.C.W.; Lu, C.H.; Lin, C.Y.C.W.; Shieh, J.Y.; Lu, F.L.; Ee, T.W.; Wu, K.W.; Lee, W.T. Evaluation of Muscular Changes by Ultrasound Nakagami Imaging in Duchenne Muscular Dystrophy. *Sci. Rep.* **2017**, *7*, 4429. [CrossRef]
84. Lin, Y.H.; Yang, T.H.; Wang, S.H.; Su, F.C. Quantitative Assessment of First Annular Pulley and Adjacent Tissues Using High-Frequency Ultrasound. *Sensors* **2017**, *17*, 107. [CrossRef]
85. Piotrzkowska-Wroblewska, H.; Litniewski, J.; Szymanska, E.; Nowicki, A. Quantitative Sonography of Basal Cell Carcinoma. *Ultrasound Med. Biol.* **2015**, *41*, 748–759. [CrossRef]
86. Rosso, G.; Guck, J. Mechanical Changes of Peripheral Nerve Tissue Microenvironment and Their Structural Basis during Development. *APL Bioeng.* **2019**, *3*, 36107. [CrossRef]

Disclaimer/Publisher's Note: The statements, opinions and data contained in all publications are solely those of the individual author(s) and contributor(s) and not of MDPI and/or the editor(s). MDPI and/or the editor(s) disclaim responsibility for any injury to people or property resulting from any ideas, methods, instructions or products referred to in the content.

MDPI
St. Alban-Anlage 66
4052 Basel
Switzerland
www.mdpi.com

Diagnostics Editorial Office
E-mail: diagnostics@mdpi.com
www.mdpi.com/journal/diagnostics

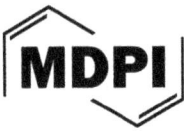

Disclaimer/Publisher's Note: The statements, opinions and data contained in all publications are solely those of the individual author(s) and contributor(s) and not of MDPI and/or the editor(s). MDPI and/or the editor(s) disclaim responsibility for any injury to people or property resulting from any ideas, methods, instructions or products referred to in the content.

www.ingramcontent.com/pod-product-compliance
Lightning Source LLC
LaVergne TN
LVHW070726100526
838202LV00013B/1182